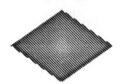

S0-DGI-380

Eating Expectantly

The Essential Eating Guide and Cookbook for Pregnancy

Bridget Swinney M.S., R.D.

Contributions by
Tracey Anderson R.N., B.S., F.A.C.C.E.
Edited by
Melinda Morris M.S., R.D.

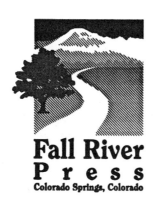

Fall River
P r e s s
Colorado Springs, Colorado

©1993 by Bridget Swinney

All rights reserved. No portions of this book may be reproduced-mechanically, electronically, or by any other means, including photocopying–without the written permission of the publisher. Exception: health professionals in a non-profit setting and reviewers who may use selected passages for review articles, providing proper credit is given. For more information:

Fall River Press
P.O Box 62578
Colorado Springs, CO 80962-2578

Publisher's Cataloging in Publication

(Prepared by Quality Books, Inc.)

Swinney, Bridget, 1960–
    Eating expectantly: the essential eating guide and cookbook for pregnancy / Bridget Swinney with Tracey Anderson ; editor, Melinda Morris.
    p. cm.
    Includes biliographical references and index.
    ISBN 0-9632917-3-4

    1. Pregnancy–Nutritional aspects. I. Anderson, Tracey, 1957– II. Title.

RG559.S95 1992   641.563
                                  QB192–1123

Library of Congress Catalog Card Number: 92–085580

Cover design and illustration:	Pat Steinholtz, P.O. Box 9132, Denver, CO 80209
Typesetting and graphic design:	Tim Chamberlain, 9913 E. Hwy 86, Franktown, CO 80116
Selected illustrations:	Russell Stueber
Back cover photograph:	Ernie Ferguson Photography
Printed by:	BookCrafters
Nutrition analysis of recipes done with:	Nutritionist III™, N-Squared Computing, Salem Oregon

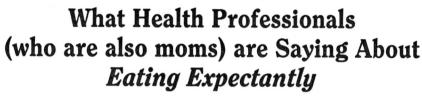

What Health Professionals (who are also moms) are Saying About *Eating Expectantly*

Eating Expectantly is an invaluable resource for the expectant mother of the 90's. Besides in-depth and practical advice about nutrition before, during and after pregnancy, you'll find a wealth of information on current issues such as food safety, vegetarianism, supplements and exercise. Tips on dining out, fast foods and saving time in the kitchen make this a great tool for today's busy parents.

Liz Marr Diemand, M.S., R.D.
Registered Dietitian
Program Manager
Western Dairy Council

What an enjoyable book! It's full of good to know facts and is written in a very readable style–sure to be appreciated by all who read it. The recipes look delicious and easy to prepare (always important!) I can't wait to make them for my family.

As an obstetrical nurse and the mother of two, (pregnant with my third!) I would not hesitate to recommend this book to any of my patients or friends.

Marilyn Prost R.N., M.S.N.
Head Nurse, Postpartum Unit

Eating Expectantly is the next best thing to having a registered dietitian in your kitchen! The author draws on her experience as a nutrition counselor and mother to provide practical answers to genuine concerns of real mothers. The sections on supplying and stocking your kitchen for health, food storage and handling, eating out (including fast food), and weight control offer information for use in all aspects of family nutrition.

Shirley K Lippincott, R.D.
Nutrition Consultant
Nutrition etc.

This book includes the latest up to date information on pregnancy and nutrition. There's something for everyone. It contains great nutrition tips, even if you're not pregnant. *Eating Expectantly* is an extensive resource book and cookbook with a personal touch! I would highly recommend this book for any pregnant woman, or for any woman considering pregnancy.

Ginny Murphy R.D.
Director, El Paso County Women, Infants and Children's (WIC)
Program, El Paso County Health Department

*This book is dedicated to the memory of two people,
my mother, Marjorie Morgan Swinney
and to my friend and mentor Robert Chambers.
It is also dedicated to the two special men in my life,
Frank and Nicolas.*

About the Contributors

Bridget Swinney, primary author, is a Registered Dietitian specializing in health communication, diabetes education and weight control. She has a Master of Science degree in Nutrition and has extensive experience in counseling pregnant women. Her goal in writing this book was to improve the health and nutrition of those starting a family by giving practical nutrition advice. Bridget lives in Colorado with her son, who was the inspiration of this book, and her very supportive husband. She enjoys cooking, traveling, reading, jazz and hiking in the Rocky Mountains.

Contributing author Tracey Anderson is a Registered Nurse and Childbirth Educator. She lives in Colorado with her husband and two young daughters. Outside of having fun being a full-time mom, Tracey can be found teaching a scripture based Lamaze series that she developed. She also enjoys teaching childbirth education classes to teens and low income moms at the Life Support Center and speaking on parenting issues to Moms of Preschoolers and other Mom support groups.

Editor Melinda Morris is a Registered Dietitian specializing in the communication of nutrition including writing, teaching college classes and counseling individuals. She is particularly interested in sports nutrition, psychological aspects of eating and maternal and child health. She enjoys cycling and running. Melinda lives with her architect husband in Boulder, Colorado.

Foreword author Michael Hambidge MD, ScD is a Professor of Pediatrics at the University of Colorado Health Sciences Center in Denver. He is also the Director of the Center for Human Nutrition at UCHSC. Dr. Hambidge served on the Subcommittee on Dietary Intake and Nutrient Supplements of the National Academy of Sciences which produced the report *Nutrition During Pregnancy*. Dr. Hambidge now serves on the Food and Nutrition Board of the National Research Council.

Acknowledgements

I would like to mention the many people who reviewed chapters or the full manuscript of this book. Their input and expertise is greatly appreciated:

Roseanne Ainscough, RD, CDE, Becky Bass MS, RD, Barb Berntsen, Mike Bolger PhD, Food and Drug Administration, Ruth Bowling, RD, Jacquie Craig MS RD CDE, Betty Crase, La Leche League International, Pat DeKam LVN, Liz Diemand MS, RD, Kathy Fraser, Maggie Garfield RN, CCE, Michael Hambidge MD, Kathy Glaaser MS, RD, Anita Hall RN, Lori Hannah RD, Janis Harsila RD, Sue Havala RD, Betty Hopkins, Pat Kendall PhD, RD, Linda Kohlman RN, CDE, Shirley Lippincott RD, Ginny Murphy, RD, Mary Peet MA, RD, Marilyn Prost RN, MSN, Gordon Silver MD, FACOG, Julie Smith RD, Leslie Weddell, Gazette Telegraph Food Editor, and DeeAnn Whitmire MS, RD.

In addition I would like to thank the individuals and organizations who assisted directly or indirectly.

Alan and Denise Fields, authors of "Bridal Bargains", The Vegetarian Resource Group, Kate Ruddon with The American College of Obstetricians and Gynecologists, Virlie Walker with the Food and Drug Administration, Kathy Fraser, Michelle Williams, Candi McNany, Wayne Valey, the staff of the Diabetes Education and Support Center, and to my other friends and colleagues who were supportive during this project. Also thanks to my family for their support.

Thanks to those who helped test recipes: Kathy Fraser, Laura Albaum, Peggy Braley and Peggy Connor; to some of my recipe tasters: Scott and Sean Fraser, Barb Berntsen, Sue Richardson, Frank and Nicolas, and to those who graciously allowed me to publish their recipes: Stella Bender, Deborah Compton, Dr. Mary Dudley, Andy Hawk, Linda Hood, Dr. R. L. Ohlsen Jr., Margo Morrow, Debbie Russell and The Vegetarian Resource Group.

Also, thanks to the American College of Obstetricians and Gynecologists, The Food and Drug Administration, The Center for Science in the Public Interest and the Vegetarian Resource Group for allowing me to reprint their documents.

Last but not least, I want to thank Pat Steinholtz, who created the beautiful cover and Tim Chamberlain who did the innovative typesetting and graphics. A picture can indeed be worth a thousand words, and putting words into print in an artistic way takes talent! I thank them both for their creativity and patience. And much thanks to Melinda Morris for editorial advice, enthusiasm and support.

Contents

Section I
Nutrition Needs, Challenges And Tips
For Eating For A Healthy Pregnancy

Chapter 1

Chapter 2

Why Prepregnancy Planning Is Best

Who Should Have Genetic Counseling?

The Importance of Good Nutrition Before Pregnancy

The Pre-Pregnancy Quiz

The Before Baby Diet

Keys For Planning A Healthy Pregnancy

Focus on Folate

Chapter 3
The Knowledgable Pregnancy

Ten Steps to a Healthy Diet

Everything You Ever Wanted to Know About
   Weight Gain During Pregnancy
   Gaining Too Fast or Too Much
   Not Gaining Enough

The Essential Guide to Vitamins and Minerals

To Supplement or Not to Supplement?

Why You May Need a Supplement

If You Take Supplements

Keeping Your Baby's Environment Safe

Travel During Pregnancy

The Positives of Pregnancy

Section II
Shopping, Cooking And Eating Out For A Healthy Pregnancy

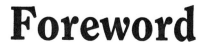

Foreword

Eating Expectantly has been written at a most favorable moment in our perception of the value of optimal maternal nutrition during pregnancy for both mother and baby. The recent report of the Food and Nutrition Board of the National Academy of Sciences entitled "Nutrition During Pregnancy" (1990) has had a special role in focusing our attention on nutrition during pregnancy and has provided a thorough, up to date review of the major issues. This report comes exactly 20 years after the Food and Nutrition Board's 1970 report on "Maternal Nutrition and the Course of Pregnancy". The convening of an expert committee, including leaders in the field of nutrition and obstetrics, to write this recent report reflects the substantial advances in our knowledge during the intervening years and the need to apply recent findings to prenatal care.

Of the many conclusions reached by this expert committee, two are especially noteworthy. The first of these is the recommendation for greater maternal weight gain than has been recommended previously. This is in recognition of the association between maternal weight gain during the second and third trimesters and the growth of the baby prior to birth. The specific recommendation is for a minimum weight gain of 25 pounds unless the mother is overweight prior to pregnancy. For mothers who are underweight prior to pregnancy, even greater weight gain is recommended.

The second recommendation of particular note is that routine micronutrient supplements be limited to a daily iron supplement of 30 mg. While other specific micronutrient supplements are advised in a number of special circumstatnces, a routine prenatal vitamin/mineral supplement is not recommended. Rather there is an emphasis on optimal diet as the source of micronutrients.

The reasons for this outstanding emphasis on the foods we eat reach far beyond the simple fact that we don't need to take supplements if we consume an adequate, nutritionally well-balanced diet. One important reason is the very real risk that we will consciously or subconsciously pay less attention to an optimal diet if we take our daily multivitamin/mineral pill. Shortcomings of the latter approach include the risk of nutrient/nutrient interactions and imbalances, an area which we continue to learn more about. "New" micronutrients that are important for human health continue to be "discovered." These will not be included in the current generation of prenatal supplements and, once again, we are dependent on a well balanced diet.

One of the most important reasons for the selection of an optimal diet rather than on a substitute pill is the fact that prenatal vitamins are not prescribed until the first prenatal visit to an obstetrician. It is uncommon still for this visit to occur prior to conception or prior to the critical early development of the baby during the first four to six weeks of pregnancy. We now know, for example that an adequate intake of folate, one of the B vitamins, in the peri-conceptional period will prevent the recurrence of about three quarters of all cases of spina bifidia and anencephaly in women who have had the misfortune to have had a previous baby with a neural tube defect. There is very strong suggestive evidence that the same protective effect applies to women who have not had a previous baby with a neural tube defect. To be protective, however, adequate folate must be taken prior to conception and in those first few weeks of pregnancy. The bottom-line message is that the emphasis on optimal diet is of the greatest importance to all women of childbearing age at all times-not only when pregnancy has been confirmed.

I commend Bridget Swinney for her timely and informative guide. You should get your copy now and not wait until you are pregnant.

Michael Hambidge, MD, ScD
Professor of Pediatrics,
Director of the Center for Human Nutrition,
University of Colorado Health Sciences Center.

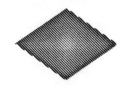

Section I
Nutrition Needs, Challenges And Tips For Eating For A Healthy Pregnancy

Why You Need This Book!

When a woman became pregnant years go, she didn't change her life that much. The health of the baby was thought to depend mostly on chance and the placenta was thought to protect the fetus from all dangerous substances.   Things are different today. We have an abundance of knowledge about pregnancy and nutrition, and the amount of research on the subject grows daily. Now we know that the placenta acts as a "screen" and many toxic substances can get through to the baby, making mom the true "gatekeeper".

You will probably find pregnancy to be much more "high tech" than just 10 years ago. But even with all the diagnostic tests and fancy equipment now available, good nutrition is still the most important factor in giving your baby a healthy start in life.

Eating Expectantly puts nutrition and health during pregnancy into perspective for the 90's. It gives you answers to questions you may want to ask, but are not quite sure *who* to ask. It's a realistic and practical approach to eating instead of theoretical advice that doesn't work in the "real world."

And *Eating Expectantly* not only gives you guidance on what to eat, it carries through with over 80 delicious recipes developed just for the stages of pregnancy. Also, over 150 menus are included to meet different needs such as Don't Feel Like Cooking Menus, Meals in Minutes, I Could Cook All Day Menus, Healthiest Fast Food Menus. and Company's Coming! Menus.

If you are vegetarian or trying to eat meatless meals more often, you'll find the vegetarian chapter helpful. If you experience one of the unexpected conditions of pregnancy, like gestational diabetes, high blood pressure or bedrest, *Eating Expectantly* will guide you though it by explaining the facts and giving eating and food preparation tips.

Eating Expectantly answers these questions...and more:

♦ What can I do **before** I get pregnant to help insure I have a healthy baby?

♦ Will **pesticides and preservatives** in foods affect my baby?

♦ What if I can't drink milk; do I really need a lot of **calcium**?

♦ I'm **vegetarian**, how can I meet my nutrient needs?

♦ Help! I was just diagnosed with **gestational diabetes**... what do I do?

♦ Should I take a **vitamin supplement**?

♦ How much **weight** should I gain?

♦ How is my **current diet**?

♦ Do I need to go on a **low salt diet** if I start to have high blood pressure?

♦ How can I eat right when I'm on **bedrest**?

♦ I don't feel like **cooking**, help!

♦ What are the best **fast food** and **restaurant** choices for me while I'm pregnant?

♦ Should I **exercise**?

This book uses knowledge and experience gathered from hundreds of pregnant women and mothers including myself. I've also gotten answers from the scientific experts; those who do nutrition research, and who work with pregnant and breastfeeding women on a daily basis.

If you have any questions or concerns about what to eat, how much to eat, or how to **practice** good nutrition--before, during or after your pregnancy, this book is a **must!** I hope you enjoy reading it as much as I enjoyed writing it. More importantly, I hope that by reading and following the advice in *Eating Expectantly*, you can give your baby and yourself the gift of good nutrition and good health!

Note: This book is not meant to take the place of medical or nutritional counseling by a qualified health professional. If you are contemplating pregnancy or are pregnant, please visit your health care provider, and if necessary, a registered dietitian.

2

Contemplating Pregnancy

What You Will Find In This Chapter:

- Why Prepregnancy Planning is Best
- Who Should Have Genetic Counseling
- The Importance of Good Nutrition Before Pregnancy
- The Prepregnancy Quiz
- The Before Baby Diet

- Keys for Planning a Healthy Pregnancy
- Focus on Folate

And answers to questions you may have:

- How will I know if I have too much lead in my tap water?
- How can I cut down on caffeine?
- How will I know if I'm healthy enough to have a baby?
- How can I stop eating junk food?

Why Prepregnancy Planning Is Best

Thinking about having a baby? If you are thinking about starting or adding to your family and are seeking information about pregnancy, you're making a smart move! It's a good idea to visit with your health care provider when you decide you'd like to become pregnant. Prepregnancy counseling is recommended for several reasons...

1. You have time to change some lifestyle habits that may affect your pregnancy like smoking, drinking, caffeine intake and your eating habits.

2. You have time to start eating a well balanced diet, start exercising regularly, and lose or gain weight, if needed.

3. You can begin to understand the importance of changing your habits before the first weeks of pregnancy. It is during the first weeks when many things can go wrong with the fetus, but when most women don't know they're pregnant.

4. If you have any chronic medical

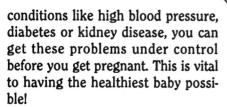

conditions like high blood pressure, diabetes or kidney disease, you can get these problems under control before you get pregnant. This is vital to having the healthiest baby possible!

5. If you have had an unsuccessful pregnancy, or have delivered a baby with birth defects, you can find out how to improve the outcome of your next pregnancy and the health of your next baby.

6. If this is your first pregnancy but you have a history of genetic defects in your family or you have a genetic condition that you could pass on to your children, you will have time to receive genetic counseling.

Who Should Have Genetic Counseling?

According to the March of Dimes, anyone who has unanswered questions about diseases in the family or who is concerned about being at increased risk of having a child with a birth defect or inherited disorder should consider genetic counseling. It is also suitable for:

Couples who have:

◆ A child with a birth defect or genetic disorder

◆ A child or relative with mental retardation

◆ An ethnic background known to have a higher incidence of specific disorders (Tay-Sach, thalassemia, and sickle cell anemia)

◆ Are first cousins or other close blood relatives

Women who:

◆ Will be 35 years or older at the time of pregnancy

◆ Have a history of miscarriages

◆ Have a history of infertility

The Importance of Good Nutrition Before Pregnancy

The importance of good nutrition and early prenatal care for a healthy pregnancy is shown in the following examples:

◆ In a landmark study done in several countries, it was found that a B vitamin called folacin (also called folate and folic acid) could prevent up to 72% of neural tube defects like spina bifida (1). Women who have had a child with this defect are much more likely to have another child with the same problem; those women should talk to their health care provider about a folacin supplement. Other women should try to get adequate amounts of folacin through the foods they eat. It has also been suggested that all women who are planning a pregnancy or suspect they are pregnant take a multi-vitamin containing folacin (2). (See page 27 about the key nutrients of pregnancy including folacin.)

◆ Women with pre-existing diabetes are several times more likely than the non-diabetic woman to have a baby with birth defects. This may be related to glucose control before conception and in the very early weeks of pregnancy (3). However, this increased risk can be reduced significantly with good control of blood sugars and early prenatal counseling.

♦ Anyone who is unknowingly pregnant might drink alcohol or take medication that could harm the fetus. Currently there is no established safe level of alcohol intake during pregnancy. Women who are contemplating pregnancy and those who are pregnant should avoid alcohol.

♦ In general, women may not get enough of some vitamins and minerals when they aren't pregnant. The Total Diet Study found that women aged 25-30 ate less than 75% of the RDA for calcium, magnesium, and iron, and only 80% of the RDA for zinc (4). A 1987 report showed that one out of four women between the ages of 25 and 34 skipped breakfast regularly. Skipping a meal can significantly cut down on needed nutrients (5). One out of five women has no iron reserves. Many women eat only half the recommended amount of calcium (6). Thus, women may be starting their pregnancy with a depleted supply of many nutrients which

play vital roles in the development of the fetus.

♦ The death rate seems to be higher for babies of overweight women then for babies of women at their ideal weight, primarily due to an increase in premature deliveries (7). The solution? If you are overweight, and especially if you are 20% or more over your ideal weight, lose weight before you conceive. See the resources section for weight control resources.

A few words of advice: make sure that you don't become pregnant while you are on a weight loss diet—your intake of certain vitamins may not be enough for the important stages of early development. Taking a vitamin-mineral supplement during the weight loss period is advisable. (See page 35)

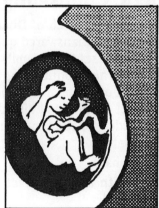

The Prepregnancy Quiz:
Is your body ready for a baby?

The following quiz will help you know if your body and lifestyle are ready for pregnancy. Add up the points in parentheses next to your answer and compare with the scores at the bottom. For more information about the question see the page number in parentheses.

1. How many servings of fruits per day do you eat? (page 9) 0 (-1) 1-2 (1) 2 (2) more than 2 (3)

2. Do you eat a vitamin C-rich food daily? (page 9) (examples include citrus fruit or juice, berries, papaya, mango, pineapple, melon, broccoli, cauliflower, tomato, vegetable juice) yes (1) no (0)

3. How many vegetables do you eat per day? (page 9) 0 (-1) 1-2 (1) 2 (2) more than 2 (3)

4. How often do you exercise? (page 172) 0 (0) 1-2 times per week (1) 3 or more times per week (2)

5. Do you smoke or live with someone who smokes? (page 39) No (0) yes, live with someone who smokes (-2) yes, 1/2 pack per day (-3) yes, 1 pack per day (-5) yes, over 1 pack per day (-8)

6. How often do you drink caffeinated beverages? (page 42) Twice a week or less (1) 1-2 caffeinated beverages per day (0) 4 caffeinated beverages per day (-2) over 4 caffeinated beverages per day (-4)

7. Do you regularly take drugs of any kind; prescription, over-the counter, herbal preparations or "street drugs"? (page 43) Yes (-5) No (1)

8. Are you constantly on a weight loss diet or have you been dieting in the last 6 months? (page 35) Yes (-2) No (0)

9. Are you regularly exposed to radiation, pesticides, herbicides, solvents, PCB's, or other chemicals? (page 9) Yes (-5) No (0)

10. Do you eat shark, swordfish or lake whitefish once a week or more? (page 211) Yes (-3) No (0)

11. Do you eat 3 balanced meals a day? (page 57) Yes (3) No (0)

12. How many servings of high calcium foods do you eat in a day? (page 61) (this includes milk, yogurt, cheese and high calcium vegetables) 3 or more (2) 1-2 (1) 0 (-1)

13. Do you generally "not eat right?" (page 9) Yes (-1) No (0)

14. Do you take a vitamin supplement of a single vitamin or mineral

The Prepregnancy Quiz:
Is your body ready for a baby?

(not a multi-vitamin) that is not prescribed or recommended by a physician such as vitamin A or C? (page 35) Yes (-5) No (0)

15. How many alcoholic beverages do you drink at one time? (page 41) You don't drink alcohol (1) 1 drink (-1) 2-4 drinks (-2) 5 or more drinks (-4)

16. Do you regularly eat raw milk, eggs, shellfish or foods that are made with these (caesar salad dressing, mousse with uncooked egg, sushi)? (page 196) Yes (-4) No (0)

17. Do you eat several servings of whole grain breads, cereals, etc. per day? (page 51) Yes (2) No (0)

18. Are you more than 20 pounds overweight or 10 pounds or more underweight? ("The Weighing Issue" on page 21) Yes (-2) No (0)

19. Do you live life in the "fast lane", often getting less than 8 hours of sleep per night, have many time commitments, and feel stressed? (page 10) Yes (-2) No (0)

20. Do you skip meals regularly? (page 57) Yes (-2) No (0)

21. Are you a vegetarian who eats no animal products and don't take vitamin B-12 or calcium supplements or eat foods naturally high or supplemented with those nutrients?

(page 85) Yes (-1) No (0)

22. Are you a vegetarian who carefully watches your diet by eating a large variety of foods including good sources of protein? (page 84) Yes (2) No (0)

How did you do?

17-21: Congratulations! You're body is ready for pregnancy!

13-17: You're doing pretty well, you have just a few things to work on to have the healthiest pregnancy possible.

9-13: Start working–it may take a few months to make the changes to have the healthiest pregnancy possible.

9 or less: Oops! Your lifestyle may need an overhaul! Talk to your health care provider before beginning a pregnancy.

If any of your answers had a negative number for a score, this indicates a habit that needs to be changed. If you're curious about any of the questions, look to the page number next to the question for more information.

How to use this book before you're pregnant...

If you're not pregnant yet, you will benefit even more from this book. You'll know how your diet should be and you'll know what to expect during pregnancy. I'd suggest that you read the whole book, skipping the chapter on high risk pregnancies (unless you already have a chronic disease like diabetes). Then, start using the menus and recipes now! This will get you used to eating right and it will be easy to keep it up when you're pregnant. Just keep in mind that you won't need to increase your calories until you are pregnant.

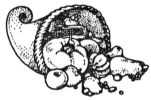

"The Before Baby Diet"

Food	Daily Servings
Grains/Starches	6 or more
Fruits	2 or more
Vegetables	3 or more
Be sure to include at least 1 vitamin C and 1 vitamin A-rich fruit or vegetable daily.	
Protein or equivalent	4-6 ounces
Dairy or calcium rich foods	3 or more

Eating at least the above number of servings will help you become a healthy future mom.   As soon as you find out you're pregnant, you can switch over to the Eating Expectantly Diet, page 47. It's not too different, so the transition will be easy. If you're wondering how to begin to eat healthy, see Chapter 13 Stocking the Pregnant Kitchen.

Keys For Planning A Healthy Pregnancy

Both you and your partner should follow the advice below several months before you become pregnant. Although men are often left out of the prepregnancy planning stage, they must also take good care of themselves since sperm can be also be affected by diet and the environment.

1. **Don't drink alcohol or take drugs.** That includes aspirin! If you take a prescription medication, ask your doctor if it is safe to take during pregnancy. He can possibly substitute a medication that is. Find out from your health care provider which over-the- counter medications are safe during pregnancy and especially during the first trimester.

2. **Don't take X rays**, unless you tell the medical personnel that you may be pregnant. Radiation can also affect sperm.

3. **Keep your environment safe.** This means avoiding exposure to pesticides and herbicides, radiation, fumes from paint, extermination chemicals and glue. Avoid exposure to lead, which can cause premature birth, brain damage, learning disabilities, kidney and liver damage. Up to

40 million people have too much lead in their drinking water. See page 39 for the important details (8).

If you smoke, try to quit or reduce your amount. Avoid or limit exposure to second-hand smoke.

4.   Both you and your partner should follow the "Before Baby Diet" –preferably for 3 months prior to pregnancy since one cycle of sperm production takes 10 weeks (9). The father's diet is often ignored when discussing pregnancy. However, current research now shows that the father's diet can affect his sperm and ultimately the fetus. A joint project at U.C. Berkeley and USDA's Western Human Nutrition Research Center have linked low dietary intakes of vitamin C to increased genetic damage in sperm, which presumably translates to a higher risk of birth defects and genetic disease (10). (See page 31 for good food sources of vitamin C.)

Study Leader Dr. Bruce Ames says, "All we know now is that if your dietary intake of vitamin C gets below a certain level–about 60 mg. per day, which is the Recommended Daily Allowance–you get into trouble." "This strongly indicates that vitamin C protects against DNA damage."

5.   If you think your diet is not adequate, take a vitamin supplement providing no more than 100% of the RDA. See page 35 for more indications of why you might need a supplement. If you choose to take one, make sure it contains folacin.

6.   Limit caffeine. Caffeine does not seem to be a factor which affects fertility. However very high caffeine intake in combination with cigarette smoking has delayed conception in one study of Danish women. A recent study of 40,000 Canadian women showed that caffeine intake during pregnancy has no adverse affect on offspring. The study investigator Dr. Alison McDonald concluded, "There's no evidence that moderate caffeine intake has adverse effects on pregnancy outcome." (11)

7.   Reduce stress or learn how to effectively cope with it. Extreme stress is thought to affect fertility. However, stress is hard to measure as all of us perceive it differently. Exercise is a good stress reliever.

8.   Avoid exposure to high temperatures. For example, sperm production is reduced in men who weld inside storage tanks, who drive a truck and literally sit on a "hot seat" for hours, and even those who regularly sit in a hot tub. Tight briefs or pants can also reduce sperm production. However, most experts believe that to have a real effect on fertility, a man's exposure would have to be continuous over a long period of time (12).

On the other hand, women who take long hot baths or sit in the hot tub or sauna can actually damage the embryo's nervous system during the first thirty days after conception.

9.   Analyze your workplace for reproductive hazards. Many occupations are dangerous to future children because of the chemicals or energy used. Much controversy surrounded a lawsuit which addressed

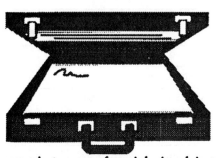

removing women from jobs involving exposure to lead because of the reproductive hazard. However, your baby or your ability to become pregnant could be affected by what you **and** your partner are exposed to at the workplace (and other places too). One study showed that the wives of men exposed to ethylene oxide, rubber chemicals, solvents used in refineries and solvents used in the manufacturing of rubber products had increased risk of miscarriage (13). Other known hazards include radiation, exposure to lead, solvents, paints, anesthetic gases, glues, exposure to copper, arsenic and cadmium, solder fumes, polyvinyl chloride, aerosol sprays, and dyes (14).

If you are exposed to any of the above or any other chemicals you are unsure of, ask your supervisor about the Material Safety Data Sheets. For more information, contact the National Institute for Occupational Safety and Health (in the phone book under Government Agencies), who can refer you to government agencies about specific health concerns. Or contact the Women's Occupational Health Resource Center, Columbia University School of Public Health, 21 Audubon Ave, NY, NY 10032.

For a copy of *Art Material Safety Alert*, send a postcard to CSPC, Washington, DC 20207.

10. Prevent Toxoplasmosis.

Toxoplasmosis is an infection that can cause mental retardation and blindness in babies exposed to the parasite (toxoplasma gondii) before birth. It is excreted in cat feces and is also found in raw meats. So avoid changing the cat litter box, keep cats off kitchen surfaces, and wear gloves while gardening. Don't feed your cats raw meat. Cook meats, especially lamb and pork to a temperature of 160° throughout. Toxoplasmosis can also be transmitted through uncooked or undercooked meat and unwashed fruits and vegetables (15).

FOCUS ON FOLATE

Folate, also called folic acid or folacin, is a B vitamin that is very important during pregnancy; it is needed for cell division and for blood cells. Folacin is water soluble and can be destroyed in cooking. Thus when you cook your vegetables, cook in as little water as possible for as short a time as possible.

People who may need more folacin in their diet are those who have been on medications such as anti-convulsants and some birth control pills. Women in a high risk group may need a folacin supplement; if you are expecting twins, you are a teen, or you have had a child with a neural tube defect. Check with your health care provider.

Best Sources of Folate

The RDA for folate during pregnancy is 400 micrograms; 280 micrograms for breastfeeding.

Food	Folate in micrograms
Chicken liver, 3.5 oz.	763
Veal liver, 3.5 oz.	752
Chicken giblets, 3.5 oz.	372
Lentils, 1 cup	358
Cowpeas, 1 cup	356
Sunflower seeds, 1 cup	317
Pinto beans, 1 cup	294
Baked beans, homemade, 1 cup	256
Navy beans, 1 cup	255
Asparagus, 1 cup	242
Spinach, frozen, drained	220
Beef liver, 3.5 oz.	217
Refried beans, 1 cup	211
Turnip greens, 1 cup	171
Pork liver, 3.5 oz.	163
Black bean soup, 1 cup	158
Hummus, 1 cup	146
Split peas, 1 cup	127
Mixed nuts, 1 cup	118
Creamed corn, 1 cup	115
Orange juice, 1 cup	109
Trail mix, 1 cup	107
Broccoli, frozen 1 cup	104
Peas, frozen, 1 cup	94
Tempeh, 1 cup	86
Boysenberries, 1 cup	84
Taco Bell Bean Tostada	75
Taco Bell Bean Burrito	73

Food	Folate in micrograms
Iceberg lettuce, 1/4 head	73
Beets, 1 cup	73
Arby's Ham and Cheese Sandwich	71
Artichoke, 1	61
Wakame, (seaweed) 1 oz.	55
Papaya, 1 cup	53
Kombu, (seaweed) 1 oz.	51
Vegetable juice, 1 cup	51
Blackberries, 1 cup	49
Melon balls, 1 cup	44

Numbers are rounded to nearest whole number; numbers are for cooked foods, as applicable.

Source: *Nutritionist III Nutrition Software*

Questions You May Have

I drink about 4 or more cups of coffee every day. Any advice on cutting down?

Caffeine is a stimulant, and as most people know, it is habit forming. It's a good idea to cut down or cut out your caffeine because it's also a diuretic. It causes your body to lose fluid, and during pregnancy your need for fluid increases. Substances found in coffee and tea also interfere with the absorption of iron; all good reasons for reducing coffee and tea. Cut down gradually to avoid side effects like headaches. You may want to substitute other lower caffeine

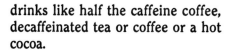

drinks like half the caffeine coffee, decaffeinated tea or coffee or a hot cocoa.

Help! I'm a junk food junkie! I eat fast food every day and actually crave it. How can I improve my diet?

Fast food can fit into a balanced diet if done right. However, if you eat fast food often, (and depending on your choices) you are likely to have decreased intakes of vitamin A, vitamin B6, vitamin C and calcium, which are all important nutrients during pregnancy (16). The other problem is that most restaurant meals are higher in fat and calories than those eaten at home.

Try switching to healthier choices like bean burritos, grilled chicken sandwiches, or salads with low fat meats. Add a salad bar or side salad with lots of fruits and vegetables. Drink lowfat or skim milk with your meal, and bring along a fruit for dessert. Be sure to eat more fruits, vegetables and whole grains at other meals to reach your totals. For more information and suggested menus from fast food restaurants, see page 220.

I've been taking the birth control pill for five years. Is there anything special I should do before I become pregnant?

Physicians usually recommend that you have at least two periods "off the pill" to make sure your hormone levels are back to normal. However, the American College of Obstetricians and Gynecologists no longer has a recommendation regarding this. They state in their book, "Using birth control pills before you become pregnant does not cause birth defects, no matter how close to conception you stop using them." (17) However, your periods may be irregular at first, which makes it difficult to determine your fertile times, or to calculate your due date when you become pregnant. If you had painful periods or heavy periods before you started taking the pill, you may experience those types of menstrual cycles again.

Nutritionally, you should make sure your diet is better than average, since any medication taken over a long period of time can affect your nutritional status. Oral contraceptives can increase your need for B vitamins including folacin. If you've had a poor diet over the past 6 months, you might consider a vitamin-mineral supplement.

I'm 38 and my biological clock just went off. Anything I can do before pregnancy to insure the health of my baby?

Make a visit to your health care provider to get a check-up and a "bill of good health." Older women in good health who have early and regular prenatal care can have perfectly healthy babies. Preparing for your pregnancy and getting into some good lifestyle habits can start your baby out on the right foot! However, there are increased risks of a few problems for older moms during pregnancy, mostly because as we get older, some conditions are more common, such as diabetes and high blood pressure. See page 121 for more information.

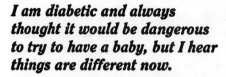

I am diabetic and always thought it would be dangerous to try to have a baby, but I hear things are different now.

You're right! The important thing is for your diabetes to be under control before you get pregnant because high blood sugar could cause birth defects in the first few weeks of pregnancy. Also, during pregnancy your insulin needs will change often and you will need close monitoring. Visit your primary physician and tell her your plan. She will probably refer you to an obstetrician who specializes in taking care of diabetic moms.

You may also want to see an eye doctor. More advice for diabetic moms-to-be is on page 103.

Before I realized I was pregnant, I drank too much at a party; what shall I do?

Your situation is not rare since many pregnancies are a "surprise." The best thing to do is don't panic. Start right now following all the above advice and try not to think about what you've done in the past. Do discuss your concerns with your health care provider, who will help you put them in perspective.

The Knowledgable Pregnancy

What Every Woman Needs to Know

What You Will Find In This Chapter:

- ◆ Ten Steps to a Healthy Diet
- ◆ Everything You Ever Wanted to Know about Weight Gain During Pregnancy
  Gaining Too Fast or Too Much
  Not Gaining Enough
- ◆ The Essential Guide to Vitamins and Minerals
- ◆ To Supplement or Not To Supplement?
- ◆ Why You May Need a Supplement
- ◆ If You Take Supplements
- ◆ Keeping Your Baby's Environment Safe

- ◆ Traveling While Pregnant
- ◆ The Positives of Pregnancy

And answers to questions you may have:

- ◆ Should I take a vitamin supplement?
- ◆ What if I'm not gaining enough weight?
- ◆ How often should I weigh?
- ◆ How much caffeine is OK during pregnancy?
- ◆ How can I reduce my exposure to lead?
- ◆ Should I take individual vitamin supplements?
- ◆ How much caffeine is in hot chocolate?

So you're pregnant–or planning to be. Congratulations! You are about to begin the most fun, tiring, challenging, and special time of your life. No doubt you will find yourself daydreaming in the months to come... what will my baby look like, how will I be as a first time (or second or third time) mom, what will he or she grow up to be—will he discover the cure to cancer, or will she be the first woman president? But your thoughts will inevitably drift back to one important question...will my baby be healthy?

Fortunately, the answer to that question mostly depends on you. Although genetics and pure chance can affect your baby's health, taking good care of yourself can give your baby the best odds of being born healthy.

If you are just considering pregnancy, you are one step ahead of the game and have time to get your body and personal habits into great shape. (See chapter 2 "Considering Pregnancy".) Pre-conception counseling seems to be the new buzz word among hopeful moms-to-be, and with good reason. Your health care provider can give you advice on eating, exercise, alcohol, etc. If you are diabetic, or have another medical condition, this type of counseling is an especially good idea.

As a pregnant or soon to be pregnant woman, you have a unique opportunity to make your health the best it can be.

The good habits you start now can be with you and your family for life- its up to you!

I've seen many a 50 year old who needed to change his or her eating habits to lose weight, reduce blood sugar, or lower cholesterol. However, it truly is tough to "teach an old dog new tricks." So if your children learn good eating habits from

the start, they will never have to worry about changing them!

Because there is so much conflicting advice on nutrition today, I've put together ten easy eating tips to follow now and after your pregnancy.

Ten Steps to a Healthy Diet

1. **Variety.** We've all known those people who eat the same thing for breakfast day after day. Variety is not only the spice of life, it's also important for good health. Not that a banana, cornflakes, and milk is a bad breakfast. Just think about all the other foods and nutrients you are missing!

2. **Moderation** is the key to an enjoyable life and also the key to good health! A recent survey of 4th-8th graders showed that 85% of them said that you should avoid all high fat foods and 77% thought that you should never eat foods that have a lot of sugar (1)! Wrong! There is not one food that you should never eat, regardless if it's high fat, high sugar or both! Just eat it in small amounts. (The exception would be diabetics who must strictly control their blood sugar. The occasional addition of a sweet is probably O.K. but you should discuss this with your health care provider or diabetes educator first.)

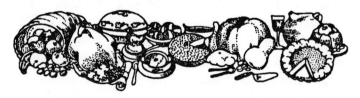

3. Balance. Did you ever meet someone on the "all fruit" diet or the "high protein, low carbohydrate diet?" They don't stay on them long, because not only are they boring, they also lack many of the important nutrients that our bodies need. We need just the right balance of nutrients to maintain good health. We achieve that by eating meals that are balanced with foods from different food groups.

4. Calcium. Pregnant women often concentrate on getting calcium in their diet, as they should. But even after pregnancy, you should try to have 2 or 3 servings a day (more if breastfeeding). Research on calcium is promising–showing that certain amounts of calcium may reduce high blood pressure and may prevent colon cancer (2; 3). Of course, cal-

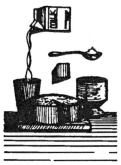

cium is well known for building bones to their maximum strength and keeping them that way, thus helping to prevent osteoporosis.

5. Iron. Many women have a hard time getting enough iron in their diets due to frequent dieting. Let's face it, some of us cut out lots of nutritious foods in order to keep our weight down. Some women cut red meat totally out of their diet, which drastically cuts iron intake. At the

risk of being repetitive, variety comes in again. Don't totally cut red meat out of your diet–simply choose lean cuts and have modest portions. There are also good vegetable sources of iron and foods which help in iron's absorption. See page 64 for more information.

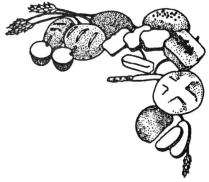

6. Complex Carbohydrates. Women often shy away from things like potatoes, pasta and bread, because they're thought of as fattening. Actually, they are the basis of a healthy diet, and should be the "headline" of the meal. They provide energy, fiber, vitamins and minerals. As far as the fattening part goes, it's generally what you put on it that adds the fat and the calories...think about it!

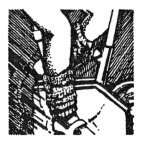

7. Exercise. We've become a nation of couch potatoes, and as the saying goes...couch potatoes breed tater tots! But that is happily changing as people realize the many benefits of exercise...stress reduction, improved endurance, lowered resting heart rate, blood pressure control, cardiovascular efficiency, improved self-esteem and body image, better sleep habits, lowered risk of heart attack, stroke, diabetes and even some types of cancer. During pregnancy, staying limber can help those aches and pains and can help reduce fatigue. It also gets you ready for the "Mother's Marathon"--labor and delivery! However, exercise should be toned down during pregnancy (see page 171).

8. **Fluids.** Our body is comprised of about 60% water, so it makes sense to drink plenty of it. Thirst is the first sign of dehydration, though it lags behind actual need. Thus, by the time you feel thirsty, you are already behind in your fluid intake! Eight to ten glasses a day are recommended during pregnancy. With your increased blood supply, amniotic fluid, and extra tissue to support, the more fluids you have, the better. You can have fluid in the form of juices, decaffeinated teas and sodas, but try to have most of it as clear, clean water!

9. **Fiber.** Most of us don't get enough fiber; 20-35 grams are recommended by the National Cancer Institute (4). During pregnancy, you'll find yourself trying to eat more high fiber foods to combat constipation. Adequate fiber in the diet may reduce risk of colon cancer, breast cancer, and during pregnancy can prevent constipation and hemorrhoids. See page 51 for for more fiber facts.

10. **Spare the extras.** As mentioned before, no food should be totally off limits. However, you can also go overboard in fat, sugar, and even artificial sweeteners if you let your tastebuds rule. The extras like candy, "junk food", and ice cream, should be eaten as a treat after you have eaten all the "must" foods. With all the extra nutrients you need during pregnancy, you can't afford to eat too many "empty calorie" ones.

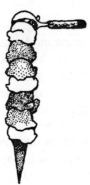

Everything You Ever Wanted to Know About Weight Gain During Pregnancy

Putting on pounds is probably every woman's nightmare, but during pregnancy, the amount of weight you gain and how you gain it may be the distinguishing factor between a normal, term baby and one that is born small and premature.

In one study, women with a low rate of weight gain were more than twice as likely to have a preterm delivery than those with an average weight gain (5). It may be tough to happily watch yourself gaining weight, but try to get used to it.

Where the Weight Goes

You have probably seen life-sized pictures of a fetus, being no bigger than a spoon and weighing no more than an ounce. So why have you gained 5 pounds?! Pregnancy weight gain is obviously more than just baby since the average birth weight is about 7 pounds and the average weight gain is 30! Your blood supply increases, your breasts and uterus enlarge, there are miscellaneous extra fluids, plus, you guessed it–FAT! The fat is there to provide additional calories for breastfeeding. During pregnancy, your body also builds additional muscle to carry the extra weight. The chart below shows where your weight goes.

Tissue	Pounds
Breast	1-2 pounds
Placenta	1 1/2 pounds
Enlarged Uterus	2 pounds
Increased Blood and Fluids	8 1/2 pounds
Baby	7 1/2 pounds
Fat stores	4-14 pounds
Total gained	25-35 pounds

Historically, weight gain recommendations have gone from one extreme to another. It was once thought that toxemia of pregnancy (now called preeclampsia) and high blood pressure could be prevented if the mom-to-be gained as little as possible. Now we know that good nutrition and increased weight gain are the keys to having healthier babies.

According to U.C. Berkeley nutritional epidemiologist Barbara Abrams, co-author of a large study which looked at weight gain in pregnant women, "Our study shows that maternal weight gain is an important factor in pregnancy outcome, especially the baby's birth weight. Since low birthweight is the major cause of infant mortality and mental and physical disability, it can be dangerous to restrict a pregnant woman's weight gains (6)."

Twenty-five to thirty-five pounds is the recommended weight gain for the "average woman," but many don't fit into the average "mold". The amount of weight you should gain depends on your weight before you were pregnant, and if you are having twins or more. (see page 126 on information for multiple births) See how much you should gain from the chart below:

Pre-Pregnancy Weight	Suggested Weight Gain
Underweight 10% below ideal body weight	28-40 pounds
Normal Weight (Average weight for height)	25-35 pounds
Overweight 20% or more over ideal body weight	15-25 pounds
Teens and African-American women should strive for gains at the upper end of the range. Women under 5'3" should gain an amount of weight at the lower end of the range.	

Source: *Nutrition During Pregnancy:* Part I, Weight Gain: Part II, Nutrient Supplements, Subcommittee on Nutritional Status and Weight Gain During Pregnancy, National Academy of Sciences

What's "Ideal Weight"? Ideal weight has different definitions. Some health professionals use insurance weight charts, some use the "rule of 5" and others use the recent Suggested Weights for Adults from the U.S. Department of Agriculture and U.S. Department of Health and Human Services. You could also define ideal body weight as the weight you feel best at.

"Rule of 5" Start with 100 pounds for 5 feet tall. Add 5 pounds for every inch over 5 feet you are. There is always a plus or minus 10% factor to account for bone and body build, etc.

Suggested Weights for Adults

Height[1]	Weight in pounds[2]	
	[3]19 to 34 years	35 years and over
5'0"	97–128	108–138
5'1"	101–132	111–143
5'2"	104–137	115–148
5'3"	107–141	119–152
5'4"	111–146	122–157
5'5"	114–150	126–162
5'6"	118–155	130–167
5'7"	121–160	134–172
5'8"	125–164	138–178
5'9"	129–169	142–183
5'10"	132–174	146–188
5'11"	136–179	151–194
6'0"	140–184	155–199
6'1"	144–189	159–205
6'2"	148–195	164–210
6'3"	152–200	168–216
6'4"	156–205	173–222
6'5"	160–216	177–228
6'6"	164–216	182–234

[1]Without shoes
[2]Without clothes
[3]The higher weight in the ranges generally apply to men, who tend to have more muscle and bone; the lower weights more often apply to women, who have less muscle and bone.

Monitoring Your Own Weight Gain

Keep in mind that it isn't just the amount of weight gain, but how you gain it or the pattern of weight gain that is also important. It should be a gradual weight gain and should somewhat follow the curves below. You should gain approximately 2-4 pounds during the first trimester, and close to a pound a week during the second and especially the third trimester, when baby grows the most. If your goal is more or less than average, adapt those numbers accordingly.

Weight Gain Chart

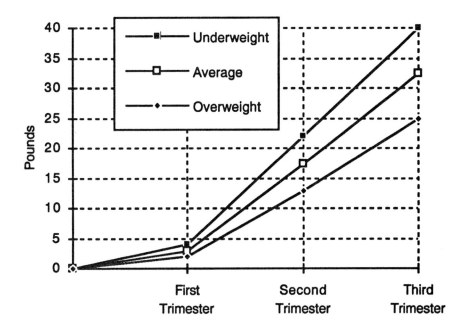

The Weighing Issue

In general, if you are eating all the right foods with just a few splurges, your weight gain will follow the right pattern for you. Remember that women have fluctuating weights which vary even more during pregnancy. A few tips for weighing are listed below.

♦ **Weigh yourself at the same time of day and under the same conditions.** For example, always first thing in the morning, after you use the restroom, naked or wearing the same nightgown.

♦ **Weigh yourself weekly, not daily!** Weighing daily could drive a person nuts! Since your weight depends on what you have had to eat and drink, how much sodium you've consumed and even your

bowel habits, you could show a 3 pound "weight gain" on Monday, and a 4 pound "weight loss" on Wednesday.

♦ **Only compare weights from the same scale.** Your health care provider's scale shows a 4 pound weight gain compared to your home scale. Don't go into a panic! Scales are often different, and all the above factors come into play too, so only compare weights from the same scale.

Gaining Too Fast or Too Much

Most women fear gaining too much, because they think it will be difficult to take off. Also, gaining too much weight can cause excessive infant size and increased risk of a C-section. However, regardless of how much you gain, **pregnancy is never the time to try to lose weight**. If you have reached your goal 30 pound weight gain by week 35, it doesn't mean you should not gain any more for the remaining 5 weeks!

Here are several explanations for gaining too much weight or gaining too fast:

♦ **Overeating** or simply eating too many high fat, high calorie foods (are you trying to truly eat for two)? See the quiz on the next page to evaluate the "extras" in your diet.

♦ **Multiple fetuses.** If you don't feel like your weight gain is related to eating, consult your health care provider about the possibility of carrying more than one baby.

♦ **Inaccurate weighing** or weighing after eating or drinking. (weighing after drinking a quart of water for example, will add two pounds to your weight!)

♦ **Preeclampsia/High Blood Pressure.** If you gain 3 or more pounds a week in the second or third trimester of pregnancy, and you also experience swelling of feet, hands, severe headache or have trouble seeing, contact your health care provider immediately! Those could be the first signs of preeclampsia, a potentially serious problem. See page 125 for more.

How To Avoid Gaining Too Much Weight

With the recommended weight gain more than it was a few years ago, you will definitely "look" pregnant!

However, there are two things that control your weight gain, and how it looks on you – your diet and your activity level. Where the weight is gained varies between women. You will hear myths about your weight gain. Some people will tell you that if you're having a boy, the weight will be all in your stomach. And if your weight gain is spread out all over, many will predict a girl! The truth is where the weight goes is controlled by your genes.

If you start or continue an exercise program, you will look and feel better since you will be well toned. Being in good overall physical shape will make you feel good about your expanding waistline. Having more lean muscle tissue will also help you lose weight after you have your baby.

An experienced mother of two says:

"I lost all my weight within a few months of having Brian. I swam regularly right up to delivery. However with Emily, I was very sick with bronchitis the last 6 weeks and spent a lot of time in bed. Overall, I was much less active when I was pregnant with Emily and it took me much longer to take the weight off after Emily was born."

Of course, your diet may need critical analysis. If you follow The Eating Expectantly Diet, you shouldn't have any problem with excess weight gain. The quiz below may shed some light on your eating habits.

◆ Will You Gain Too Much Weight? ◆ Quiz:

1. Do you eat sweets 4 times a week or more?

2. Do you snack on chips, nuts, nachos, french fries etc. 4 times per week or more?

3. Do you pile on the margarine, salad dressing, sour cream, and cheese?

4. When you cook, do you pour more than 1 teaspoon of oil per serving cooked into the pan?

5. Do you regularly eat the skin on the chicken, fat on your steak, etc.?

6. Do you eat "typical" fast food or fried food regularly?

7. Do you often eat when bored, depressed, angry or happy, but not hungry?

8. Do you usually eat while doing something else like reading, watching T.V. etc?

9. Do you eat snacks like regular ice cream and regular cheese?

If you answered yes to 3 or more, you have a good chance of gaining too much weight (or too much fat) during your pregnancy. Keeping an eye on fat intake will help you now and later when you are trying to lose your "baby fat."

All About

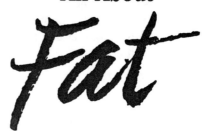

There are several reasons why watching your fat is important--for the short term and long term.

1. Ounce per ounce, fat has more than twice as many calories as carbohydrate or protein.

2. Fat calories are stored easier than calories from other sources, so it is actually better to eat more starches and less fat. Meaning the more fat you eat, the more fat you wear!

3. A high fat intake is implicated in certain types of cancer especially breast and colon cancer (7).

4. A high fat diet, or eating fried foods can aggravate the nausea of early pregnancy and heartburn later in pregnancy.

To put your own fat intake in perspective, it should be about 30% of your calories. If you are trying to gain weight, your fat intake may be more, but try to make it from vegetable sources (such as avocado, nuts, peanut butter, vegetable oils, etc.). Most health organizations recommend that we eat 30% or less of our calories from fat. A specific guideline for pregnancy hasn't been established, but somewhere around 30% fat is a prudent recommendation. The *average* pregnant woman needs 2200-2400 calories and 30% of those calories would work out to be about 70-90 grams of fat. This may sound like a lot. Are you savvy about fat? Look at the following diet and guess how much fat it contains.

How Much Fat?

Breakfast

Cereal with 1 cup 2% milk
2 Slices of Toast with
2 tsp. margarine
Fresh fruit

Snack

1 oz. cheese
10 wheat crackers

Lunch

Deluxe Cheeseburger
Fries
Side salad with 2 Tb. dressing

Snack

2 Tb. peanut butter on melba toast
1 1/2 cups 2% milk

Dinner

6 oz. fish sauteed in olive oil
Baked potato with 2 Tb. sour cream
and 2 tsp. margarine
Fresh steamed spinach
Tomatoes and cucumbers with 2 Tb.
vinaigrette

Snack

Ice Cream
Chocolate chip cookie

Believe it or not, the above menu has 160 grams of fat, or double that recommended during pregnancy. Let's change a few things and see how the fat adds up in our modified menu:

Breakfast

Cereal with 1 cup skim milk
2 Slices of toast with 1 tsp. margarine, 2 tsp. fruit spread, banana

Snack

1 oz. lowfat cheese
8 wheat crackers

Lunch

Grilled chicken sandwich
Side salad with pasta salad,
lite vinaigrette
Peaches and pineapple
1 cup 2% milk

Snack

2 Tb. peanut butter
1/2 bagel
Vegetable juice

Dinner

6 oz. fish baked with Parmesan /
crumb topping, 1 tsp. margarine
Boiled new potatoes with 2 tsp.
margarine
Fresh steamed spinach
Melon balls
Skim milk

Snack

Frozen yogurt
Graham crackers

We've cut the fat in half with just a few changes! It now has under 80 grams of fat, a much better number.

You can check the vitamin and mineral aspect of your diet out by taking the nutrition quiz on page 67 or send in the Nutrition Analysis form at the back of the book.

Not Gaining Enough

There are as many reasons for not being able to gain as there are for gaining too much. Not gaining enough weight, though it may seem a blessing to some, can cause major problems for your baby. Women who don't gain enough are more likely to deliver their babies before they are due and their babies are likely to be smaller. Newborn death is more related to prematurity and low-birth weight than any other cause (8). So if you fall into this category, be sure to find the reason below and do something about it.

♦ **High metabolism.** Those who were underweight before pregnancy may just burn calories more quickly. You may need to closely analyze your diet for ways to increase calories–and may need individual help from a registered dietitian.

♦ **You can't eat much** because of nausea, heartburn, stress or other problems. First you need to get to the root of the problem. Nausea usually goes away after the first trimester. The other problems may have simple solutions. Psychosocial stress has been known to decrease weight gain and you may need help from a counselor or social worker. Ask your health care provider for assistance.

♦ **You go a mile a minute.** Some moms-to-be have a very active lifestyle and don't slow down for pregnancy. This could result in burning too many calories, or not taking the time to eat enough. Either scenario leaves fewer calories left for baby to grow on. If your lifestyle is interfering with your weight gain, you may need to look at slowing down your activities and exercise, increasing calories or both.

♦ **You're not into the mindset of gaining weight.** If you have ever had a weight problem or a history of eating disorders, it might be difficult to actually gain weight "on purpose". Your health care provider or a counselor may be needed to help you come to terms with this situation

♦ **You smoke.** Smoking is associated with reduced weight gain as well as placenta previa (9). Do your best to cut down or quit.

What You Can Do If You Are Not Gaining Enough Weight

1. Make sure your diet is like The Eating Expectantly Diet on page 47.

2. Slow down!

3. Increase fat intake. This is the easiest way to increase calories without increasing the bulk–thus is the best way to add calories if you are too full to eat. Unsaturated fats are the best types to add, like vegetable oils, salad dressings, mayonnaise and margarines, nuts, seeds, avocado, and peanut butter.

4. Increase what I call "Healthy Junk Food" or all those things that have some nutritive value, but can have extra calories too–like milkshakes, frozen yogurt, pudding, egg custard. You might want to add a food supplement like Instant Breakfast to your milk to add calories.

5. Don't forget snacks. If you're eating just 3 meals a day, chances are that you're not eating enough. Most women need a few snacks a day to fit in all the nutrients and calories they need for pregnancy.

See page 241 for snack ideas for high energy moms.

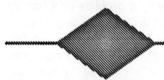

Changing Your Mindset for Pregnancy

Up to now you've been the perfect model of health. You don't eat eggs, you work out 5 times a week and you haven't eaten red meat in years. Now you're craving a steak, don't feel like exercising (or doing much of anything for that matter) and eggs seem to go down real well. What's a woman to do? First, let's set a few things straight.

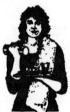

True, the average American diet contains too much protein, but eating red meat in moderation is fine. You just need to choose lean cuts like top round, eye of round and flank steak. In fact, several studies have shown that cutting red meat from the diet doesn't necessarily reduce cholesterol. Red meat has lots going for it too! It has plenty of iron, and it also helps your body absorb iron from non-meat sources. It is also a good source of zinc, an important nutrient during pregnancy.

The same goes for eggs, which have been looked down on in the past. Eggs supply perfect protein, even if high in cholesterol. Even the American Heart Association allows 3-4 egg yolks a week in their Eating Plan for Healthy Americans(10). So don't feel bad about eating extra eggs--just watch the accompaniments (bacon, sausage, biscuits, hash browns etc.).

Your body is going through a tremendous amount of change (no kidding!) and it's normal not to feel quite as energetic as you used to. You also may not feel as comfortable about the size or look of your "body with baby", which may make it difficult to get into an exercise outfit or bathing suit. Try to keep up some exercise, even if it's just walking around the neighborhood. It will help keep muscle tone, and will make you feel good--mentally and physically. (see chapter 11 for more on exercise)

Lastly, remember that pregnancy doesn't last forever, even though sometimes it feels like it might!

◆ The Essential Guide to Vitamins ◆ and Minerals

The body needs many different nutrients every day. All vitamins and minerals play an important, if minor, role in the making of a healthy baby.

The Energy Releasing Nutrients:

You have probably heard people say, "vitamins give me more energy." Actually vitamins have no calories; but you must have them to be able to use the energy in your food.

Thiamin-(Vitamin B-1)

RDA for pregnancy: 1.5 milligrams; for breastfeeding: 1.6 milligrams.

Functions: Energy metabolism, appetite and nervous system function.

Note: thiamin is unstable in heat and light. Vegetables high in thiamin and other water soluble vitamins, should be cooked minimally with as little water as possible.

Best Sources: Pork, green peas, collards, lima beans, dried beans, sunflower seeds.

Riboflavin (Vitamin B-2)

RDA for pregnancy: 1.7 milligrams; for breastfeeding, first 6 months: 1.8 milligrams; for second 6 months: 1.7 milligrams.

Functions: Helps release energy from food, maintains normal vision and skin health.

Best Sources: Liver, milk, yogurt, cheese.

Niacin (Vitamin B3)

RDA for pregnancy: 1.7 milligrams; for breastfeeding: 20 milligrams.

Functions: Helps release energy from food, supports health of skin, nervous system, and digestive system.

Best Sources: Meat, poultry, whole and enriched grains, legumes and nuts.

Pantothenic acid

The estimated safe and adequate daily dietary intake is 4 to 7 milligrams.

Functions: Helps release energy from food; involved in antibody production.

Best Sources: Widespread in many foods.

Biotin

The estimated safe and adequate daily dietary intake is 30 to 100 micrograms.

Functions: Helps release energy from food; assists in fat synthesis and carbohydrate storage.

Sources: Widespread in many foods.

The Building Nutrients

These nutrients are responsible for helping to build bone, muscle tissue, hormones, and other tissues.

Calcium:

RDA for pregnancy and breastfeeding: 1200 milligrams.

Functions: Principal material of bones and teeth; vital in muscle con-

The Essential Guide to Vitamins and Minerals

traction, nerve functioning, blood clotting, blood pressure and immune defense. Research shows a possible relationship between adequate calcium in the diet and reduced risk of hypertension (11) and colon cancer. Adequate calcium over the life-span can protect against osteoporosis.

Best Sources: Milk and milk products, small fish with bones, blackstrap molasses, tofu that has calcium added during processing, greens, legumes, some seaweed and sea vegetables.

Vitamin B12 (cobalamin)

RDA for pregnancy: 2.2 micrograms; for breastfeeding: 2.6 micrograms.

Functions: Helps in new red blood cell production, helps maintain health of nerve cells.

Best Sources: Liver, muscle meats, fish, eggs, milk and milk products and fortified foods.

Note: Only foods of animal origin and certain fortified foods contain Vitamin B12. Check the label of foods to see if B12 is added. For more information see page 85.

Phosphorous:

RDA for pregnancy and breastfeeding: 1200 milligrams.

Calcium and phosphorous make up 3/4 of the total weight of minerals found in the body. Unlike calcium, a deficiency of phosphorous is rare.

Functions: Used in building bones and teeth; needed in every cell membrane, in genetic material, as part of energy production, and in the body's buffering system.

Sources: All animal protein, preservatives.

Note: excess phosphorous may draw calcium out of the body.

Primary sources of phosphorous in the American diet are animal protein, and carbonated sodas.

Magnesium

RDA for pregnancy: 320 milligrams; for breastfeeding, first 6 months: 355 milligrams; for second 6 months: 340 milligrams.

Functions: Bone mineralization, protein building, enzyme action, muscle contraction, transmission of nerve impulses, maintenance of teeth.

Best Sources: Nuts, legumes, whole grains, dark green vegetables, seafood.

Vitamin A

RDA for pregnancy: 800 retinol equivalents; for breastfeeding, first 6 months: 1300 retinol equivalents; for second 6 months: 1200 retinol equivalents. One retinol equivalent is equal to 1 microgram of vitamin A or 6 micrograms of beta carotene. Beta carotene is converted in the body to vitamin A.

Functions: Helps in cell growth and development; formation of bones and teeth; needed for healthy skin and mucous membranes and cornea of the eye; reproductive health.

Carotenoids such as beta carotene are pre-cursors of Vitamin A and are

◆ The Essential Guide to Vitamins ◆ and Minerals

found in vegetable sources. Very promising research is going on regarding beta-carotene, cancer and heart disease.

Best Sources:

Vitamin A: Fortified milk, cheese, eggs, liver. Fish liver oils are also good sources. Because toxins tend to accumulate in the fat of fish, fish oils are not recommended during pregnancy.

A Word of Caution: Excess Vitamin A is very toxic to the fetus, so if you are taking an individual supplement of Vitamin A or a high potency multi-vitamin containing several times the RDA for the vitamin, STOP IMMEDIATELY and consult your health care provider. Also, if you are trying to conceive or are already pregnant, you should not be taking any medication containing Vitamin A such as Retin-A.

Beta Carotene

The body converts beta carotene to Vitamin A as needed, so there is no worry in having too much beta carotene in the diet. However, people who have consumed large amounts of carrots or carrot juice have had their skin turn orange! The skin returns to normal after a moderate diet is resumed.

Best Sources: Spinach and dark leafy greens, broccoli, deep orange fruits like apricots, peaches, canteloupe, and orange vegetables like squash, carrots, sweet potatoes, pumpkin.

Vitamin K

RDA for pregnancy and breastfeeding: 65 micrograms.

Functions: Synthesis of blood clotting proteins.

Note: Vitamin K is made in the digestive tract, though infants are given a dose at birth before their own production starts.

Sources: Seaweed (dulce and rockweed), green tea, soybean oil, turnip greens, lettuce.

Vitamin D

RDA for pregnancy: and breastfeeding: 10 micrograms or 400 International Units (IU).

Functions: Bone mineralization through control of calcium and phosphorous in the body.

Best Sources: Sunshine, fortified milk, fortified cereals, egg yolks, fish liver oil, liver.

Note: The best source of Vitamin D is sunlight! Your skin produces it's own vitamin D when it is exposed to sufficient sunlight. People who develop deficiencies generally have very dark skin, or spend little time in the sun. In fact, dark skinned people may need 6 times more sun exposure than fair skinned people to produce the same amount of Vitamin D (12).

The climate where you live can also affect how much Vitamin D you produce. For example, the winter sunlight in Britain, Alberta, Canada, and Massachusetts is not enough to cause vitamin D production in the

◆ The Essential Guide to Vitamins ◆ and Minerals

skin (13). If you drink no milk and spend little time in the sun or live in an area where there is little sunshine in the winter, you probably need to eat more foods with Vitamin D or take a supplement.

Don't take a Vitamin D supplement unless your health care provider prescribes it because Vitamin D is toxic in large doses.

Vitamin B-6 (Pyridoxine)

RDA for pregnancy: 2.2 milligrams; for breastfeeding: 2.1 milligrams.

Functions: Used in amino acid and fatty acid metabolism; helps to make red blood cells. B6 is needed in amounts proportional to the amount of protein in the diet.

Best Sources: Green and leafy vegetables, meats, fish, poultry, shellfish, legumes, fruits, whole grains.

Note: Women--pregnant and not, don't seem to have enough B6 in their diet. Some women who take birth control pills may have a slightly increased need for the vitamin. Deficiency of the vitamin can cause anemia, irritability and abnormal brain wave pattern.

Folate (folacin, folic acid)

RDA for pregnancy: 400 micrograms; for breastfeeding, first 6 months: 280 micrograms; for second 6 months: 260 micrograms.

Functions: Needed for all new cell production and use of amino acids. Needed for some enzymes

Sources: Cooked spinach, leafy green vegetables, liver, black-eyed peas, lentils, red kidney beans, broccoli, brussel sprouts, beets, okra, green peas, asparagus, legumes, orange and grapefruit juice, fortified cereals.

Note: The need for folacin during pregnancy more than doubles, due to vast increases in the number of new cells being made. Folate can be easily destroyed in cooking. Certain medications such as oral contraceptives, anticonvulsants, aspirin, chemotherapy drugs and antacids can affect your folate status. Alcohol and smoking can also increase the need for folate (14)

If you take any of the above medications, smoke or drink regularly or if you did just prior to pregnancy, your need for folate is probably greater than average. You will need to choose your diet more carefully or you may need a supplement. If you are not taking a prenatal vitamin and don't have an adequate diet, you may also need a folacin supplement. Contact your health care provider.

A landmark study done in several countries showed that folacin supplementation at around the time of conception could prevent close to 3/4 of recurrent neural tube defects. The Center for Disease Control has released recommendations for women who have previously had a baby or fetus with a neural tube defect (15). For those women plan-

The Essential Guide to Vitamins and Minerals

ning a pregnancy, or who are already pregnant, they should contact their health care provider immediately about taking a folacin supplement.

The research showed how supplementation could prevent recurring neural tube defects, but whether increased folate could also prevent first time occurrences is unsure, though there is a good chance it will. Since adequate folate intake before and at conception is vital, all women should be wary of their folacin intake, whether they are at the first weeks of pregnancy or are just planning.

Iron:

RDA for pregnancy: 30 milligrams; for breastfeeding: 15 milligrams.

Functions: Part of the blood protein hemoglobin, which carries oxygen in the body; part of muscle protein; necessary for the use of energy in the body.

Best Sources: Clams, red meats and organ meats, eggs, chicken, fish, legumes, iron fortified cereals and breads.

Note: Iron deficiency anemia is still a public health problem in the U. S. This may be due to a decrease in eating red meat and an increase in caffeine containing beverages, which decreases the absorption of iron. In the 1985 Continuing Surveys of Food Intakes of Individuals (CSFII) only 4% of women met or exceeded the RDA for iron (16).

Zinc:

RDA for pregnancy: 15 milligrams; for breastfeeding, first 6 months: 19 milligrams; for second 6 months: 16 milligrams.

Functions: Promotes normal growth of tissues and bones; needed for the normal development of a fetus, involved in making genetic material, in immune reactions, taste and smell perception, and wound healing. Zinc is also required for sperm production.

Zinc deficiency during pregnancy can cause lowbirth weight, increased pregnancy complications and premature births. A deficiency during fetal brain development could cause fetal brain injury (17).

Best Sources: Shellfish (oysters), meat, poultry, whole grains, dried beans and nuts.

Vitamin C (ascorbic acid)

RDA for pregnancy: 70 milligrams; for breastfeeding, first 6 months: 95 milligrams; for second 6 months: 90 milligrams.

Functions: Needed for thyroid hormone, collagen synthesis and for the production of amino acids. Strengthens resistance to infection, helps in the absorption of iron and acts as an antioxidant to protect cell membranes.

Best Sources: Papaya, citrus fruits, melons, peppers, berries, green leafy vegetables, tomatoes, broccoli, cauliflower, cabbage.

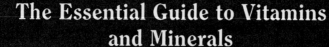

The Essential Guide to Vitamins and Minerals

The Support Nutrients

These nutrients help all the other nutrients with their functions.

Vitamin E (tocopherol)

RDA for pregnancy: 10 milligrams; for breastfeeding, first 6 months: 12 milligrams; for second 6 months: 11 milligrams (all based on alpha-tocopherol equivalents).

Functions: Strong antioxidant, meaning it breaks down oxidants, or free radicals, which can be destructive to cell membranes. Promising research is being done with Vitamin E and cancer.

Best Sources: Wheat germ and wheat germ oil, sunflower oil, safflower oil, almond oil and almonds, hazelnuts, mayonnaise and salad dressings made with the above oils.

Sodium

There is no RDA for sodium; estimated minimum requirement during pregnancy is 570 milligrams; 635 milligrams for breastfeeding.

Functions: Maintains normal fluid balance. It is needed for nerve impulse transmission.

Note: Historically, pregnant women lowered their salt and sodium intake during pregnancy to reduce water retention, and sometimes to prevent toxemia or preeclampsia. Now, moderation rather than restriction is the key for pregnant women.

Potassium:

There is no RDA for potassium; estimated minimum requirement during pregnancy is 2,000 milligrams; 2,500 milligrams for breastfeeding.

Functions: Needed for many reactions such as protein production, fluid balance, transmission of nerve impulses, and muscle contractions.

Sources: Fruits, vegetables, meats, milk, grains, legumes.

Note: A high intake of potassium has been linked to a reduced incidence of high blood pressure in certain populations (18).

In the 1985 Continuing Survey of Food Intakes of Individuals, women's intakes of potassium was well below the Estimated Safe and Adequate Daily Dietary Intake (19).

Other Trace Elements

Zinc and iron are considered trace elements, but they are so important during pregnancy, they were included in the other sections. Other trace elements include copper, iodine, selenium, fluoride, manganese, chromium and molydenum. According to the Subcommittee on Dietary Intake and Nutrient Supplements, there is no persuasive evidence that routine supplementation of trace elements during pregnancy is warranted, with the exception of iron.

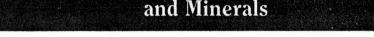

The Essential Guide to Vitamins and Minerals

Copper:

The estimated safe and adequate daily dietary intake for adults is 1.5 to 3 milligrams.

Functions: Helps in red blood cell production, is found in nerve coverings, and connective tissue. It also assists in energy production and in respiration. Copper deficiency during pregnancy is unknown.

Best Sources: Whole grains, shellfish, liver and kidney, raisins, nuts, peas and beans.

Iodine:

The RDA for pregnancy is 175 micrograms; for breastfeeding: 200 micrograms.

Functions: Is essential component of the thyroid hormone thyroxine, which is responsible for regulating the metabolic rate (the amount of energy the body needs at rest). Iodine deficiency during pregnancy can cause disorders in the fetus including stillbirth, birth defects and neurological impairment. However, there is no evidence of iodine deficiency in the U.S.

Best Sources: Seafood, iodized salt, and food grown in ocean areas which contain iodine rich soil.

Selenium:

The RDA for pregnancy: 65 micrograms; for breastfeeding: 75 micrograms.

Functions: As an antioxidant, selenium works to protect body compounds from oxidation. Promising research links selenium and other antioxidants with reduced cancer risk.

Best Sources: Seafood, meats, grains.

Fluoride:

The estimated safe and adequate daily dietary intake for adults is 1.5 to 4 milligrams.

Functions: Bonds calcium and phosphorus in bones and teeth. Prevents cavities in teeth. Though some research shows that fluoride supplementation may prevent cavities to a greater extent in baby, this has been challenged. The subcommittee concluded that there is insufficient evidence to recommend fluoride supplements during pregnancy.

Best Sources: Water that naturally contains fluoride or water that has fluoride added.

Manganese:

The estimated safe and adequate daily dietary intake for adults is 2 to 5 milligrams.

Functions: Is part of enzymes which are active in many cell processes. Also is a component of an important antioxidant.

Best Sources: Whole grains, beans, peas and nuts.

Chromium:

The estimated safe and adequate daily dietary intake for adults is 50-200 micrograms.

The Essential Guide to Vitamins and Minerals

Functions: Associated with insulin; needed for the release of energy from glucose. Deficiency symptoms are diabetes–like from inability to use glucose. There is some concern that increased refinement of foods such as whole grains could lead to decreased intake of this trace mineral.

Best Sources: Whole grains, meat, mushrooms, asparagus, brewers yeast.

Molybdenum:

The estimated safe and adequate daily dietary intake for adults is 75 to 250 micrograms.

Functions: Is a component of enzymes used in many body processes.

Best Sources: Legumes, cereals, organ meats.

Of Special Concern

Studies of pregnant women's diets have shown that intakes of Vitamin B6, D, E, folate, iron, calcium, zinc, and magnesium were below the RDA's. Look above and see if you have sources of these nutrients in your diet.

Selected Nutrients in Various Cuts of Meat

All animal proteins are not equal; they provide varying amounts of zinc, iron, vitamin B6 and B12. The table below shows why you should eat a variety of meats.

Source: Modified from *A Good Start; Nutrition During Pregnancy*, National Livestock and Meat Board, and Food Values of Portions Commonly Used, 15th Edition.

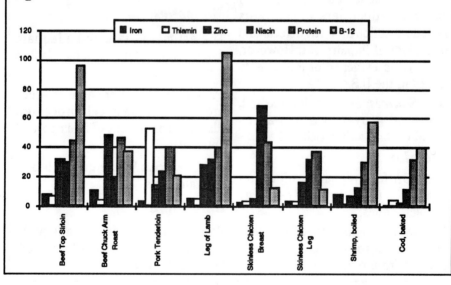

To Supplement or Not to Supplement?

The need for vitamin/mineral supplements has been controversial for years, and their use during pregnancy also has two sides.

Prenatal vitamins have generally been prescribed across the board for most pregnant women. However, a National Academy of Sciences subcommittee recommends in it's report, *Nutrition During Pregnancy*, that prenatal vitamin supplements should be prescribed on an individual basis based on the woman's current nutritional status (20).

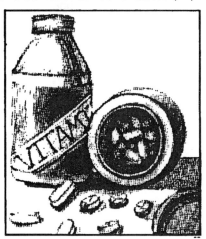

The reason for the concern over supplementation is that certain nutrients in large doses can be toxic to the fetus including iron, zinc, selenium, Vitamins A, B6, C and D. Moreover, an increase in the amount of one nutrient may negatively affect how other nutrients are absorbed and used (21).

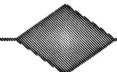

"Dietary Supplements should not replace dietary counseling or a well-balanced diet..."Subcommittee on Dietary Intake and Nutrient Supplements during Pregnancy, National Academy of Sciences (22).

There are several exceptions. Iron is needed in an amount that can't be obtained from food, so a 30 mg. supplement is recommended. Recently it was found that a folacin deficiency right before or during the first weeks of pregnancy is related to neural tube defects. If you have had a baby with a neural tube defect like spina bifida, chances are a folacin supplement may prevent the same problem in your next baby (23). Other women should examine their own diet for an adequate intake of folacin or may want to take a multi-vitamin supplement containing folacin.

Why You May Need a Supplement

There are some situations that alter your food intake or increase your need for nutrients. If any of the conditions listed below apply to you, then you may need a multi-vitamin and mineral supplement. The need for a supplement should be discussed with your health care provider along with the help of a registered dietitian.

♦ You have a limited income or inadequate access to food.

♦ You avoid certain foods because you can't tolerate them, or because of cultural practices or religious taboos.

♦ You are a total vegetarian.

♦ You have a lifestyle that doesn't allow you to acquire, prepare or eat the right foods for pregnancy such as a hectic job or family responsibilities.

♦ You are unhappy about being pregnant.

♦ You eat or crave non-food items like clay or starch.

♦ You are a smoker.

♦ You are a teen.

♦ You are carrying twins or more.

♦ You are anemic.

♦ You drink substantial amounts of alcohol, you smoke, take illegal drugs or have taken prescription medication over a long period of time.

♦ You are restricting certain foods in your diet to control your weight gain.

♦ You are substantially overweight or underweight.

♦ You have been on a strict weight reduction diet or fad diet just before pregnancy.

♦ You eat or drink only one dairy product or calcium rich food per day.

♦ You live in a northern city that has little sunshine in the winter and you don't drink milk.

Source: Modified from *Nutrition During Pregnancy*; Part I Weight Gain, Nutrient Supplements p 251)

If you feel that none of the above applies to you, but think that your own diet leaves something to be desired, a prenatal vitamin may be warranted. Some researchers believe that women should be on a prenatal vitamin supplement during pregnancy or if you're planning to become pregnant. According to Margie Profet, a research associate at the University of California, Berkeley, "Our modern fast-food diet is very different from that of our hunter- gatherer ancestors and many people aren't getting proper levels of vitamins and minerals (24)."

If You Take Supplements

Once you visit your health care provider, you can make the decision together about taking a prenatal vitamin. However, most women don't make their first visit to the doctor until the tenth or twelfth week of pregnancy, after much of the organ development has taken place. If you feel you need to take a supplement before you visit your health care provider, you may want to call him or her before your first appointment. Here are some words of advice about taking vitamin supplements:

1. If you take a supplement, take a multi-vitamin/mineral supplement that contains no more than 100% of the RDAs. This information is found on the label. Although nutrient needs for pregnancy are higher, your food can make up the difference until you decide with your health care provider if a more potent supplement is needed.

2. Remember that a vitamin-mineral supplement is no substitute for a healthy diet!

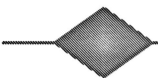

"The bottom-line message is that the emphasis on optimal diet is of the greatest importance to all women of the child bearing age at all times – not only when pregnancy has been confirmed."

Michael Hambidge, M.D., Sc.D., Director of the Center for Human Nutrition, University of Colorado Health Sciences Center.

3. Make sure your supplement contains iron and folacin. However, you should not take individual supplements of these nutrients unless your health care provider recommends it.

4. DO NOT take any individual nutrient supplements, especially vitamin A or vitamin D unless prescribed by your health care provider. Some individual supplements can be toxic to the fetus and cause birth defects, or can create imbalances competing with other nutrients for absorption.

5. If you are already taking single nutrient supplements, discontinue their use until you discuss it with your health care provider.

6. If your health care provider suggests a supplement, but it makes you nauseated, consider taking them before you go to bed with a light snack.

Calcium Supplements

Calcium is vital during pregnancy for the health of your baby and especially for your future bone health. Preliminary research also shows some correlation between increased calcium in the diet and reduced incidence of high blood pressure during pregnancy (25; 26; 27).

Yet so many women, both pregnant and not, don't have enough calcium in their diet. Women often think about osteoporosis around the time of menopause, but they should actually consider their bone health all their lives; bone continues to grow until age 25 and gradually starts losing mass after age 35. (For information on how to sneak calcium into your diet see page 62.)

Another good reason to have enough calcium in your diet; recent research shows that as your bones lose calcium to make up for the calcium that is missing from your diet, lead stored there is also released. You are exposed to small amounts of lead over a lifetime from drinking water and other sources and it is stored in your bone. During times when the bones lose calcium, (during pregnancy, lactation, and after menopause, in women), lead is released into the bloodstream.

Adequate dietary calcium is essential in preventing or keeping to a minimum the turnover of bone. For women who had a substantial lead exposure earlier in life, (such as living in a house with lead pipes or eating leaded paint chips as a child), adequate calcium is even more important to prevent possible lead poisoning of yourself and your child (28).

If your are under 25 and your diet contains less than 600 mg. of calcium in a day, (found in 1 serving of dairy products plus other nondairy foods), a calcium supplement is recommended (29).   Ask your health care provider about the specifics.

If you are currently taking a calcium or iron supplement, there are a few things you should consider about the way you take them:

Type of calcium:

Calcium is best absorbed from calcium citrate and calcium carbonate. Many women take Tums® because they contain calcium carbonate. However, since calcium carbonate acts as an antacid, this form of calcium, if taken in large amounts, can cause the stomach to "rebound" and make even more acid. Increased stomach acid can lead to heartburn. Therefore, calcium citrate or a supplement containing several kinds of calcium are better sources to use during pregnancy. Oyster shell calcium and dolomite should be avoided due to possible lead and heavy metal contamination.

What you take it with: Calcium is best absorbed when taken with food; iron is best absorbed on an empty stomach.

However, if you take an iron supplement along with calcium citrate or calcium phosphate (types of supplements) on an empty stomach, the amount of iron you absorb may be decreased (30).

The solution:

If you take both iron and calcium, take them at different times. Take your iron supplement on an empty stomach (or with a light snack when you are not having a dairy product.) Take your calcium supplement with a light snack. Registered Pharmacist Nellie Whaley suggests that if you take calcium and iron, take the calcium at least 2 hours after or 1 hour before you take the iron.

Some women find that iron or prenatal vitamin supplements make them nauseated. Taking them right before bedtime or with a snack usually helps. Whenever you decide to take your supplements, make sure to make it a ritual; calcium or iron left in the bottle won't bring you any benefit!

Keeping Your Baby's Environment Safe

You knew they were coming, "the don'ts". A physician who specializes in high risk pregnancies once told me, "You have only one chance to give your baby what it needs. Why not do everything you can to help your baby along–it's only 9 months." It's easy to give advice, but may not be as easy to follow it. If you are hav-

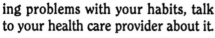

ing problems with your habits, talk to your health care provider about it.

Smoking

The first trimester, and before pregnancy, if possible, is a good time to kick some bad habits and pick up some good ones. Kiss your cigarettes good-bye, because babies of smokers weigh an average of 1/2 pound less that those of non-smokers. Research shows that to quit smoking is the single most important thing you can do to improve the growth and long-term health of your baby.

Other adverse affects of smoking while pregnant include higher risk of preterm delivery, early infant death and possible long term growth problems, problems with intellectual performance and behavioral development. After your baby is born, he or she will also suffer the ill effects of second hand smoke (31; 32; 33).

Smokers may need extra nutrients such as vitamins B12 and C, amino acids, , folate, and zinc, and thus may need a multi-vitamin mineral supplement (34).

For more information about quitting smoking call the Cancer Information Service at 1-800-4CANCER

Lead Exposure

Although lead may not be something that you consume consciously, you probably do receive a regular dose of lead either from your drinking water, lead crystal or pottery with lead containing glaze. According to the Environmental Protection Agency (EPA), as many as 40 million people may have too much lead in their drinking water. Pregnant women and children run the highest risk of problems from lead exposure. Lead exposure can cause increased rates of miscarriage and still births and long term effects such as learning disability, brain damage, hyperactivity, high blood pressure and kidney disease (35). You may have exposure to too much lead if:

♦ Your home was built between 1978 and 1988. Lead solder was used in home plumbing during those years. In older homes with lead solder, minerals usually coat the pipes and keep the lead from leaching out.

♦ Your home was built before 1930. These homes often used lead pipes instead of copper ones. Also water companies installed lead pipes underground to bring water to homes built during the first part of the century.

♦ You have "soft" or acidic water. Soft or acidic water can strip away the coating or the solder on the inside of water pipes. If no lead was used either in pipes or in the service pipes carrying water to your home, you are safe, even if you have soft water.

To be safe, you should have your water tested for lead; this costs from $15-25. Beware of scam artists who provide free lead testing and then sell you a treatment system you don't really need. The EPA suggests you take steps to purify your water if your water has over 20 parts per billion of lead. A reverse-osmosis or distillation system can remove the lead, but can be expensive and waste resources. Less expensive treatments are available; make sure that the equipment is certified by Water Quality Association or the National Sanitation Foundation.

◆ To decrease the lead in your water until you can do further testing or treatment, run the cold water for several minutes before using. (Instead of wasting the water, consider saving it to water plants, wash windows, etc.) If you usually use hot water to make coffee, tea or cook with, use cold instead.

Other possible sources of lead exposure include leaded crystal decanters, ceramic pottery (especially imported) and lead based paint that is chipping or being removed. (Paint applied before 1978 contains lead.) Stripping lead paint from your home should only be done by a professional since the fine lead particles can circulate in the air and home environment if not removed properly. Hot, acidic drinks such as coffee can cause lead to leach from leaden glazed mugs. Don't store fruit juice or acidic foods in crystal decanters because lead can be leached into the food or drink. Also choose seamless cans or welded seam cans instead of soldered seam cans, which may have lead. If you eat canned imported foods regularly, their cans often contain lead solder (36).

For More Information:

Water Quality Association: 4151 Naperville Rd., Lisle, IL 60532

(Can inform you which types of water filters handle lead removal.)

National Sanitation Foundation: P.O. Box 1468, AnnArbor, MI 48106

(This organization sets the standards for water treatment systems.)

Environmental Protection Agency (EPA) Safe Drinking Water Hotline

1-800-426-4791 (202-382-5533 in Washington D.C.)

The EPA can give you a list of state-certified testing labs and can answer questions about the water supply.

Frandon Enterprises: 1-800-359-9000 Makes two inexpensive lead-testing kits; one for water and one for ceramic ware, crystal and even children's toys.

If you think your job is exposing you to dangerous amounts of lead contact the nearest office of the Occupational Safety and Health Administration (OSHA-listed under US Department of Labor in the phone book) or call OSHA's Office of Information and Consumer Affairs at 202-523-8151.

Illness During Pregnancy

Though no one plans on getting sick or being exposed to illness during pregnancy, knowing the facts can help.

Fever: If you have a fever during pregnancy, contact your health care provider immediately. Temperatures over 102.5 may increase the risk of certain birth defects.

Rubella: Between 1988-1990, the number of rubella cases doubled. Rubella during pregnancy can cause stillbirth and birth defects. However, if you happened to receive a rubella vaccine before or during the first 3 months of pregnancy, chances are your baby will not have any of the problems associated with the disease. However, the March of Dimes recommends that women be tested for immunity to rubella before pregnancy (37).

Toxoplasmosis: The parasite that causes it is passed in cat feces and it can also be transmitted in uncooked and undercooked meats and unwashed fruits and vegetables. (See page 11 for more details)

Warning: alcohol may cause birth defects

"Think before you drink" is a slogan that the March of Dimes has used to remind women of the risk of drinking alcohol when pregnant. Fetal Alcohol Syndrome (FAS) and a variation, Fetal Alcohol Effect (FAE) describe children who are scarred by the drinking habits of their mothers during pregnancy. It is estimated that FAE affects as many as 3% of all infants, making it the leading known cause of mental retardation, learning and behavior problems (38). Some milder cases of FAE cause irritability, impulsiveness and learning disabilities and aren't diagnosed for years; many kids affected by FAE end up dropping out of school.

Alcohol is now recognized as a potent teratogen (a substance capable of causing birth defects) that can cause growth retardation (both in the womb and after birth) and facial abnormalities. Chronic alcohol abuse has been defined as more than two drinks per day. One drink per day has been shown to decrease birth weight (39). Since alcohol freely crosses the placenta, the fetus's blood alcohol level is equal to the mother's. So one drink in a day might not be risky, but a single drinking binge, on a critical day of development could damage the fetus.

According to the Public Health Service, as many as 86% of women drink once during pregnancy; women with a higher level of education appear to drink more. Some women may be genetically susceptible to having a child with FAS. It has been reported in one study that black women are seven times more likely to have a child with the syndrome than white women with the same drinking habits (40).

The good news is that if you are a drinker, whenever you stop, you increase your chances of having a healthy baby. Women who stopped drinking before their seventh month of pregnancy had healthy babies with no symptoms of FAS (41).

What about an occasional drink? Research concerning low levels of alcohol consumption is limited and inconsistent. To feel totally safe, becoming a "teetotaler" (someone who totally avoids alcohol) is probably best except for a rare sip of alcohol to bring in the new year or an anniversary. Consult your health care provider on his or her opinion about this issue

Caffeine

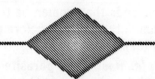

Caffeine Content of your Favorite Beverages and Foods

You may be one of those people who "aren't worth a darn before your first cup of coffee!" Although there is evidence that caffeine can cause birth defects in animals, there is not convincing evidence that the same is true in humans (42). In a 1988 review article of caffeine's effect on pregnancy, Dr. Alan Leviton summarized in the Journal of Reproductive Medicine, "No evidence has yet been offered that caffeine consumption at moderate levels by pregnant women has any discernible adverse effect on their fetuses (43)."

The Food and Drug Administration continues to advise pregnant women to consume caffeine in moderation. Since caffeine is a central nervous system stimulant, is addictive, and acts as a diuretic, it's best to cut down or cut out your coffee (the beverage with the most caffeine) and look for beverages that contain less or no caffeine. Moderation, a word you will read often when it comes to advice during pregnancy, is also the key word in caffeine consumption.

Drink/Food	Caffeine in mg.
Soft Drinks (in 12 oz.)	
Mountain Dew	54
Mellow Yellow	52
Diet cherry cola, Slice	48
Coke classic, cherry coke, diet coke	46
Tab	46
Pepsi Cola	38
Diet Pepsi Light	36
Sprite, 7-up, Slice reg or diet	0
Any decaffeinated sodas	0
Coffee	
6oz brewed	103
Instant (1 tsp. rounded)	57
Instant decaffeinated (1 tsp. rounded)	2
Coffee Drinks (2 rounded teaspoons)	
Orange cappucino	75
Cafe Amaretto	60
Cafe Vienna	60
Cafe Francais	50
Suisse Mocha	40
Dutch Chocolate Mint	30
Viennese Chocolate Cafe	25

Drink/Food	Caffeine in mg.
Tea	
6 oz. brewed 3 minutes	36
Instant tea (1 tsp.)	31
Herb teas	0
Cocoa drinks	
Chocolate flavor mix in milk (2-3 heaping tsp.)	8
Chocolate syrup in milk (2 Tb.)	6
Hot cocoa (1 oz. packet)	5
Miscellaneous	
1 oz. milk chocolate (Cadbury)	15
1/4 cup chocolate chips	12
1/2 cup Jello chocolate pudding	5
Jello chocolate pudding pop with chocolate coating	3

Source: *Food Values of Portions Commonly Used*, 15th edition, Jean Pennington, and General Foods.

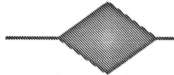

About Herb Teas

Many people turn to herb teas to cut their caffeine intake. However, you should stay away from tea containing coltsfoot, sassafras or comfrey, which are suspected carcinogens (46). Many herbal preparations, whether they be sold as teas or quasi-medications, can act as drugs because they contain natural active chemicals, that can be harmful to the fetus. Remember that many of our modern day drugs first came from herbs, flowers and trees. Before taking any herbal preparation, whether tea or otherwise, check with your health care provider or a pharmacist as to their safety during pregnancy. To be safe, stay with name brand decaffeinated teas.

Drugs–Prescription, Over the Counter and Otherwise

All drugs, legal and illegal have the potential to seriously harm your baby...even something as seemingly harmless as aspirin. So let your health care provider know if you are taking any kind of drug regularly. Also, ask what is safe to take for a cold, flu or bad headache. It's best to avoid all medications when pregnant especially during the first trimester. However if you must take something, make sure it's something your health care provider approves of.

Just because you are pregnant doesn't mean you are immune to headaches, colds, flu and other problems which you might ordinarily take medication for. You may be on vacation like I was, and suddenly have a bad case of hay fever. For these times, it's great to have a list of over the counter medications that your health care provider has given the OK for.

Cocaine

It has been estimated that over half the people addicted to crack cocaine are women (47). Three studies done

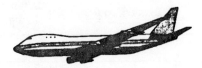

in urban areas showed that between 10-17% of women registered for prenatal care showed evidence of cocaine use (48).

Cocaine addiction is of course, harmful to the mother, but can have lifelong effects on a baby. Cocaine may take up to 6 days to leave the fetal blood supply. This increased exposure to the drug can result in premature separation of the placenta, growth retardation of the fetus, decreased birth weight, length, and head circumference, and premature delivery. Cocaine may also cause miscarriages, birth defects and increases neurological and behavioral problems which may last a lifetime (49).

If you are addicted to cocaine or any other drug, seek help through your local health department or drug treatment center.

(If you'd like to read further about Drugs and Pregnancy, there is an excellent handbook entitled *Drugs, Vitamins and Minerals in Pregnancy* by Ann Karen Henry, Pharm D. and Jil Feldhausen, M.S., R.D., Fisher Books, 1989.)

Travel During Pregnancy

Chances are that during the nine months of pregnancy, you will travel somewhere. Traveling while pregnant may offer yet another challenge or it may be "business as usual." Traveling can affect your exercise schedule and the types and amounts of food that you eat.

In the Plane

1. Request an aisle seat so that you can get up to walk and stretch or go to the restroom.

2. Drink plenty of fluids before and during your flight if your flight is a long one such as cross-country or overseas. Flying can dehydrate you.

3. Get up and walk around several times during the flight. Or you may want to go to the back of the plane and just stand or stretch for a while. While sitting down you can do isometric exercises, which can improve circulation.

4. Request a special meal, if desired. You can ask for a vegetarian, seafood, diabetic or any number of special request meals. Generally, you need to call the airline at least 24 hours before your flight to arrange special meals.

5. Since airline food often doesn't include fresh fruit, bring a few of your own. Or bring a baggie of prunes or other dried fruit for snacks.

6. Instead of eating all of the food on your tray, you may want to save a few things for a snack.

7. Avoid taking heavy carry on luggage unless someone else can carry it for you. This can make back pain worse.

8. If you have a layover between flights, use it as exercise time. Walk to your gate instead of using moving sidewalks or a bus.

In the Car

1. Bring along a small cooler that you can keep yogurt, cheese, milk, fruit and other snacks in. You can even bring the makings of a sandwich, which can save you money on restaurant food. If you forget a cooler, you can always stop at a grocery along the way and pick up fruit, dried fruit and ready-to-eat raw vegetables.

2. Instead of eating regular sized meals when you stop, order appetizer size meals, or eat just half a portion. Sitting in the car for extended periods of time will decrease your energy needs and may increase indigestion.

3. Drink plenty of fluids. Lack of activity can slow your digestion down and increase constipation. Having to make "pit stops" will allow you to get out and stretch, which can prevent back pain and increase circulation.

4. Plan "adventure stops". Try to include enough time in your itinerary to make extended stops to see something of interest. Use this as your exercise time to walk and stretch.

At Your Destination

1. If you are traveling to a foreign country, talk to your physician before making your reservations. There may be vaccinations normally required that you can't take while pregnant. Or you may need to eat especially carefully to avoid bacterial poisoning or "turista". You may want to take some non-perishable foods with you to snack on if familiar foods aren't available where you are going, or if food safety may be an issue. A friend of mine who went to an Asian country lived on peanuts and beer because it was the only foods she felt were safe. Thankfully, she wasn't pregnant.

2. If you are staying at a hotel, try to get a room with a mini-fridge or kitchenette. You can keep your own snack foods as well as high fiber cereals for breakfast or snacks.

3. Try to make wise food choices when eating out. When most meals are eaten out, diets tend to be lower in fiber, calcium vitamin C, and folacin, and high in fat and sodium (50). See page 225 for advice on eating out.

4. If you are staying with friends or relatives, pick up a few of the foods you usually eat before you arrive, such as high fiber cereal, milk and extra fresh or dried fruit. This way your diet won't be lacking and you won't be embarrassed about asking your host to buy special foods for you.

5. Make sure you pack non-perishable snacks in your bag for those hectic tourist schedules. Good ones are cheese or peanut butter crackers, boxes of raisins, wheat crackers, fiber bars, apples or bananas and individual bags of pretzels. Don't forget to drink! Juice boxes pack well.

The Positives of Pregnancy

There are many positive aspects of being pregnant. Some women feel at their best when they're pregnant. Some women with chronic medical problems go into remission or have decreased symptoms. We usually only hear the negatives. By concentrating on the good things that occur during these nine months, life will be a lot more pleasant. Here are just a few of the good things about being pregnant. Try to think of them often!

♦ Thick shiny hair.

♦ That warm, healthy glow of pregnancy.

♦ People open the door for you.

♦ Finally, a larger bra size!

♦ Weight gain without guilt!

♦ You don't have to tuck your blouses in.

♦ You have an excuse now for being tired.

♦ You feel great all over.

♦ You feel good about taking care of yourself.

♦ You have a great reason for starting a walking program and for eating right.

♦ You are the designated driver for the next nine months.

♦ Your husband brings you breakfast (or lunch or dinner) in bed.

♦ You're too tired to clean house!

♦ Finally, a long vacation to look forward to (maternity leave).

♦ Your other kids learn how to help around the house.

♦ The love for your yet-to-be-born baby abounds.

♦ You don't have to worry about forgetting your birth control pill.

♦ You can wear "one size fits all" clothes.

♦ You will become a member of the clan of "Universal Motherhood"

♦ You are part of a miracle.

♦ You have a special new friend living close by.

♦ This is an experience you have only once or several times in your life, so enjoy it!

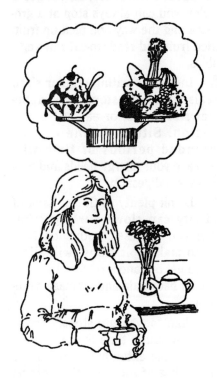

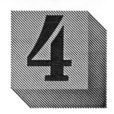

The First Trimester

What You Will Find In This Chapter:

- The Eating Expectantly Diet
- Weight Gain/Energy Needs
- Protein Needs
- Protein Content of Food Groups
- Focus on Fiber
- First Trimester Challenges
- How Baby is Growing
- First Trimester Menus

And answers to questions you may have:

- How much weight should I gain?
- I've read that I should eat 100 grams of protein; how much is that?
- How much protein is in an egg?
- How else can I get protein in my diet if I don't feel like eating meat?
- What can I do about morning sickness?
- How can I avoid constipation?

The Eating Expectantly Diet

10 or more servings of starches/grains

One serving is 1 slice of any type bread, 1 flour tortilla, 1/2 cup pasta, 1/3 cup rice or legumes, 6 crackers, 1/2 cup of potato.

3 or more servings of fruit

One serving is 1 medium piece of fresh fruit, 1/2 banana, 1/2 cup canned fruit in it's own juice, 1 cup melon or berries, 2 plums or nectarines.

3 or more servings of vegetables

One serving is 1/2 cup of any cooked non-starchy vegetable or 1 cup of lettuce.

(Be sure to include at least 1 fruit or vegetable that is a good source of vitamin A and 1 servings high in vitamin C.)

6 or more ounces of protein or equivalent

(Increase your protein intake one ounce for each serving of milk that you don't drink)

One protein equivalent is 1 ounce of lean meat, 1 ounce reduced fat

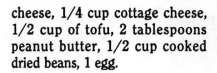

cheese, 1/4 cup cottage cheese, 1/2 cup of tofu, 2 tablespoons peanut butter, 1/2 cup cooked dried beans, 1 egg.

4 or more servings of dairy products

One serving is 1 cup of any type milk or yogurt, preferably skim or lowfat.

3-5 or more servings of fat

One serving is 1 teaspoon margarine or butter, or 2 teaspoons reduced fat margarine, 1 teaspoon mayonnaise, or 2 teaspoons reduced fat mayonnaise, 1 slice bacon, 1/2 oz. cream cheese, 1 tablespoon sour cream, 1/8 avocado, 10 peanuts, 5 olives.

And here is an example of a "real" meal plan:

Breakfast:

Raisin Bran with strawberries
Whole wheat bagel with light cream cheese
Milk

Snack:

Vegetable juice
Rye crackers
Low-fat cheese

Lunch:

Ham sandwich on wheat bread
Raw vegetables with dip
Melon balls
Sugar cookies
Milk

Snack:

Popcorn

Dinner:

Grilled salmon steak
Grilled corn on the cob
Spinach salad with tomato and mushrooms
Roll
Fresh orange
Milk

Snack:

Peanut butter and graham crackers
Yogurt with dried fruit

Weight Gain/Energy Needs

Are you one of those people who received a "special license to eat" because you are pregnant? Well your license was just recalled because "eating for two" is a bit of a misnomer. You do need larger amounts of many nutrients during pregnancy, but eating twice as much food and calories is not needed, especially in the first trimester.

The Subcommittee on Nutritional Status and Weight Gain During Pregnancy of the National Academy of Sciences recommends that you gain about a pound or less per month during the first trimester. That translates into 135 extra calories (or less) per day (1). Uh oh, there go the visions of dancing chocolate sundaes in your head! Later in this chapter we'll talk about how to make your diet a winner without gaining too much weight!

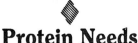

Protein Needs

Protein is essential during pregnancy because it is used in building each new cell for your baby. It is also needed for the placenta; your baby's lifeline which brings nourishment from you to your baby. Protein helps make new blood cells and muscle tissue that supports your baby. To top it all off, protein is used to make all the hormones that are playing havoc in your body right now!

In the first trimester, your protein needs don't increase very much; only about 1.3 grams extra each day or the equivalent of 1/6 of an ounce of meat. The RDA for protein throughout pregnancy is 10 grams higher than non-pregnant needs (2). This translates to about 1.5 ounces of animal protein, 1 1/4 cups of legumes, 1 1/2 eggs, or 1 1/4 oz. of cheese.

Protein Content of Food Groups

Food/typical serving	Protein per serving
Dairy Products (1 cup milk, 1 oz. cheese)	8-12 grams
Legumes(1/2 cup)	7-11 grams
Meat, Poultry, Fish (1 oz.)	6-10 grams
Vegetables (1/2 cup)	2-3 grams

Food/typical serving	Protein per serving
Fruits & Juice (1 medium/1/2 cup)	0-1 gram
Bread/Cereal(1 slice/1 oz.)	2-4 grams
Fat/Oil	0

Other things influence your protein needs and the way your body uses protein. Your total calorie or energy intake must be adequate in order for your body to use protein to build new tissues, etc.

Let's say you eat 10 ounces of chicken and fish every day. However, you aren't very hungry, so mostly you fill up on water, rice cakes and salad. If you do this, your calorie intake won't be enough to meet your baby's demands for energy, and thus the protein you eat is used to supply energy instead of supplying building materials.

Also, you won't have enough glucose or blood sugar to supply your brain with energy, so your body will start breaking down fat into fragments called ketones. Ketones are a sign that your body can't complete the metabolic process. If made in large amounts (usually only in diabetics) it can be harmful to your body. Avoid the production of ketones by having enough calories and carbohydrate in your diet.

Another thing which affects your body's use of protein is the quality of it.

Protein needs are calculated by determining the need for high biological value or high quality protein. High quality protein is highly digest-

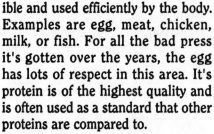

ible and used efficiently by the body. Examples are egg, meat, chicken, milk, or fish. For all the bad press it's gotten over the years, the egg has lots of respect in this area. It's protein is of the highest quality and is often used as a standard that other proteins are compared to.

Lower quality proteins found in vegetable sources are needed in greater quantities to meet protein needs. Vegetarians don't despair! You can meet your protein needs without meat, though you must look at your intake of certain nutrients carefully.

For more information on vegetarian sources of protein, see page 87.

As a rule, Americans eat about twice as much protein as they really need. Pregnant women are no different, eating an average of 75 to 110 grams per day–well above the 60 grams per day recommended by the Food and Nutrition Board. However, some health care providers and birthing programs recommend up to 100 grams of protein, especially for high-risk pregnancies. A diet that contains approximately 100 grams of protein would, for example, contain 4 servings of dairy product, 6 oz. of animal protein or the equivalent, 3 vegetables, 2 fruits and 8 servings of starch or bread.

If you are typical of most of us, you won't have a problem meeting protein needs. In fact, the National Academy of Sciences advises pregnant women not to use specially formulated high protein supplements, protein powders or high protein beverages because some evidence suggests possible harm from using these supplementary protein products (3).

Why You May Need to "Work" to Meet Your Protein Needs

You might not be able to meet your protein needs if you:

♦ don't drink milk or eat dairy products

♦ have nausea or vomiting which prevents you from eating much of anything

♦ just don't have the desire to eat meat

If you drink the recommended 4 servings of dairy products each day, you will be meeting half your protein needs. If you don't, you'll need to increase protein from other sources.

If you just don't feel like eating meat, you are not alone. Most women have some food aversion; some stomachs turn at the thought of eating what used to be their favorite food. For example, I loved shrimp and scallops before my pregnancy. When I was pregnant, I couldn't stand the smell of them cooking or the taste of them!

If your favorite high protein foods turn your stomach off, you can eat more dairy products, which are also good sources of protein, or you can turn to other sources. Many of the women I've talked to could tolerate eggs and cheese well, even if they couldn't eat meat. There are many vegetarian sources of protein that you may easily tolerate; a list is found on page 60. Experiment with what works for you...

If you can't eat much of anything due to first trimester morning sick-

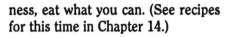

ness, eat what you can. (See recipes for this time in Chapter 14.)

If the condition persists to the point that you are losing weight, make sure your health care provider is alerted. He may want to treat your nausea more aggressively, or may refer you to a registered dietitian for individual counseling.

Focus on Fiber

After "lowfat", "high-fiber" may be the catch word of the 90's. Fiber is one of those things most people don't have enough of even though there are new studies every day which cite its benefits.

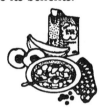

The old saying, "An apple a day keeps the doctor away" may well relate to an apple's fiber content. Here's why:

♦ Adequate fiber can reduce the risk of colon cancer.

♦ New research shows that wheat fiber may play a direct role in preventing breast cancer (4).

♦ Soluble fiber has been shown to reduce cholesterol, thus reducing risk of heart disease.

♦ Soluble fiber also helps control blood glucose, which is particularly beneficial to diabetics (5).

♦ Fiber fills you up not out!

♦ Fiber keeps your bowels moving, which can help prevent constipation and hemorrhoids.

Eating Your Oats and Bran

Before we get into the specifics of fiber, there are a few simple ways to make sure you get enough fiber every day...

♦ Follow the National Cancer Institute's slogan "Five a Day for Better Health" and you're on your way to having adequate dietary fiber.

♦ Choose whole wheat bread, crackers and pasta.

♦ Eat brown rice or bulgur instead of white rice.

♦ Start your day with a high fiber cereal (containing at least 5 grams per serving).

♦ Snack on other high fiber foods such as bran muffins, dried fruit, fresh fruit, vegetables and whole grain crackers.

♦ Add wheat bran, whole wheat flour or oatmeal to baked goods in place of part of the flour.

If you follow the advice above, you will be sure to get the recommended 20-35 grams of fiber currently recommended by the National Cancer Institute (6). But if you want to really key in to the specific amounts of fiber found in foods, look below.

If your diet is normally low in fiber, make sure to increase the fiber in your diet gradually. Adding a lot of fiber to your meals all at once can result in bloating and gas.

Remember to drink plenty of fluids while eating high fiber foods, or the extra fiber may make matters worse.

Fiber Content of Foods

(Listed from most to least fiber content)

Fruits

Food/Amount	Dietary Fiber in Grams*
Figs, 5	12
Prunes, 5	8
Blackberries, canned 1/2 cup, solid & liquid	7
Raspberries, fresh, 1/2 cup	5
Dates, 5	4
Pear, fresh with skin	4
Nectarines, fresh	3
Orange, fresh	3
Raisins, 1/4 cup	2
Pineapple, fresh 2 slices	2
Strawberries, 1/2 cup	2

Most other fruits contain between 1-3 grams of fiber per serving.

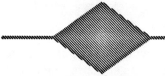

Snack Tip

The fig may be the best kept nutrition secret! Not only do figs have the highest amount of dietary fiber of any common fruit, nut or vegetable, they are also higher in potassium than bananas and are considered a good calcium source!

Pack this sweet and healthy treat as a between-meal snack.

Stuffed Figs

Make a large slice in fresh or dried fig. Fill with lowfat or fat-free cream cheese, or puree cottage cheese in the blender until it's the consistency of cream cheese. You can flavor the cheese with cinnamon or nutmeg for more flavor.

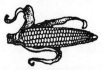

Vegetables

Food	Dietary fiber in grams*
Spinach, cooked, 1/2 cup drained	6
Corn, canned, 1/2 cup	5
Broccoli, chopped, 1/2 cup cooked	4
Sweet Potato, baked in skin, 1 medium	3.5
Rhubarb, cooked, 1/2 cup	3
Tomato, fresh, 1 medium	2
Carrots, cooked, 1/2 cup	2

Cereals, Grains and Legumes

Food	Dietary fiber in grams*
Baked beans, canned, 1/2 cup	6-8
Wheat bran, unprocessed, 1/4 cup	7
Refried pinto beans, canned, 1/2 cup	5
Barley, light pearled, 1/2 cup	4
Black beans, 1/2 cup	4
Aunt Jemima Whole Grain Wheat Frozen Waffle, one waffle	3
Corn tortillas, 2	3
Bran Muffin	2-5
Whole wheat bread	1-2
Rye crisp, 1/4 of large square	2
Brown rice, instant, 1/2 cup	2
Popcorn, 3.5 cups	1
White rice, 1/2 cup	1

Compiled from *Nutrients in Foods*, Leveille, Zabik and Morgan, 1983, *The Complete Book of Food Counts* by Corrine Netzer, 1991, and Manufacturer's labels.
*Numbers rounded off to nearest whole number.

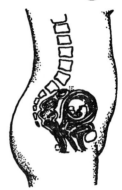

First Trimester Challenges

Nausea or Morning Sickness

Some women feel this malady was misnamed since it can occur any time of day or night and unfortunately for some women, it does! One possible cause of the nausea is sudden surges in hormone levels; queasiness can also be worsened by low blood sugar. The same hormones that cause morning sickness slow down the digestive process so that more nutrients can be absorbed for your baby.

According to research done by Margie Profet, U.C. Berkeley Research Associate, women are offended by smells given off from the natural toxins in food. Smells are especially offensive during the third to the eighth week of pregnancy, when the embryo is developing it's major organs and is most susceptible to deformities from certain toxins and chemicals. The top 10 foods likely to turn your tastebuds off? Coffee, onions, garlic, herbs and spices, barbecued foods, fried foods, fish, chili peppers, mustard and canned fish or meats. Very fresh fish shouldn't be offensive–a fishy smell indicates bacterial growth, which could be harmful. Ms. Profet has done research on morning sickness and its effects on nutrition (7). Some researchers believe morning sickness is actually a characteristic passed down from our ancestors that protects us from toxins in food.

What you can do...

◆ Get up slowly when you awake in the morning.

◆ A dry "pre-breakfast" snack sometimes helps prevent nausea. You can leave crackers beside your bed at night, or let Dad get involved and serve you dry toast in bed. (This is a good habit to get into!) Many women feel better if they eat before they ever lift their head off the pillow!

◆ Avoid getting very hungry. Eat small frequent meals with snacks in between, especially those which contain protein–this keeps your stomach from being completely empty (see page 240 for creative snack ideas).

◆ Drink fluids between instead of with meals. To avoid dehydration it is important not to forget to drink, especially if you are vomiting. Appealing ways to improve your fluid intake: jello, broth, popsicles or frozen juice bars, slushy drinks, fluid packed fruits like watermelon, frozen grapes and frozen melon balls.

◆ Avoid greasy, fried, highly seasoned foods and any foods that

have an unpleasant or strong smell. Some women find cold, somewhat bland foods more appealing at this time. See page 238 for meal ideas.

◆ Have your partner do the cooking and take that time to go for a walk or take a catnap. This will help you avoid cooking odors and can give you time to do other important things.

If your nausea or vomiting becomes severe, notify your health care provider. Never take any medications without approval.

Frequent Urination

This may give you the first hint that you're pregnant. It seems like in those first few months, you make a path in the carpet to the bathroom! Your baby, within the uterus, sits right above your bladder. As your uterus engorges with blood and baby increases in size, there is more pressure and less space for storing urine.

What you can do...

◆ DON'T decrease your total fluid intake! However, you may want to slightly decrease your intake of fluids in the evening if you're getting up several times during the night to use the restroom.

◆ Lying on one side may help relieve pressure on the bladder.

◆ Kegel exercises can be started now and continued during and after your pregnancy. This tones up the muscles that "hold" in urine. Have you ever sneezed or coughed and felt like you nearly emptied your bladder? This can happen more frequently during the third trimester and again later

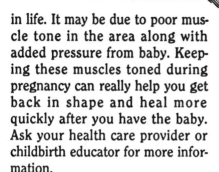

in life. It may be due to poor muscle tone in the area along with added pressure from baby. Keeping these muscles toned during pregnancy can really help you get back in shape and heal more quickly after you have the baby. Ask your health care provider or childbirth educator for more information.

If urination is painful, contact your health care provider.

Fatigue

You may feel like you could sleep for the rest of your pregnancy. During the first trimester, when your hormones are playing tag and "you're it," fatigue is common.

What you can do...

♦ Accept your need for rest and slow down your lifestyle.

♦ Eat regular, balanced meals that are high in the essential nutrients. (see page 27 for more information) Your diet could be partly to blame if you're not eating enough calories or not getting enough essential nutrients. During the first trimester, your health care provider will probably check the amount of iron in your blood. Iron-deficiency anemia can cause fatigue and is fairly common in pregnancy due to the greatly increased need for the mineral. Adequate dietary iron before and during pregnancy can prevent anemia; see page 65 for good sources of iron.

♦ Exercise regularly. Even though you may not feel you have the energy for it, you'll be glad you did afterward. (see Chapter 11 for Fitting Fitness In)

Breast Changes

Often, breast enlargement and sensitivity are another of the first noticeable changes in pregnancy. In this first trimester, the fat layer of your breast is thickening and the number of milk glands is increasing. The veins close to the surface become larger due to the increase in blood flow within your body. Your nipples and areolas (the dark area around your nipple) will enlarge and probably get darker.

What you can do...

♦ Find a good supportive bra, preferably one with flexible straps. If you plan to breastfeed, you may find that a nursing bra suits your needs now and later.

♦ Large busted women might want to sleep in a lightweight bra.

Teeth and Gum Changes

Hormones and increased blood flow affect many areas of your body, including your gums. They can soften and become more prone to developing gum infections.

What you can do...

♦ Good nutrition is the first defense against gum disease. Eat a balanced diet which contains plenty of vitamin C.

♦ Don't neglect teeth and gums during pregnancy. Continue regular flossing and brushing. Have a dental checkup during your pregnancy. However, be sure your dentist knows that you are pregnant before your visit. If you are planning a pregnancy, visit your dentist first for a check up or cleaning.

How Baby Is Growing

Good nutrition is vital in the first three months for your baby's development. Babies born to poorly nourished mothers are more susceptible to infections in early life and to birth defects.

Many miraculous events are taking place within your body in just 12 weeks.

At the end of 1 week

For the first 7 days after the sperm fertilizes the egg, the group of cells is traveling down the fallopian tube towards the uterus. It is now called a "zygote." Although the zygote is no larger than the tiniest speck of sand, it carries all the genetic material (DNA) necessary for development. It implants in the uterine wall 7-8 days after fertilization; then it is known as an "embryo."

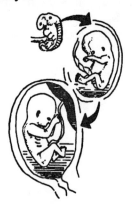

During the first week, the cells are rapidly dividing into what will become organs, skin, hair, bones and muscle. Even though the DNA and cells "know" the sex of the baby, there is no genital formation yet, so we refer to the baby as "it".

The mass of cells that includes the embryo and what will become the placenta is only about the size of a blueberry.

At the end of 4 Weeks

By this time, you may be confirming your pregnancy and may be experiencing some of the tell-tale signs. The embryo is no bigger than a grain of rice, and its heart is beating by the 25th day. The digestive system, backbone, and spinal cord are all beginning to form. Tiny limb buds are appearing which will become the arms and legs. The next 4 weeks are vitally important as development rapidly occurs.

At the end of 8 weeks

The embryo is now about the size of your big toe or a little over one inch long. All the major organs and systems are formed yet some are not completely developed. The embryo clearly looks like a human. The long arm and leg bones are beginning to form and are visible under the embryo's thin skin. The brain has taken shape and the embryo has a face. The embryo weighs only 1/4 of an ounce!

At the end of 12 weeks

From the 9th week on, the "embryo" is now called a "fetus". The nails are developed and the fetus can suck it's fingers and curl it's hands into a fist. The kidneys are beginning to form

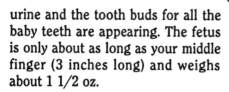

urine and the tooth buds for all the baby teeth are appearing. The fetus is only about as long as your middle finger (3 inches long) and weighs about 1 1/2 oz.

Although you may be just starting to buy maternity clothes or adjust your belt to the next notch, most of your baby's organs and tissues are already formed.

Questions you may have:

What if I skip meals–is that bad for the baby?

Yes, and for you too! During pregnancy, your baby depends entirely on you for energy. When you don't eat, it makes it difficult for your baby to have the energy it needs. When you skip meals, you often eat much more food later to make up for it, and you may store those extra calories as fat. Try to avoid the "Feast or Famine" approach by taking the time to eat regular meals and snacks.

I'm in the habit of eating fast food for lunch every day. How can I eat more nutritiously?

Planning ahead and taking the time to shop and cook is the solution for too many meals eaten on the run. Eating "typical" fast food is expensive–both in dollars and to your diet. It provides lots of calories but not too many nutrients. On the other hand, fast food is improving and it's getting easier to eat nutritiously while on the run. See page 296 for Meals in Minutes, and "The Most Nutritious Fast Foods" on page 226 for The Most Nutritious Fast Foods.

What if I just can't eat much at all? My "morning sickness" occurs all the time.

As noted earlier, extra calories aren't a priority in the first trimester; keeping your baby's environment safe and having an adequate intake of some vitamins is. The baby will draw on your stored nutrients if you aren't able to eat much. However, make your calories count. When you are able to eat, eat the most nutritious foods you can and when your "morning sickness" has subsided, eat well to re-stock your body's nutrient stores.

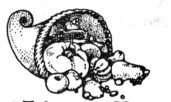

First Trimester Menus

The menus and recipes on page 237 were designed with the first trimester in mind. This is probably the time in your pregnancy when eating can present the biggest problem. So, the menus are practical and realistic for what you may face.

Menus

◆ Don't Feel Like Eating Menus
◆ Don't Feel Like Cooking Menus
◆ Don't Feel Like Eating or Cooking Menu
◆ Feel Like Staying in Bed but Can't Menus
◆ Feel Great Menu
◆ Blender Breakfasts (or Snacks to Go)
◆ Snack Ideas
◆ High Energy Mom Snack Ideas

5

The Second Trimester

◆

What You Will Find In This Chapter:

- ◆ Energy Needs
- ◆ Protein Needs
- ◆ Protein Content of Common Foods
- ◆ Focus on Minerals: Calcium and Iron
- ◆ Twelve Ways to Sneak Calcium into Your Diet
- ◆ "How's Your Diet?" Quiz
- ◆ "Thrive on Five"
- ◆ Smart Snacking

- ◆ Second Trimester Challenges
- ◆ How Baby is Growing
- ◆ Second Trimester Menus

And answers to questions you may have:

- ◆ Isn't there enough calcium in my prenatal vitamin?
- ◆ Which foods are high in iron?
- ◆ What's a good snack?
- ◆ What about chocolate milk?
- ◆ Is there more calcium in milk or yogurt?
- ◆ When will I feel my baby move?

You made it through the first trimester–congratulations! The second trimester includes the 13th through the 26th week and is usually when most women feel their best. During this time, you'll have lots of energy, especially if you are eating right and exercising. You'll mark the halfway point of your pregnancy and you'll feel your baby move!

Energy Needs

During the last two trimesters of your pregnancy your body needs about 300 more calories per day than you ate before you were pregnant. Eating at this level will result in a 25-35 pound weight gain–considered optimal for a healthy baby. However, many things will affect your energy needs including pre-pregnant weight, your activity level, and your current weight. Some women are less active during the last half of pregnancy; others remain active and burn even more calories due to their increasing weight.

From now on, you should try to gain about 1 pound per week (1). Remember that much of the extra energy and protein you are eating is working towards creating a healthy environment for your baby to live in until birth. The extra nutrients are required for increased blood volume, increase in placenta size, increase in fat storage, increase in breast tissue, production of amniotic fluid, as well as providing the building materials for your growing fetus!

In the next few weeks--usually between 16 and 20 weeks gestation, you should feel a small fluttering in your uterus--this is your baby moving! It's a very exciting feeling and also a good reminder that during these special months, you must take good care of yourself by eating right, exercising moderately, and trying to improve other lifestyle habits.

This is a good time to take a personal inventory of diet and health habits. A diet and health survey follows and you will also find a few more in this book to help keep you on your toes!

Protein Needs

Your body's need for protein starts increasing now and doesn't stop until your baby is born! Protein is used for the growing tissue of the fetus and placenta, expanding blood volume, as well as growing tissues in your own body.

All protein is not equal... Proteins are made of amino acids and all the essential amino acids must be present in a food in certain amounts and proportions to be used most efficiently. The term "complete protein" describes protein which has all the "essential" amino acids (amino acids which your body can't produce) in the amounts needed to build proteins. "Incomplete proteins" are missing one or more amino acids or they are found in small amounts. This is important for people who don't eat animal protein. It used to be thought that we needed to "combine" incomplete proteins at the same meal to have all the needed amino acids. Now, we know that eating a variety of different protein sources throughout the day is adequate (2). For more information see page 83, Vegetarian Eating.

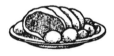

Examples of foods containing complete protein include beef, poultry, fish, milk, eggs, and cheese. Foods considered incomplete protein sources include beans, rice, grains, peanut butter, nuts, pasta, and some vegetables. (Fruit contains very small amounts of protein.) The variety of protein sources supply different nutrients and sources of fat, so eat a variety of complete and incomplete protein containing foods.

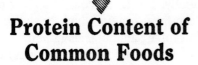

Protein Content of Common Foods

The RDA for Pregnancy is 60 grams; 65 grams for breastfeeding (3).

Complete Protein Foods	Protein in grams
(Per 3 oz. serving unless specified)	
Lentils, 1 cup cooked	16
Beef chuck arm roast	28
Pork, center loin	27
Turkey	27
Chicken breast	26
Flounder	25
Tuna fish, canned & drained	24
Beef, lean ground	22
Scallops	16
Cottage cheese, 1/2 cup	15
Ham	15
Eggs, 2 large	12
Shrimp	11
Yogurt, 1 cup	8
Milk, any type, 1 cup	8
Cheddar cheese, 1 oz.	7
Hormel Light & Lean Hot Dog, 1	6
Frankfurter, beef, 1	5
Quinoa (a high quality grain), 1/2 cup	4

Incomplete Protein Foods	Protein in grams
Vegetarian Chili, 2/3 cup canned	11
Tofu, 1/2 cup	10
Turkee Slices, 2 slices (Worthington)	9
Split pea soup, 1 cup	9
Green Peas, 1 cup	9
Bulgur, 1 cup cooked	8
Peanut Butter, 2 Tb.	8
Vega Link, 2 (Worthington)	8
Egg noodles, 1 cup cooked	7
Soy milk, 1 cup	7
Brown Rice, 1 cup cooked	5
White rice, 1 cup cooked	4
Bread, whole wheat, 1 slice	3

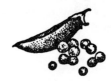

Numbers rounded off to nearest whole number Source: *Value of Foods Commonly Used*, 15th Edition, by Jean Pennington, *The Complete Book of Food Counts*, by Corrine T. Netzer, and manufacturer labels.

If you just aren't much of a meat eater, you can eat smaller amounts of the higher protein meats or eat more vegetable sources of protein. See Chapter 7, Vegetarian Eating, for more information.

Focus On Minerals; Calcium and Iron

Calcium

Calcium is a mineral that is vital for your baby's bone development. Unfortunately, it's a mineral that adults often delete from their diet when they cut down on dairy products. An intake of 1200 mg. per day is recommended (4); if you drink milk, this amount is found in 4 cups of milk. Milk and dairy products also provide important nutrients like protein, magnesium, vitamin D and riboflavin. Calcium is thought to be best absorbed from milk.

Calcium Content of Foods and Beverages

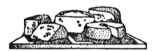

The RDA for Pregnancy and Breast-feeding is 1200 mg.

Food	Calcium in mg.
Animal Sources	
Carnation instant breakfast, strawberry, with 8 oz. 1% milk	500
McDonald's lowfat milkshake	350
Yogurt fruit flavored, w/ nonfat dry milk, 8 oz.	314
Alba chocolate flavored milk drink, 8 oz.	310
Lowfat 1% milk, 8 oz.	300

Food	Calcium in mg.
Lactaid milk, 8 oz.	300
Frosty frozen dessert, small	300
Cheese pizza, 2 slices	29
Whole milk 3.5% fat, 8 oz.	288
Buttermilk, cultured, 8 oz.	285
Chocolate milk 2% fat, 8 oz.	284
Swiss cheese, 1 oz.	272
1 taco	200
Cheddar cheese, 1 oz.	204
Macaroni and cheese, 1 cup	200
1 Taco Bell Beefy Tostada	200
Cottage cheese, lowfat 2% fat, 1 cup	155
Salmon, canned with bones, 3 oz.	133
American processed, 1 oz.	124
McDonald's yogurt cone	100

Source: *Food Values of Portions Commonly Used*, 15th Edition, Jean Pennington
See page 225 for fast foods highest in calcium.

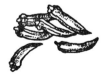

Food	Calcium in mg.
Vegetarian Sources	
Agar, dried, 3.5 oz.	625
Collard greens, 1 cup	357
Cooked rhubarb, 1 cup	348
Firm tofu made with calcium sulfate, 4 oz.	250-765
Regular tofu made with calcium sulfate, 4 oz.	120-392
*Cooked spinach, 1 cup	278
Blackstrap molasses, 2 Tb.	274
Cooked turnip greens, 1 cup	249
Sesame seeds, 2 Tb.	176
Okra, 1 cup cooked	176
Tortillas, corn, 2	196
Kombu, raw, 3.5 oz.	168
Wakame, raw, 3.5 oz.	150
Tofu made with nijari, 4 oz. (calcium sulfate and nijari are processing agents)	80-146
Kale, 1 cup	79
Nori, raw, 3.5 oz.	58

Foods are cooked unless noted otherwise.

*Spinach contains oxalates, which can significantly cut down on calcium absorption.

Source: *Simply Vegan*, Debra Wasserman and Reed Mangels, The Vegetarian Resource Group, and *Food Values of Portions Commonly Used*, 15th Edition, Jean Pennington.

Twelve Ways To Sneak Calcium Into Your Diet

If you don't like milk, the following foods or recipes contain a good source of calcium, yet they don't taste like milk. If you think creatively, you can sneak calcium into your diet in dozens of ways. Here are just a few ways to increase the calcium in your diet. Recipes marked with a * and page number indicate location of the recipe later in the book.

1. Make creamy soups (homemade or canned) with milk or evaporated milk.

2. Use evaporated milk (which has twice the calcium) in food preparation such as when making mashed potatoes, pudding, cream sauces, etc.

3. Eat dairy based desserts such as pudding, frozen yogurt, milkshakes and Yogurt Fruit Parfait* (page 262).

4. Add reduced-fat cheese to your mashed potatoes, vegetables, pasta, sandwiches and sauces.

5. Substitute cheese for meat in your lasagna or stuffed shells. (Spinach Stuffed Shells* page 331)

6. Add molasses to homemade quick breads, cookies and pancakes (or add to your mix.) Sesame seeds and tahini (sesame seed butter) are also high in calcium and can be added to snack bars, cakes, vegetables and dips (See Favorite Snack Cake* page 315 and Quick and

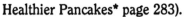

Healthier Pancakes* page 283).

7. Add nonfat milk powder to prepared soups, pancake mix, milkshakes, and yogurt shakes.

8. Make dip out of yogurt or herbed cheese spread from yogurt cheese* (page 282). Add your own herbs and spices or use a packaged mix. Or use tofu that contains calcium for your dips.

9. Eat fish with small bones. Salmon Paté* (page 252) contains both salmon and fat-free cream cheese.

10. Prepare quiche, (Crustless Quiche* page 312) or egg custard, which contain milk. Eat more vegetables which are good sources of calcium.

11. Instead of buying regular orange juice choose Citrus Hill Plus Calcium Orange Juice. It contains 225 mg. of calcium in 6 ounces. Unlike other calcium sources, this form of calcium doesn't significantly affect iron absorption from a meal (5).

12. Add powdered nonfat milk to your pancake and cake batter, to your cream sauces, and to milkshakes.

Questions You May Have

I can't tolerate milk! What can I do?

Many African-Americans, Asians, Native-Americans, and Hispanics have lactose intolerance, meaning they have trouble absorbing and digesting lactose, or milk sugar. The result is uncomfortable gas, stomach aches and in some cases diarrhea. Don't throw out the milk bottle forever! Research shows that as pregnancy progresses, especially in the third trimester, women who are lactose intolerant can break down much more lactose. This may be a compensatory effect since calcium is needed in large amounts in the third trimester (6).

Lactase, the enzyme that is lacking, can be purchased in drop form to put into milk or in pill form to take directly before drinking milk. It's sold over the counter in pharmacies as "Lactaid" "Lactrace" and "Dairy Ease." You can also purchase Lactaid milk which is 2% milk that has reduced lactose content.

Some people can tolerate milk with food and especially one containing fiber such as milk over raisin bran at breakfast (7). Cocoa may stimulate the body to produce more lactase, thereby increasing the tolerance of chocolate milk or hot cocoa (8). I've found that some women tolerate whole milk better than skim or lowfat. This may be because the fat slows digestion of the milk and improves digestion of the lactose. For those who can use the extra calories and sugar, chocolate milk is an option that will increase calcium in the diet. Other low lactose dairy options are yogurt, buttermilk, sweet acidophilus milk, and cheeses.

If none of the above solutions work for you, the last resort is to take a calcium supplement. More about calcium supplements on page 37.

What about drinking chocolate milk?

Until recently, it was thought that the calcium in chocolate milk was not absorbed well because of another element in the milk, oxalate. However, it has been found that the amount of calcium absorbed from chocolate milk is similar to that absorbed from whole milk, yogurt and cheese (9). The amount of calcium found in chocolate milk is also similar to that found in regular milk–284 mg. in 8 oz.

Another concern about drinking chocolate milk has been its caffeine content. You'll be happy to know that 8 oz. of chocolate milk contains only 5 mg. per 8 oz.–or about the amount found in 5 oz. of decaffeinated coffee. If you prefer chocolate milk to white milk, and can afford the calories (179 for 8 oz. of 2% lowfat chocolate milk compared to 120 calories for plain 2% milk), then drink and enjoy!

Isn't there enough calcium in my prenatal vitamin?

No, though the pill seems big enough! If it did contain all the calcium needed, you really *wouldn't* be able to swallow it! Most prenatal vitamins contain only a small percentage of the RDA for calcium. You must obtain the majority of calcium you need from your diet.

Iron

Some time during the 24th through to the 28th week, your health care provider will probably again have your blood tested for anemia, which is somewhat common during pregnancy. Because your blood volume expands up to 50%, you need twice as much iron than before you were pregnant. Knowing a few things about iron will help you prevent anemia and improve your iron status if you are anemic.

Iron is best absorbed from animal sources like beef, eggs, etc. If you are not a big meat eater, combine a small amount of animal protein with vegetable protein. This helps you absorb more iron from the vegetable foods. For example, mix a small amount of ham in with your pinto beans, or chop a hard boiled egg into your cooked spinach or spinach salad.

You can increase the amount of iron your body absorbs from food by eating a vitamin C food along with it. For example, have an orange, melon or berries for dessert after a meal, or have raw or cooked tomatoes, tomato juice, broccoli, cabbage, greens, cauliflower, or bell pepper as your veggie. Or drink citrus juice, vegetable or tomato juice, or vitamin C fortified apple juice with your meal.

Iron Content of Foods
Good Sources of Iron

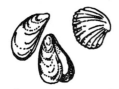

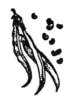

The RDA for pregnancy is 30 mg.; 15 mg. for breastfeeding.

Food	Iron in mg.
Animal Sources	
Clams, 3 oz.	24
Pork liver, 3 oz.	15
Oysters, 3 oz., (also a great source of zinc)	11
Beef liver, 3 oz.	6
Mussels, 3 oz.	6
*Canneloni with spinach and veal, 8 oz.	4
Roast Beef Sandwich	4
*Chili, 1 cup	4
*Stuffed Green Pepper with beef and crumbs	4
*Spaghetti & meatballs, with tomato sauce, 1 cup	4
Shrimp, 3 oz.	3
Egg McMuffin	3
*Green Pepper Steak, 10 oz.	3
*Beef and vegetable stew, 1 cup	3
Cheeseburger, fast food	3
*Chicken ala king, 1 cup	2.5

Food	Iron in mg.
Vegetarian Sources	
Soybeans, 1 cup cooked	9
Tofu, firm 4 oz.	7-13
Molasses, Blackstrap, 2 Tb.	6
Chick peas, 1 cup cooked	5
Quinoa, 1 cup cooked	5
Pinto beans, 1 cup cooked	4
Prune juice, 8 oz.	3
*Spinach, 1 cup cooked	3
*Potato, 1 medium	3
Peas, 1 cup cooked	3
Soy yogurt, 1 cup plain	3
Figs, 5 medium	2
Bulgur, 1 cup cooked	2
*Watermelon, 1/8 medium	2
Bok choy, 1 cup *cooked	2
Green beans, 1 cup cooked or *Broccoli	1
*Tomato juice, 8 oz.	1

*Also contains a significant amount of vitamin C which helps absorption of iron.

Numbers are rounded off. Numbers are for cooked foods, as applicable.

Source: *Food Values of Portions Commonly Used*, 15th Edition, Jean Pennington

Factors which inhibit the absorption of iron

◆ Coffee
◆ Tea
◆ Calcium supplements
◆ Antacids
◆ Dairy products
◆ Soy protein
◆ Wheat bran
◆ Fiber

Factors which aid in absorption of iron

◆ **Vitamin C** Other vitamin C foods include tomato, greens, cabbage, citrus, peppers, pineapple, mango and papaya.

◆ **Cooking with an iron skillet.** The iron content of about 3 ounces of spaghetti sauce increases from 3 mg. to 87 mg. of iron when cooked in an unenameled iron skillet (10).

"How's Your Diet?" Quiz:

First write down everything you've eaten during the last day or on a typical day. Then using the checklist, make a tally for each serving eaten next to each food. Compare your totals for the day with those recommended.

Breakfast

Snack

Lunch

Snack

Dinner

Snack

How Did You Do?

Your diet should contain at least the following:

10 Servings Starches/Grains

Best choices: whole grain bread and cereal, sweet potatoes, winter squash, potatoes, dried beans, peas, corn, wheat crackers, popcorn.

3 Servings Fruits

Best choices: papaya, mango, melon, berries, apricots, peaches, grapefruit, orange, kiwi.

3 Servings Vegetables

Best choices: broccoli, cauliflower, carrots, spinach, cabbage, romaine and leaf lettuce, greens, sweet peppers, tomatoes.

Note: Don't forget to eat at least one vitamin C-rich and one vitamin A-rich fruit or vegetable every day!

6 ounces Protein or equivalent

Best choices: lean beef, dried beans and legumes, shellfish, lean lamb, tofu, fish, lean pork, chicken, turkey. Be sure to eat a variety!

4 Servings Dairy Product or high calcium equivalent

Best choices: Skim and lowfat milk and yogurt, lowfat cheeses, nonfat or lowfat frozen yogurt or dairy desserts.

3-5 Servings of Fat

Best choices: Avocado, nuts, seeds, canola or olive oil, margarine, salad dressing or mayonnaise made from canola, sunflower or safflower oils. Remember that there are many hidden fats in baked goods, fried foods, whole milk products and desserts. Fat has twice as many calories as carbohydrate or protein.

8-10 Cups of Fluid

You should be drinking to thirst, or at least 8 cups of fluid per day, most of it from water.

"Thrive on Five"

The National Cancer Institute is using the slogan "Thrive on Five" and "Five a Day for Better Health" to encourage Americans to eat more fruits and vegetables.

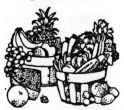

Why? Fruits and vegetables are great sources of vitamins, minerals and fiber. And when you fill up on them, you are less likely to eat things like chips, cookies and other less nutrient dense foods. Of course, you don't want to eat the same things day after day–variety is important.

Do five fruits and vegetables a day sound like a lot of food? Here are a few easy tips for adding fruits and vegetables to your meals.

Breakfast:

♦ Add mashed banana, dried fruit or applesauce to pancake batter. Top pancakes and waffles with strawberries or other fresh fruit.

♦ Add dried fruit, peaches, strawberries, blueberries or other fresh fruit to your cereal.

♦ Whip up a fruit shake. (recipe page 252).

♦ Eat a fruit or some juice before you have anything else.

Lunch:

♦ Add apple, pineapple, or mandarin orange slices to your chicken, tuna, or tossed salad.

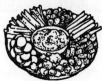

♦ Have a salad or raw veggies before your meal.

♦ Drink vegetable or tomato juice with your meal or as a pre-meal "cocktail".

♦ Add sprouts, leaf lettuce, spinach and tomatoes to your sandwiches.

♦ Stuff leftover veggies or salad in a pita pocket with cheese for lunch.

Dinner:

♦ Do a stir-fry for dinner. You can even buy the vegetables cleaned, chopped and ready to go!

♦ Zip up your spaghetti sauce with bell pepper, zucchini, carrots or eggplant. Shred or chop finely and they will cook quickly. If you have picky children at home, you can puree the cooked vegetables and they'll never know they're there!

♦ Start dinner with a vegetable based soup or a fruit soup (recipes page 314).

♦ Make a fruit salsa to accompany your grilled chicken or seafood. (recipe page 308).

Dessert:

♦ Top angel food or pound cake with fresh or canned fruits.

♦ Try a fruit sorbet.

♦ Have a frozen yogurt layered with fruit.

- How about a frozen banana or frozen grapes?
- A mixed fresh fruit salad makes a great finish.
- Grilled fruit kabobs to top off a grilled dinner.

Snacks:

- Snack on dried or fresh fruit. Since dried fruits are concentrated, they are a great source of vitamins, minerals and fiber. You can also keep them in your purse or desk drawer.

- Keep raw vegetables ready to eat in your refrigerator. You can buy them ready to eat. Some McDonald's now carry VegiSnax, carrots grown just for snacking!
- Heat up leftover vegetables.
- Drink fruit or vegetable juice, fruit juice mixed with club soda, or a fruit smoothie.

Smart Snacking

When I ask my clients if they snack, they usually look embarrassed. You would think that SNACK is a four letter word, since most people think of snacking as "eating foods they shouldn't" or "cheating." Actually, snacking can be healthy, and it's a must during pregnancy. Snacking helps you get all the nutrients you need when you can't eat much at a meal. It also gives you more energy during those times when baby seems to have sapped it all.

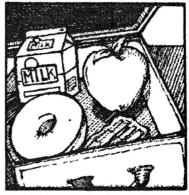

Keep Your own "snack stash" at work!

What are the best snacks?

The best snacks are those that offer the most nutrition for the fewest calories. What comes to mind first is fruits and vegetables– they offer lots of nutrition, virtually no fat and few calories. An added plus is their fiber and fluid content.

The Center for Science in the Public Interest, publisher of Nutrition Action Healthletter recently published a list of the healthiest fruits, based on their nutrient and fiber content. Here are the "Top Fifteen:" papaya, canteloupe, strawberries, oranges, tangerines, kiwis, mango, apricots, persimmons, watermelon, raspberries, red or pink grapefruit, blackberries, dried apricots, and white grapefruit (11).

Don't despair if your favorite fruit isn't on this list–just try to include the above fruits more often to get the most nutrition out of your fruit.

Second on our list of good snacks would be other high carbohydrate foods. Again they provide energy, little fat, and contain fiber. Of course, they must also taste good! Lastly, we have the dairy and protein food combinations. Try to have a variety of snacks during the day.

Healthy Snack Options

♦ Health Valley Granola Bars (I like these because they are sweetened with fruit and are high in fiber)

♦ Fibars (contain added sugar and fat)

♦ Raisin bran or other high fiber cereal

♦ Rice or popcorn cakes (for a sweet tooth, Quaker Caramel Corn Popcorn Cakes are my favorite!)

♦ Popcorn (choose the one with the least fat or pop your own)

♦ Rye or wheat crackers

♦ Graham crackers

♦ Fig Newtons

♦ Guiltless Gourmet™ No Oil Tortilla Chips

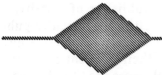

At Last, A Lowfat Chip

As I write this, I'm snacking on tortilla chips that aren't fried–and they taste great! Guiltless Gourmet Inc. did what was thought to be impossible; made tortilla chips as well as black bean and pinto bean dips, salsas and queso dips without added

fat! 1 oz. of chips also provides 80 mg. of calcium.

But beware, if you like spicy, the "spicy" dips are pretty hot; mild is also available. They are widely available in health food stores and are gradually entering grocery stores. You can call 512-443-4373 to find where they are available locally or order direct from the distributor at 1-800-878-8486.

And don't forget the dairy foods!

♦ Milk

♦ Yogurt

♦ Cheese

♦ Dip made with cottage cheese or fat free cream cheese

♦ Milkshake made with fresh fruit (see "Shakes" on page 253 for yogurt shakes)

Add other protein foods for a hungry appetite. Eating a snack that contains protein before you go to bed at night can also prevent low-blood sugar in the morning.

♦ Tofu spread on whole grain bread

♦ Peanut butter on crackers or with banana or apple

♦ Cheese and apple

♦ Tortilla rolled up with ham and cheese

♦ Cottage cheese and fruit

♦ Fat-free cheese on celery, carrots and broccoli

♦ Tortilla chips and refried beans (vegetarian)

♦ See page 240 for other snack ideas.

Second Trimester Challenges

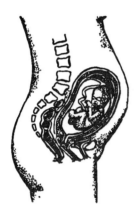

Vaginal Discharge

Increased discharge is considered normal in pregnancy. It is usually whitish and is the result of an increased supply of blood and glucose to the vaginal walls and increased production of mucus by the endocervical glands. The acid level of your mucus changes in pregnancy making you more susceptible to vaginal infections. If you have severe itching and irritation and a foul odor, contact your health care provider.

What you can do...

♦ Continue to bathe daily.

♦ Wear cotton underwear.

♦ Avoid feminine deodorants, powders and bubble baths.

Constipation

Progesterone, a pregnancy hormone, slows down the movement of food in your intestine, causing more water and nutrients to be absorbed and constipation is often the result. The pressure of the growing baby on your intestines and rectum can also cause this problem. An iron supplement can further worsen it.

What you can do...

♦ Drink plenty of fluids–at least 8-10 glasses daily, mostly from water.

♦ Eat high fiber foods (see Focus on Fiber, "Focus on Fiber" on page 51).

♦ Exercise regularly.

♦ Some people are constipated when they eat certain foods such as cheese and bananas.

♦ Avoid caffeine, since it can cause a loss of even more fluid which can make the stools hard.

Hemorrhoids

Hemorrhoids are swollen or enlarged veins in the rectum. Hormones once again play a role in this problem as does straining during a bowel movement. As the baby grows, greater pressure from the uterus displaces intestines which can lead to constipation and then hemorrhoids.

What you can do...

♦ Prevent constipation.

♦ Discuss hemorrhoids with your health care provider. He may advise a stool softener or high fiber laxative like Metamucil. (If you do take a stool softener, keep in mind that they can take as long as 3 days to work. Don't take more than one type of stool softener at the same time.)

♦ DON'T take over the counter laxatives, stool softeners or hemorrhoid treatments without your health care provider's approval.

♦ Taking warm baths and sitting on soft pillows can relieve the pressure.

♦ Avoid heavy lifting, pushing and standing for long periods of time.

Stress

We all live with stress. If stress isn't managed, it can lead to chronic medical problems such as ulcers and heart disease. Pregnancy offers it's own special stresses. Just wondering if you are doing "all the right things" for your baby is a stress. You may be debating about working after you have the baby or preparing another child for your "new arrival". You may be trying to figure out how you'll pay for the delivery or all those baby things you need to buy. The hormones of pregnancy can cause mood swings and can cause you to cope less effectively with stress.

According to the March of Dimes, there are some studies that show that extreme stress can play a role in low birthweight.

What you can do...

♦ Make realistic goals. You probably can't physically do what you did before pregnancy. You also need to take more time for yourself; time to exercise, time to rest, time to plan and prepare good meals. This can put a time crunch on an already busy schedule. Try to plan for it and take it in stride.

♦ Use relaxation techniques like biofeedback and meditation. There are many audio and video tapes with relaxing music and scenery- this can help you take a mental vacation.

♦ Try to find support in your spouse, friends and co-workers. Other new moms are especially empathetic to your needs. Remember that your spouse will be feeling his own stresses and probably needs your support too.

How Baby is Growing

At this time, all the major organs and systems are started or completely established. From now on the fetus will start to gain more weight. Your body is producing more blood in order to nourish your baby. You need to be drinking plenty of fluids, preferably 10 cups per day of water, milk, juice, or soup. Anything with caffeine can cause you to lose your needed fluids.

At the end of 16 weeks- 4 months

Your baby is quite active even though you might not feel it yet. Making facial expressions, swallowing, rotating feet, kicking, sleeping, waking and even listening to you are all part of the daily routine. Fine downy "lanugo" hair much like peach fuzz is developing on the head. The fetus is now six to seven inches long and weighs six to seven ounces; the weight of a big red apple.

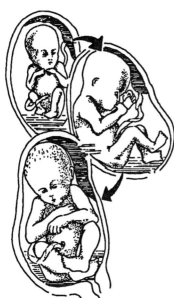

respond to external noise and music. The distinct fingerprints and footprints are formed; even identical twins have different fingerprints. The alveoli in the lungs are just beginning to develop. If the baby is born at this time, it would need extremely specialized care.

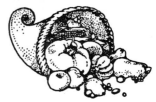

At the end of 20 weeks- 5 months

A growth spurt has occurred within the last month. The fetus now measures between eight and twelve inches long and weighs about 1 pound. Lanugo hair now covers the whole body and the hair on the head is getting thicker. Eyebrows and eyelashes are developing. Moms are beginning to sense the baby's movements as their muscles develop and they become stronger at turning and rolling.

At the end of 24 weeks- 6 months

Baby is now about 11-14 inches long, averaging the length of a ruler. Your baby now weighs between $1\frac{1}{2}$- $1\frac{3}{4}$ pounds The fetus looks like a wrinkled old man with skin covered in vernix, a thick creamy lotion, that protects it while in the amniotic fluid. The eyes are opening and closing and baby can hear and

Second Trimester Menus

Most women feel their best during the second trimester, and the menus and recipes in Chapter 15 reflect this. Your appetite may be robust, so the menus are a little heavier. Some recipes will take a little more time in case you feel like spending more time in the kitchen.

◆ A Month of Breakfast Ideas
◆ Menus for a Hungry Appetite
◆ I Could Cook All Day Menus
◆ Company's Coming! Menus

6

The Third Trimester

◆

What You Will Find In This Chapter:

- Weight Gain/Energy Needs
- Other Nutrient Needs
- Focus on Vitamin B6 and Zinc
- Tip For Keeping Your Energy UP!
- Third Trimester Challenges
- How Baby is Growing
- Third Trimester Menus

And answers to questions you may have:

- What if I have gained too much weight?
- I feel so tired; what can I do?
- What can I do for heartburn?
- I can't sleep; any advice?
- I have hemorrhoids, what can I do?

The third trimester is an important time for many reasons. It's the "home stretch," so to speak; a time when you will be making last minute preparations for your baby's arrival. Likewise, your baby will be making strides in its growth to prepare for its birth into the world.

Weight Gain/Energy Needs

During the last three months of your pregnancy, you will probably gain a large proportion of your total weight. Just when you think you can not gain another pound, or expand your stomach another inch, you do! Remember that in all your prepara-

tion for the baby's arrival, you still need to eat, and make wise food choices.

You should continue to gain about a pound a week during this time. Remember that if you are overweight or underweight, your weight gain should be adjusted accordingly. If you find that you have exceeded your goal weight already, discuss this with your health care provider. He will still want you to continue gaining weight, but perhaps at a slower rate. **Caution: never try to lose weight while pregnant, no matter how much weight you have gained.** Your baby needs you to eat adequately so that it can grow and develop enough to survive on its own in our world!

Many women find that their "get up and go has got up and went!" Regular exercise (even a simple walk around the block) will improve your endurance and you won't feel like a couch potato! If you find that you are much less active than in previous months, you may not need the entire 300 extra calories recommended earlier. However, you still need all the added nutrients, so if you do cut down on food intake, you must make your food choices with even more care!

On the other hand, you may find that with the thought of your baby's arrival just around the corner, you have renewed energy! You may need to increase your calories. See the snack ideas for "High Energy Moms" page 241.

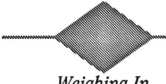

Weighing In

Are you one of those weight conscious women who weigh daily? Don't! It is a good idea to be aware of your weight, however during the third trimester, you are more prone to water retention and fluctuations in weight gain. So when you panic, thinking you've gained a pound in 2 days, it may be that your body is just retaining fluid. Develop a healthy attitude about weighing by weighing just once a week, and at the same time of day under the same condi-

tions. This will give you a truer idea of how your weight is progressing...

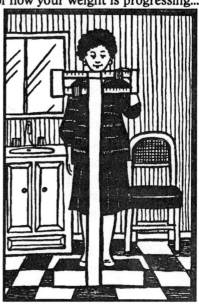

(NOTE: If you do find that you have gained 2 or more pounds in 2 days of if you notice extreme swelling in your hands, face or feet, or have headaches or trouble with vision, notify your health care provider. This may be a sign of preeclampsia. For more information, see page 125.

Other Nutrient Needs

Your need for vitamins and minerals during the third trimester remains essentially the same as the second trimester. Keep in mind that certain water soluble vitamins such as thiamin, riboflavin, and niacin are required in amounts relative to your calorie intake. Thus if you increase your calories, make sure your diet contains foods rich in these vitamins. Also, vitamin B6 is needed in amounts proportionate to your protein intake. So if you're eating many high protein foods, you may want to be sure that you have some good sources of B6 in your diet.

Women who follow strict vegetarian diets (no animal protein) should take a supplement of vitamin B-12; 2.2 micrograms per day (1)

Research data show that pregnant women's diets contain less than the RDA for vitamin B-6, vitamin D, vitamin E, folate, iron, zinc, calcium and magnesium (2). How does your diet stack up?

Take the following Diet Analysis to find out. Answer yes or no:

1. I eat a variety of foods daily.

2. I eat a dark green or orange vegetable daily.

3. I eat a citrus fruit or fruit or vegetable high in vitamin C daily.

4. I eat 2-3 servings of protein food daily.

5. I eat poultry, fish, beef and pork weekly.

6. I eat whole grains as often as possible.

7. I eat 5 fruits and vegetables on most days.

8. I eat 4 servings of dairy product or high calcium food daily.

9. I am gaining about 1 pound per week.

10. I avoid caffeine, alcohol and drugs.

If you answered yes to 7 or more questions, you're doing pretty well. Less than that? Well, you know what you need to work on.

Focus On Vitamin B6 and Zinc

Good Sources of vitamin B6

The RDA for pregnancy is 2.2 mg.; 2.1 mg. for breastfeeding.

Food	B6 in mg.
Animal Sources	
Beef liver, 3 oz.	0.77
Light meat chicken, 3 oz.	0.51
Pork loin, 3 oz.	0.40
Halibut, 3 oz.	0.34
Ham, 3 oz.	0.39
Tuna, light, 3 oz.	0.32
Vegetable Sources	
Mustard Greens, 1 cup	1.62
Soybeans, 1 cup	0.85
Potato, medium baked with skin	0.7
Banana, 1 medium	0.7
Bran flakes, 3/4 cup	0.6
Prune juice, 1 cup	0.6
Lentils, 1 cup	0.57
Chickpeas, 1 cup	0.54
Sweet potato, 1 cup	0.51
Pinto beans, 1 cup	0.50
Brown rice, cooked, 1 cup	0.5
Dates, dried, 10	0.42
Wheat germ, 1/4 cup	0.3

Values represent cooked foods, as aplicable.

Source: *Food Values of Portions Commonly Used*, and *The Nutrition Challenge for Women*, Louise Lambert-Lagace'.

Good Sources of Zinc

The RDA for pregnancy is 15 mg.; 19 mg. for breastfeeding.

Food	Zinc in mg.
Animal Sources	
Oysters, 3 oz.	154.0
Crab, Alaska, 3 oz.	6.4
Pork or beef liver, 3 oz.	6.0
Beef top round, 3 oz.	4.7
Veal roast, 3 oz.	3.7
Lamb chop, 3 oz. lean	3.0
Pork roast, 3 oz.	2.6
Lobster, 3 oz.	2.5
Clams, 3 oz.	2.3
Shrimp, 3 oz.	1.3
Trout, 3 oz.	1.2
Vegetarian Sources	
Wheat germ, toasted, 1/4 cup	4.7
Green peas, 1 cup	2.0
Bran flakes, 3/4 cup	1.9
Spinach, 1 cup	1.4
Bran muffin, 1 medium	1.1

Values represent cooked foods, as applicable. Source: *Food Values of Portions Commonly Used,* and *The Nutrition Challenge for Women,* Louise Lambert-Lagace'.

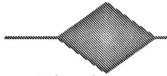

What about sugar?

Sugar has gotten knocked around a lot in the past 10 years. There are still many myths circulating about it. Here are "just the facts".

1. Sugar doesn't cause diabetes, though it does cause the body to produce more insulin in order to use the sugar. This happens with any carbohydrate food, but the effect is more pronounced with simple sugars.

2. Sugar doesn't appear to cause hyperactivity. Studies have shown just the opposite–sugar actually has a calming effect when given to children (3; 4). Often the increased activity in children after eating a sugary food may be from the caffeine, as in a cola. Another possibility may be the activities that generally surround the eating of a lot of sweets, such as a birthday party. However, there are sometimes individual reactions to any food.

3. Sugar does cause tooth decay, as do many other carbohydrate foods.

4. High sugar foods are often low-nutrient foods. They can also be high in fat, so if your diet has a lot of sweets in it, your diet may be too high in fat and calories and lacking in important nutrients.

5. Sugar in moderation helps your food taste good, though many of us have too much sugar in our diets. It is estimated that total sweetener consumption in the US is 18% of the diet; the American Dietetic Association recommends limiting sugar in the diet to 10-15% of total calories (5).

You may have heard that the third trimester and especially the last month, is a real challenge. You feel like you can't possibly get bigger. It is sometimes tough to get out of your chair or bed (especially if you have a waterbed!) and your energy level may need a boost. On the other hand, many women feel energetic and get sudden bursts of energy (often called the nesting syndrome) when they want to get everything done! The following tips will help you feel at your best during the last months of pregnancy.

Tips For Keeping Your Energy Up!

◆ Put up your feet from time to time. Some swelling in the feet and legs is considered normal these last few months. Keep in mind that the extra 20 to 30 pounds you are now carrying is putting a lot of pressure on legs, knees and feet. Wear flat, supportive shoes; support hose may also be a good idea.

◆ Take catnaps at lunch if you can, but after you've eaten! (I remember several times taking naps on my boss's couch during lunch!)

◆ Let the housework go! It's good practice for the first few months with baby. Start putting your feelings first and the housework second. Do only what has to be done (like laundry) or enlist the help of your spouse or other children.

◆ Don't forget those in between snacks--they help boost your energy. Keep a "snack stash" in your drawer-peanut butter crackers, dried raisins, figs, apricots and prunes, graham crackers, granola bars.

◆ Keep up with your exercise program. Exercise is probably the last thing you want to do when you feel tired, but it really will help in the long run. I don't really like to swim but when I attended a water exercise class for pregnant women, I loved it. You see, you feel weightless in the water and that was a nice feeling! After a long work day, being in the water left me feeling refreshed.

"Baby Pick Me Up"

A High Energy Drink

Two servings

1 frozen peach or nectarine (or 1/2 cup canned) (freeze for 45 minutes or more)

1/2 banana

1/2 cup frozen strawberries

1 cup plain yogurt or 1 cup milk

2 Tb nonfat dry milk

Honey, molasses or sweetener to taste

Blend all in blender. Makes approximately 2 cups. If you don't have frozen fruit, add ice for desired consistency. This will increase the volume.

Nutrient analysis per serving:
　　141 calories
　　9 g protein
　　0 g fat
　　6 g fiber

Percentage of RDA for pregnancy:
　　47% vitamin C
　　39% vitamin B12
　　31% potassium

Third Trimester Challenges

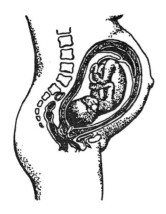

Backache

As pregnancy progresses, there is an increased curvature in the spine as the uterus enlarges. Hormones also cause the pelvic joints to loosen and relax. You may notice that the way you walk is a bit different than before you were pregnant. This may be due to expansion of joints and an adjustment in posture to compensate for carrying a big "front load."

What you can do...

♦ Practice good body mechanics and posture.

♦ Avoid bending over and lifting heavy objects (including older children if possible). Bend at the knees and keep your back straight.

♦ Wear low heeled shoes.

♦ Learn to do pelvic tilts–this will relieve pressure on the back and stretch and tone muscles. Ask your health care provider or child-birth educator for instructions or see page 179.

♦ Bend your knees slightly when standing in place.

Edema/Swelling

Many women experience ankle swelling in the last trimester. This is because it becomes more and more difficult for blood and fluids to return to the heart from the lower extremities. Let your health care provider know if you have swelling in your hands or face; this could be a sign of preeclampsia.

What you can do...

♦ Elevate your legs as often as possible to the level of your hips.

♦ Avoid standing for long periods of time.

♦ If you must sit for long periods, try to stand up, stretch and move around a bit to improve circulation.

♦ **Don't restrict fluid intake!**

♦ Avoid anything that will restrict circulation; stockings with tight bands, tight slips or pants, tight knee highs, etc.

Heartburn

As the baby grows, she compresses your stomach leaving minimal space for food. The hormones that slow down your digestion also relax the sphincter which keeps food in your stomach. These changes cause stomach acid to back up into your esophagus, causing a burning sensation that feels like it's around your heart.

What you can do...

♦ Eat small frequent meals.

- Avoid gassy foods, spicy and greasy foods. Avoid overeating.
- Avoid eating and lying down immediately afterward.
- Keep your head slightly elevated when in bed.

Sleepless Nights

As your body gets larger, you may find that getting comfortable in bed is quite a chore. The baby kicking, heartburn, and anxiety about the arrival of the new person in your life can add to sleeplessness.

What you can do...

- Try a bedtime ritual; warm bath, decaffeinated mint tea or warm milk and soft jazz or easy listening music.
- Support yourself with pillows.

"Our bed was a virtual oasis of pillows! I used two behind me to support my back, one between my knees to also relieve back pressure and one for my head."

...a new mother

- Practice the relaxation and breathing techniques that you learned in childbirth class.
- Continue regular exercise; it has a calming effect and can help with insomnia.

"My husband and I enjoyed a leisurely walk every evening after dinner. It gave us quiet time to talk and helped me to sleep better at night. Of course there were always other things we could do like clean house, or pay bills, but we made our walk together a priority."

...a new mom

How Baby Is Growing

Your baby is now rapidly filling your uterus. He will be turning flips less often, yet you might feel rhythmic movements that are hiccups!

At the end of 28 weeks- 7 months

A baby born at this time is considered able to live outside the uterus, though the lungs still are not mature. Your baby did a lot of growing in the last month and should weigh about between 2 1/2 and 3 pounds and is 14-17 inches long. Calcium is now being stored and the bones are hardening. Many babies now find they fit better upside down and start to position themselves for birth. Your health care provider can determine if the baby is positioned with his head down.

At the end of 32 weeks- 8 months

All your baby needs to do now is develop lung surfactant (which enables the lungs to inflate and deflate properly) and store some fat. Baby is beginning to store minerals like iron, calcium and phosphorous. The kicks are strong and vigorous and many women can feel a heel, fist or elbow through their abdomen. Your baby now weighs between 4 1/2 and 5 pounds and is 16 1/2-18 inches long.

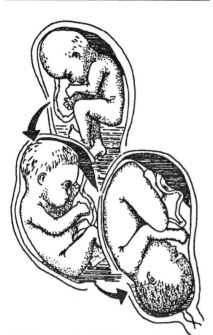

At the end of 36 weeks-
9 months

Baby is now making great strides in growth and is gaining close to 1/2 pound per week. The bones in the head are soft and ready for delivery. Lanugo hair and vernix are disappearing. Fat deposits under the skin help fill out the body and eliminate the wrinkling of the skin. Baby will settle lower into your pelvis and often seems to slow down in activity level. No day should ever pass without you noticing baby's presence. You should feel your baby move at least 10 times in a 12 hour period. If you don't–contact your health care provider.

At the end of 40 weeks-
10 months

Your baby is not considered "full term" until 38 weeks. At this time, he has a well established sleeping pattern and individual styles of

responses. He will continue to gain weight until the time of delivery. These last few weeks can be tiring as you wait for the arrival and meeting of your new little one. Congratulations!

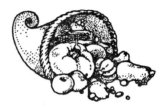

Third Trimester Menus

The main problems with eating during the last months of pregnancy are:

1. You get full quickly.

2. Fatigue may prevent you from wanting to cook.

3. Heartburn may restrict the variety or amount of food you eat.

4. You may be so busy getting ready for the baby that you neglect your own nutrition needs.

The third trimester menus are designed with the above in mind. Now is also a good time to prepare some foods to freeze for those first few days or weeks with your new baby. You may be trying to cut food expenses since you are buying many expensive necessities for the baby. So, there are some budget menus too.

- ◆ Menus from the Grocery Deli
- ◆ Using Leftovers With Flair
- ◆ Meals in Minutes
- ◆ Feel Full Menus
- ◆ Vegetarian Budget Menus

Vegetarian Eating

◆

What You Will Find In This Chapter:

◆ Vegetarians–The Healthy Minority?

◆ The Pregnant Vegetarian

◆ Nutrients of Special Concern

◆ Sample Vegetarian Meal Plans

◆ Vegetarian Shopping List

◆ Vegetarian Fast Food Choices

◆ Vegetarian Convenience Food Choices

And answers to questions you may have:

◆ How can I get enough calcium in my diet if I'm vegetarian?

◆ I'm diabetic, how do vegetarian foods fit into my diet?

◆ How can I get vitamin B12 in my diet if it is only found in animal foods?

◆ Must I buy special vegetarian foods to have a good diet?

If you've been keeping up with the news in the last few years you probably know that the country's major health organizations have set a few nutrition guidelines for us. In fact, the U.S. Department of Agriculture recently released it's Food Pyramid–a graphic designed to show us how to eat right. All those recommendations tell us to reduce fat and saturated fat, increase whole grains and complex carbohydrates, and increase consumption of fruits and vegetables. This sounds suspiciously close to a vegetarian diet!

For a long time, vegetarian eating was limited to a small group of people. Now vegetarianism enjoys a new popularity. Everyone does it to a certain extent, without even thinking about it. The teen who picks up a bean burrito is doing it, the mom who makes pasta with marinara sauce and cheese is doing it, and of course the practicing vegan who eats no animal products is doing it too. They all do it for a variety of reasons; because it's healthier, because they're concerned about the environment or animal rights, or simply because it's cheaper. Whatever the reason, vegetarianism is definitely catching on!

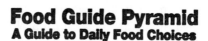

Food Guide Pyramid
A Guide to Daily Food Choices

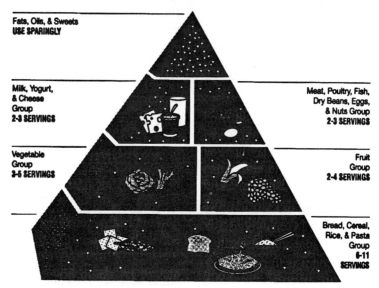

Fats, Oils, & Sweets
USE SPARINGLY

Milk, Yogurt,
& Cheese
Group
2-3 SERVINGS

Meat, Poultry, Fish,
Dry Beans, Eggs,
& Nuts Group
2-3 SERVINGS

Vegetable
Group
3-5 SERVINGS

Fruit
Group
2-4 SERVINGS

Bread, Cereal,
Rice, & Pasta
Group
**6-11
SERVINGS**

Not everyone wants to or will cut animal products totally out of their diet. You can receive some of the benefits of a vegetarian diet simply by cutting down on animal products and by increasing everything else–what I call "leaning toward vegetarian."

Vegetarians – The Healthy Minority?

Many people would like to have the health record that vegetarians do. Fewer vegetarians die from heart disease than do meat eaters (1; 2). Total serum cholesterol is generally lower too (3; 4). Vegetarians generally have lower blood pressures and lower rates of Type II diabetes than do non-vegetarians (5; 6). Vegetarians are generally closer to their ideal body weights than are non-vegetari-

ans. Some studies show that vegetarians have lower rates of osteoporosis, cancer, kidney stones, gallstones, and diverticular disease (7; 8; 9).

Good genes? Not necessarily. Most vegetarian diets are low in saturated fat, which can prevent high cholesterol levels and heart disease. They eat many fruits and vegetables which increases their intake of beta carotene and fiber–both of which are thought to be cancer fighting. Lacto-ovo vegetarians have a good amount of calcium in their diet, which may be protective against colon cancer. Vegetarians may also have beneficial lifestyle habits like regular exercise and abstinence from tobacco and alcohol, which contribute to good health. Maintaining ideal body weight can reduce the risk of heart disease, high blood pressure and diabetes. But even a vegetarian diet can be unhealthy if full of too much fat, sugar, or if not varied. If you are currently a vegetarian to some degree, your diet is probably on its way to meeting the dietary guidelines. If you are contemplating becoming vegetarian or leaning towards it, you can become part of the "healthy minority" too!

The Pregnant Vegetarian

Some women turn to vegetarian foods because they don't tolerate meat very well during pregnancy. Sometimes eggs and cheese, or black beans go down a lot easier than a steak! Of course many women are practicing vegetarians before they become pregnant.

There are several levels of vegetarianism.

1. **Lacto-ovo vegetarian:** This person eats no meat, poultry or fish, but does eat dairy products and eggs. These vegetarians have little trouble meeting nutrient needs for iron, calcium, B-12, or vitamin D.

2. **Vegan:** This person is the "true" vegetarian. Since she eats no animal products whatsoever, she should be sure to include reliable sources of vitamin B-12 which is found only in animal products or fortified foods. The vegan's need for calcium is actually less than meat eaters who consume larger amounts of protein. However, an effort may have to be made to consume enough vegetable sources of calcium. Like meat eating pregnant women, vegan

women may also have a problem with iron. Women living in Northern latitudes and those who have very little exposure to the sun in winter may have a problem producing enough vitamin D, which is made in the skin after exposure to sunlight, and is also found in dairy products.

3. **No Red Meat Vegetarian:** This person is someone who avoids red meat but does eat dairy products, fish and/or chicken. Although people who eat no red meat may call themselves vegetarians, they are not regarded as vegetarians by vegetarian organizations. These types of "vegetarians" generally will have no problem meeting nutrient needs except possibly for iron, which is found in lesser amounts in the white meats.

Nutrients of Special Concern

How does pregnancy impact vegetarians? Except for a few exceptions, pregnant vegetarians can expect to meet or exceed their nutritional needs. In fact, a study which looked at the intake of vegetarian women vs. their meat eating counterparts found that vegetarian non-pregnant women ate more of most nutrients than meat-eaters (10). The following table shows the results:

Comparison of vegetarian and non-vegetarian diets of women aged 19-34, Expressed in percentage of the RDAs

	Vegetarians	Non Vegetarians
Calcium	103	74
Iron	61	60
B6	62	58
Vit C	144	119
Vit A	101	109
B12	150	134
Magnesium	87	69

For vegetarians eating a variety of foods, there are just a handful of nutrients that they should pay particular attention to. They are vitamin B-12, iron, calcium and vitamin D. Since vitamin B-6 and zinc are nutrients lacking in all women's diets they are included here too.

Vitamin B-12

You should make sure that you have a source of vitamin B-12 in your diet since it is only found in animal products and fortified foods such as commercial breakfast cereals. Since formulations often change, it's best to check the nutrient label. According to Suzanne Havala M.S., R.D., Nutrition Adviser to the *Vegetarian Resource Group*,

"Some vegetarian specialty foods thought by many to be good sources of vitamin B-12, such as tempeh and spirulina, are in fact not reliable sources. Food labels listing the vitamin B-12 content of these foods include forms of the vitamin that are not active for humans and may compete for absorption with cyanocobalamin, the form we use."

If your diet contains neither animal products or foods fortified with vitamin B-12, a vitamin supplement is probably needed. Ask your health care provider.

Vitamin B-12 Fortified Foods

These cereals are currently fortified with at least 2.2 mg. of vitamin B12 per serving. However, since formulations often change, read the label to make sure the product still contains added vitamin B12.

Product 19
Total
100% Bran
Grape Nuts
C.W. Post (with raisins, plain and granola)
Post Raisin Bran
Maypo hot cereal
Ralston Bran Flakes
Bran Chex
Post Bran Flakes
Post Bran Flakes
Wheat Chex
Team
Nutri-Grain Wheat
Nutri-Grain Corn
Source: *Nutritionist III*, Version 7.2

Iron

It's possible that even though intakes for iron are about the same for vegetarians and non-vegetarians, the type of iron that vegetarians eat is less well absorbed than the iron in meat. However, vitamin C consumed with non-heme iron (the form of iron found in plant foods) helps increase the absorption of the mineral. Vegetarian diets are usually high in vitamin C.

Although anemia is no more common among vegetarians than meat-eaters, anemia can occur in any woman due to the high requirement for iron during pregnancy (11; 12). Thus, a supplement of 30 mg. of ferrous iron is recommended for all pregnant women. Look on page 66 for vegetarian sources of iron.

Calcium

Calcium won't be a problem for you unless you are a vegan, are lactose intolerant, or just don't like milk! Since vegetarians generally have less protein in their diet, it is thought that they will lose less calcium through their urine than people with a high-protein diet. Although the RDA for calcium is 1200 mg., the vegan's need for calcium is less than average; the World Health Organization's guideline of 1000-1200 may be a more appropriate estimate (11). The calcium content tables on page 61 will give you an idea of other foods high in calcium besides dairy products. If you are lactose intolerant, see page 63 for information. If you don't like milk by itself, but do eat other dairy products, see page 62 for tips on "sneaking calcium into your diet."

Some sea vegetables are good sources of calcium and other minerals. If you eat sea vegetables regularly, you should be aware that if they come from polluted waters, they could contain heavy metal pollutants. You should make sure the source of your seaweed is controlled, as from a sea vegetable farm in the U.S.

Certain minerals in green leafy vegetables (oxalates and phytates) have been thought to decrease absorption of calcium. Research in this area is ongoing, but it seems like the amount of these minerals in the American diet is not significant enough to change calcium absorption dramatically (12). However, if vegetables are your main calcium source, you might want to concentrate on eating those low in oxalates; broccoli, collard greens, kale, mustard and turnip greens.

Another option is to take a calcium supplement. Talk to a registered dietitian about increasing the calcium in your diet or ask your health care provider about a supplement.

Vitamin D

The need for supplemental vitamin D is rare because the body can usually produce all that it needs from exposure to sunlight. Few foods are naturally high in vitamin D; dairy products are fortified with it in the U.S. If you are strictly vegan and you either live in a northern latitude or have very limited exposure to the sun, you may need a supplement of not more than 100% of the RDA.

Brief, casual exposure of the face and hands to sunlight is thought to be equivalent to 200 IU of vitamin D (the RDA for pregnancy is 400 IU). The location, time of year, atmospheric conditions, clothing, amount

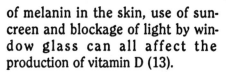

of melanin in the skin, use of suncreen and blockage of light by window glass can all affect the production of vitamin D (13).

Vitamin B-6

All women seem to have a problem getting enough vitamin B6. This vitamin is needed in proportion to your protein intake, so if your diet is especially high in protein foods, you may need even more B6. See page 76 for a list of vegetarian sources of B6.

Zinc

Zinc is a very important nutrient in the developing fetus. It is widespread in foods including legumes, shellfish, whole grains, and cheese. Many people don't have enough zinc in their diet.

One study which evaluated the diets of vegans and of lacto-ovo vegetarians found that neither group met the RDA for zinc. The mean intake for vegan women was only 13% of the RDA, while lacto-ovo vegetarian women's average intake was 71% of the RDA. The women's food choices in this study were mostly low zinc foods such as fruits, salads and vegetables (14).

Factors which may affect absorption of zinc include fiber, phytates, and some minerals. To obtain an adequate amount of zinc, vegetarians and especially vegans must make careful food choices. Consult the list on page 77 to see how much zinc your diet supplies.

Protein

Protein is important during pregnancy, and although vegetarians have just a little less protein in their diets than do non-vegetarians, their intake still exceeds the RDA. The list of foods below will give you an idea of foods that will supply you with the 10 extra grams of protein needed daily during your pregnancy. Keep in mind that it is important to eat a variety of protein foods throughout the day so that your body can utilize the protein for building material.

Vegetarian foods that contain 10 grams of protein

Black beans (or any legume), 3/4 cup
Brown rice, 2 cups
Cashews, 1/2 cup
Peas, 1 1/4 cup
Peanut butter, 2 1/4 Tb.
Quinoa, 1 cup
Soy yogurt, 1 cup
Tofu, 2 oz. firm

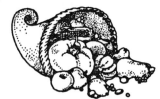

Sample Vegetarian Meal Plans

Daily Diet for Vegans

These are meant as guidelines only–eating a variety of high nutrient foods will provide the nutrition you need without following a structured diet.

Plan I

6 or more servings grains, cereals or breads (1 serving is a slice of bread or 1/2 cup cereal or grain)

3 or more servings milk or meat analogs (1 serving is 1 cup soymilk)

2 or more servings nuts, seeds or

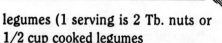

legumes (1 serving is 2 Tb. nuts or 1/2 cup cooked legumes

4 or more servings fruits (1 serving is 1 fruit or 1/2 cup canned fruit)

4 or more servings vegetables--Include some high calcium vegetables. (1 serving is 1/2 cup cooked or 1 cup raw)

3 or more servings fat

Plan II

4 or more servings legumes

4 or more servings milk or meat analogs

8 or more servings fruits and vegetables

6 or more servings of grains, cereals or breads

Source: *Simply Vegan*, by Debra Wasserman and Reed Mangels, *Vegetarian Resource Group*.

Sample Vegan Menu:

corresponds with Plan I

Breakfast:

Wheat Chex (vitamin fortified)
Banana
Soy milk
Whole wheat toast
Margarine

Snack:

Bran muffin
Juice

Lunch:

Olé Kale & Tofu Soup (recipe page 323)
Cornbread
Margarine

Fruit salad
Decaffeinated tea

Snack

Wheat crackers
Raw veggies
Hummus dip

Dinner

Colorado Stuffed Bell Peppers (page 311)
Tossed salad
Homemade tortilla chips
Soy milk-fruit shake

Snack

Soy milk
Graham crackers
Dried fruit

Lacto-Ovo Vegetarian Daily Diet

4 or more servings dairy products

1 egg or egg substitute (optional)

2 or more servings legumes or nuts

6 or more servings fruits and vegetables

6 or more servings grains, cereals or breads

Sample Lacto-ovo Vegetarian Menu

Breakfast:

Maypo Hot Cereal
Banana
Milk

Snack:

Cheese
Rye crackers
Raw veggies

Lunch:

Three bean & pasta salad
Tomato, lettuce
Bell pepper
Low-calorie ranch dressing

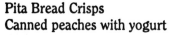

Pita Bread Crisps
Canned peaches with yogurt

Snack:
Peanut butter
1/2 whole wheat bagel
Juice

Dinner
Crustless Spinach quiche
Carrots
Oven baked fries
Margarine
Sorbet
Milk

Snack
Milk
Graham Crackers

Complementary Proteins–
An Old Myth

A myth that has been passed down for years is about complementary proteins. Even recently, vegetarians have been advised to eat the traditional legume with grain, grain with dairy or nut and grain to have "complete protein." Current thinking is that as long as a vegetarian eats a variety of foods with enough calories, she will have enough of all the amino acids. According to a position paper of the American Dietetic Association,

> "Mixtures of proteins from grains, vegetables, legumes, seeds, and nuts eaten over the course of the day complement each one another in their amino acid profiles without the necessity of precise planning and complementation of proteins with each meal, as the recently popular "combined proteins theory" has urged (16)."

Vegetarian Shopping List

Now that you are pregnant, you are probably much more aware of what you buy at the store. This handy shopping list can be reproduced and used weekly. For more information about shopping and label reading see page 184.

Produce/Tofu

tofu
asparagus/artichokes
broccoli, brussel sprouts
beets/cabbage/carrots/cauliflower/
celery/corn/eggplant/garlic/green
beans/lettuce: romaine leaf, boston/
mushrooms/onions: white, red/pep-
pers: green, red, yellow /potato:
sweet, white new/rhubarb/ruta-
baga/spinach/summer squash/swiss
chard/tomatoes/turnips/winter
squash/zucchini squash
apples/bananas, blueberries/can-
teloupe/cherries/grapes/grape-
fruit/honeydew melon/lemons/
oranges/pears/peaches/plums/
pineapple/rasberries/strawberries/
watermelon

other: _____

(foods that aren't in season fresh, should be bought frozen)

Dry Staples

whole wheat flour/wheat pastry flour
brown rice (instant/reg)
dry legumes_____
pasta (wheat, regular)
barley/quinoa/wheat germ
sugar: brown, white/molasses
honey/nutritional yeast
dry fruit: raisins, dates, apricots,
prunes, mixed
nuts: almonds, cashews, peanuts
walnuts, sesame seeds

Canned Goods/Jar Goods/ Packaged Items

tomatoes: sauce, paste, whole/
spaghetti sauce/beans: black/pinto/
chickpeas/kidney/navy bean soup/
other _____
peaches/pears/pineapple
nonfat evaporated milk
veggie burger mix
vegetarian specialty foods: _____

_____

peanut butter
tahini spread, tempeh
fruit spread
chutney

Breads

whole wheat/ rye/pita
tortillas: corn, flour
bagels/english muffins
crackers/pretzels
popcorn cakes
other:_____

Dairy Case:

soy milk/lowfat/skim milk
soy yogurt/soy cheese
cheese: mozzarella, lowfat cheddar,
american, swiss, other_____
lowfat cottage cheese
margarine, butter

eggs/fresh pasta/biscuits
Oils/Condiments
oil: olive, canola, walnut
lowfat salad dressings _____
low-sodium soy, teriyaki sauce
flavored vinegar: _____
mayonnaise/mustard
spices:_____

Frozen Foods:

meat analogs _____
fruits_____
vegetables _____
frozen dinners _____
pancakes/waffles _____
sorbet/tofutti/frozen yogurt/sherbet

Snack Foods

rice cakes/crackers _____
pretzels/graham crackers
granola bars, cookies, crackers
Other:_____

Drinks:

frozen juices_____
bottled juices _____
vegetable juice/club soda
decaf coffee, tea
other: _____

Non-Food items

soaps _____
paper goods _____
toiletries_____
misc:_____

Vegetarian Menus

In Chapter 16, you will find two weeks of budget menus, modified to fit pregnancy needs, from *Vegetarian Journal Reports*.

Vegetarian Fast Food Choices

Since more people are going meatlesss, even on an occasional basis, more restaurants are catering to vegetarian needs. The *Vegetarian Resource Group* is currently compiling information on restaurants across the country that offer vegetarian foods.

The article below is an excerpt from *The Vegetarian Journal*.

Please keep in mind that over 100 companies were surveyed by mail for menu information, but only 18 responded. Exclusion of any restaurants here doesn't mean they don't carry vegetarian selections.

What's in Fast Food?

Arby's

Arby's is now using vegetable oil for its fried foods. Their buns contain eggs or milk derivatives. Some of Arby's restaurants have salad bars, but most have converted to prepared salads. Arby's offers a baked potato and they are presently testing vegetable pita pockets which contain broccoli, carrots, cauliflower and celery. The milkshakes contain animal gelatin and the cheese contains animal rennet (an enzyme from calves which most cheeses contain.) Arby's seems sincere in their efforts to improve the selection of healthy alternatives and confirmed that they are investigating other meatless options. They have typically offered lowfat products and are phasing out the use of MSG in all their products.

Bob's Big Boy

Bob's Big Boy, part of Marriott Corporation's family restaurant division, contains a decent selection for vegetarians, though they are limited in options for vegans. For breakfast there are cereal, potatoes, pancakes, french toast, bagels, toast muffins, and a wide selection of fresh fruit. Bob's has recently switched from instant oatmeal to good old fashioned hearty kettle oatmeal from Quaker.

Another pleasant surprise at Bob's is a Garden Lasagna, which is a vegetarian lasagna containing cheese, spinach, carrots, and onions. Bob's has offered a vegetable stir-fry in the past but it did not sell well enough and so they decided upon chicken stir-fry, which is presently on their menu. This is a good example of how support by vegetarians could make a difference in determining whether or not vegetarian options are offered. Other vegetarian items on Bob's menu are French fries, onion rings, baked potato, and coleslaw. The Marriott Corporation certainly seems open to offering more vegetarian options if the demand is there.

Bonanza

Their restaurants are individually franchised. Because menu items vary among regions and are purchased from a wide listing of manufacturers and distributors, any nutritional evaluation or ingredient listing done on one unit's products may well be invalid for the rest. Vegetable items, salads, and desserts on their salad bars are purchased locally. The national headquarters recommends the use of vegetable oil, but they stated there is no guarantee it is used in every restaurant. Ask at each restaurant.

Burger King:

Burger King now uses only vegetable oil for their fried products. Their national headquarters stated that it is standard procedure for fries, French toast, onion rings and hash browns to be fried in oil separate from the 'food' products, meaning the chicken and fish. However, this conflicted with what was actually occurring in at least one Burger King restaurant that was surveyed. To be sure, ask at the restaurant you are visiting.

In addition to fried foods, vegetarian options at Burger King include the garden and side salads, croissants, bagels, blueberry muffins, and apple and cherry pies. Burger King actually has a Veggie Whopper listed on their cash register which is cheese on a bun with whatever condiments and toppings you'd like. They will also make it without cheese. The Whopper buns may contain animal shortening. The oat bran bun contains dairy products. Their bagels are made with vegetable shortening, but contain egg whites. Onion rings contain whey, but their hash browns appear to be vegan. At fast food restaurants it is often hard to tell if the salad dressings are vegan. Burger King probably has the best quality salad dressings of the fast food chains since they use Paul Newman's dressings, which avoid using preservatives and artificial ingredients. These come in individual packets which usually include ingredient listings. The French, Reduced-calorie Italian and Oil & Vinegar dressings are all vegan. Their garden salad contains cheese. The side salad lists only lettuce, tomatoes, cucumber, celery and radishes. Burger King is successfully marketing a Spicy Bean Burger in the U.K. and is reportedly considering vegetarian items for the U.S.

Carl's Jr.

French fries, onion rings, zucchini and other fried foods at Carl's Jr. are cooked in vegetable oil. Their onions rings and zucchini contain dairy derivatives. Bread products which contain no animal shortening, eggs or dairy derivatives include the breadsticks, hot dog bun, plain bun, flour tortilla, English muffin, and kaiser bun. None of their baked goods contain animal shortening. They have an all you can eat salad bar, as well as macaroni, potato, and pasta salads in some stores. They also offer a Lite Potato with margarine on the side. Carl's Jr. is making efforts to remove MSG from those foods in which it has been used in the past.

Chi-Chi's

As of July, 1991, all Chi-Chi's restaurants are phasing out the use of lard in their refried beans. They list the following items as being vegetarian: Chips and Salsa, Cheese Nachos, Guacamole, Chili Con Queso, Quesadilla, and Mexican Salad. However,

their cheese does contain rennet. Although they use vegetable oil for all their fried foods, meat products are fried in the same oil as vegetarian products. Their vegetable oil is not vegan, since it contains natural butter flavor, one percent of which is derived from animal sources. The oil is listed as "Kosher Dairy." They have a luncheon buffet, which is a food bar containing salad and some vegetarian items.

Church's Fried Chicken

Church's said that they fry their okra in all-vegetable shortening, but it is the same oil in which they fry their chicken nuggets.

Dairy Queen

The use of animal shortening in Dairy Queen/Brazier stores has been phased out, and they are presently using only vegetable shortening. Ingredients in buns and onions rings depend on the local supplier. They offer a Garden Salad, which contains eggs, and a side salad which is apparently vegan. Some stores might also carry a pasta salad with lettuce.

Denny's

Although we have been unable to obtain current information regarding their ingredients, they last stated that their deep fried items are cooked in soybean oil, though their refried beans are canned and have been prepared with lard. Grilled items, when cooked with added fat, are fried in soybean oil or butter.

Dominos

There are four different ingredient groupings for Domino's pizza crust, and any one of these might be used at your local units. Only one of the recipes is apparently vegan. The rest contain whey, and may contain egg, butter, buttermilk, cheese, and other dairy derivatives. None of these recipes use lard. Their sauce appears to be vegan. The enzymes in their cheese are listed as being either of vegetable or animal origin.

El Chico

El Chico's uses only vegetable oil for frying. Their refried beans reportedly do not contain lard, but you may want to check at your local restaurant.

Hardee's

Hardee's uses vegetable oil to cook all fried products. They offer pre-made salads including a garden salad which contains cheese, and a side salad which is vegan. Other vegetarian possibilities at Hardee's include pancakes, hash browns, egg and cheese biscuit, blueberry and raisin oat bran muffins, coleslaw, mashed potatoes, yogurt, and fries. Hardee's biscuits contain buttermilk and their gravy is sausage-based. Their Crispy Curls and French fries are fried separately from their fried meat products. Their mashed potatoes are instant and appear to be vegan except for the natural flavoring which is questionable. Hardee's is also willing to make a cheese sandwich with toppings on a roll.

Jack in the Box

They have a pamphlet which lists the ingredients for all their products. They claim to cook with only 100% vegetable oil blend, but the ingredients for this blend include natural butter flavor, one percent of which is animal derived. Bread products which appear to be vegan include their English muffins, hamburger buns, rye bread, sesame breadsticks, sour dough bread, tortilla bowl (wheat), tortilla shell (corn), and pita bread. The Cheesesteak Rolls contain whey, lecithin, and parmesan cheese, and the croissants contain nonfat dry milk and butter. The onion rings contain whey and egg yolk solids, and the apple turnover contains animal and/or vegetable shortening. Hashbrowns and guacamole appear to be vegan, but the hashbrowns are fried in the vegetable oil blend mentioned above. Jack in the Box offers a side salad which is vegan. Their reduced-calorie French dressing contains nonfat yogurt. The cheese used at Jack in the Box contains animal rennet. Their secret sauce contains egg yolks and Worcestershire sauce.

Kentucky Fried Chicken

KFC, as they prefer to be called these days, uses only vegetable shortening in all its frying procedures. Their bread products contain dairy products and whey. Some stores carry packaged salads including a small garden salad which is vegan. Other vegetarian options include corn on the cob, coleslaw, fries, plain buttermilk biscuit, and mashed potatoes, which contain butter and milk.

Little Caesar's

Little Caesar's claims that at present the cheese used in their Maryland stores uses only vegetable enzymes, but this does not necessarily apply to restaurants in other states. Most mainstream cheese companies use animal rennet. Apparently their dough is vegan, containing no whey or other dairy derivatives. You can order Little Caesar's pizza without cheese. Other options include a Veggie Sandwich, Greek Salad (contains feta cheese), Tossed Salad, Crazy Bread, and Crazy Sauce. Items that are vegan are the Crazy Sauce, Crazy Bread without parmesan cheese, Tossed Salad, and Greek Salad without feta cheese.

Long John Silver's

All their fried foods are prepared in partially hydrogenated soybean oil. They do not have a salad bar, but do offer prepared salads, corn on the cob, coleslaw, hush puppies, baked potatoes, and mixed vegetables.

McDonald's

At the beginning of 1991, McDonald's began phasing out the animal/vegetable shortening mixture it was using for frying and is replacing it with vegetable oil. Fries, hash browns, and other fried items are supposed to be prepared in separate vats from those used for meat. McDonald's offers a garden salad which includes cheese, and a side salad which is vegan. Beware that their Red French Reduced-calorie dressing lists Worcestershire sauce which contains anchovies. Their only dressing that appears to be vegan is the Lite Vinaigrette. For breakfast, vegetarian options include hash browns, danish, cinnamon rolls, blueberry or apple bran muffins, and cereal. McDonaldland Cookies contain lecithin which may be an animal

or soy product, but they contain no other animal products. The chocolate chip cookies contain dairy products and the apple pie contains margarine, lecithin and natural flavors, which may be animal derived. Some McDonald's restaurants are carrying Orange Sorbet, a newly approved frozen dessert product that appears to be vegan. It contains sugar and corn syrup. McDonald's is making efforts to measure the public's interest in healthier options as they are presently testing the sale of carrot and celery sticks in some stores. McDonald's claims that they are always looking into new products and mentioned pasta salad as one option. Sooner or later, with a little encouragement, they'll have to offer a McVeggie burger!

Nathan's

Their thick French fries are cooked in corn oil. Corn on the cob is also available.

Pizza Hut

Pizza Hut Pan Pizza Crust contains whey, but the Thin 'n Crispy Crust and Hand Tossed Crusts are vegan. Their sauce contains cheese flavor from natural Parmesan, and MSG.

Ponderosa

Ponderosa has a large food bar which typically contains plain vegetables as well as a salad bar, fruit, and fried foods. Ingredient listings were not available, but it seems possible to come up with a decent vegan meal at Ponderosa. The new product testing department for Ponderosa did state that they are working on some vegetarian options!

Rax

Rax is now using only Crisco, an all vegetable shortening for their fried foods. Their beans are first cooked with lard. Their crackers and croutons may contain animal shortening and their buns contain milk powder. Some of their pasta is vegan, but the rainbow rotini contains egg whites. Their spaghetti noodles appear to be vegan and their sauce contains Parmesan cheese. The Rax salad bar has the regular salad bar offerings, plus macaroni salad, and occasionally a three bean salad which appears to be vegan.

Round Table Pizza

The cheese used on Round Table Pizza contains animal rennet. They have a good variety of vegetable toppings including black olives, garlic, mushrooms, pineapple tidbits, tomatoes, green peppers, onions and jalepeno peppers. Their dough contains whey powder and nonfat dry milk.

Roy Rogers

All Roy Rogers's Restaurants are being converted to Hardee's. Please see previous paragraph on Hardee's.

Sbarro

This Italian fast food chain, is often located at travel rest areas and inside shopping malls. Their pizza crust is made with vegetable oil and their marinara sauce appears to be vegan. The baked ziti and mostaccioli are made using egg pasta.

Shakey's

Shakey's uses vegetable oil for frying, and all of their dough contains vegetable shortening. We were unable to determine whether or not their dough contained dairy products or if their cheese contains animal rennet. They have a salad bar.

Shoney's

Shoney's has a breakfast bar with fruit, cakes and muffins. Other breakfast items include cereals, home fries, pancakes, hash browns, grits and toast. Shoney's also has various prepared salads, a salad bar and soups.

Skipper's

While many eating establishments seem to have little or no knowledge about the ingredients in their foods, speaking with the Quality Assurance Manager at Skipper's allayed such fears with regard to Skipper's restaurants. She definitively answered questions and had access to the sources of ingredients in their food. Skipper's uses soybean oil for frying all their menu items. Their bread and breadsticks contain dairy products, but their crackers do not contain any animal products. They offer a garden salad which includes mixed greens, cucumbers, tomatoes, and carrots. Other vegetarian foods include baked potatoes, zucchini slices, and coleslaw with mayonnaise. They also have onion rings which are made with a beer-based batter that is vegan. They seemed very open to suggestions for new items. With a little encouragement and support, more vegetarian options might be offered.

Taco Bell

No lard or tropical oils are used in any of their products or frying processes. Their guacamole contains sour cream. Both the corn and wheat tortillas are vegan according to their main office. The Heat Pressed Tortilla contains nonfat dry milk. Their pita bread contains honey, but no dairy derivatives. Their Twists are vegan, containing only wheat, rice flour, corn flour and salt. MSG is not found in any Taco Bell menu item and they are currently testing a new line of salads.

Taco John's International

The only information obtained from Taco John's was that their refried beans are made with vegetable oil.

TacoTime

TacoTime uses vegetable oil for their deep friers. Their Refritos are made with vegetable shortening. Tortillas are made with vegetable margarine. Vegetarian dishes available at TacoTime include: Soft Bean Burrito, Crisp Bean Burrito, Refritos (bean, sauce, cheese), Nachos, and Mexi-Fries.

T.G.I. Friday's

Though this is more of a regular restaurant, we included it here because they presently have "real" vegetarian options on their menu including a vegetarian burger called a Garden Burger. Apparently, public response has been overwhelmingly positive to this venture, and they are very interested in expanding their vegetarian selections. The Garden Burger does have some dairy in it. Other options include a Fresh Vegetable Baguette which contains cheese and is served with yogurt, and the Garden Cob which is their number one selling salad containing artichokes, green peppers, squash, and other veggies.

They also have a Vegetable Medley, which is steamed vegetables served with rice and a dinner salad. Beware that the brown rice pilaf currently served with it contains chicken base. Order a baked potato as a substitute and you'll have a filling, vegan meal.

Wendy's

Wendy's SuperBar has one of the best salad bars in the fast food arena, but some items contain surprising ingredients. Apparently Wendy's has two suppliers for their meatless tomato sauce, one of which contains natural beef flavor. On the other hand, their Reduced-calorie Bacon & Tomato dressing appears to be vegan since the bacon granules are made from soy and vegetable protein. Their Italian Caesar dressing contains anchovy paste, as well as eggs and cheese. Aside from preservatives and colorings, the only other questionable ingredient in the French, Sweet Red French, Golden Italian and Reduced-calorie Italian Dressing is the natural flavor. Their croutons contain whey, but the chow mein noodles appear to be vegan.

At the Mexican Fiesta, the refried beans contain lard. Their Spanish rice contains liquid margarine, natural flavorings, and MSG. Their taco chips, taco sauce, and taco shells appear to be vegan. The flour tortillas contain shortening and margarine, which may or may not contain animal products. Wendy's Garden Spot Pasta Salad contains cheese and egg whites, but their Superbar Pasta Medley and Rotini appear to be vegan. Their Superbar Fettucine contains eggs, and their garlic bread contains dairy derivatives. Other vegetarian options include their Alfredo sauce, cheese ravioli, French fries, potatoes, cottage cheese, fruit, vegetables, cheddar chips, potato salad and pudding. Their buns contain whey. Wendy's has reportedly tested a Grain Burger and they are looking into other vegetarian possibilities. Their consumer department was very helpful and they definitely seem open to new ideas. Let's encourage them to follow up on a veggie burger!

Mrs. Winner's

Their potatoes are fried only in vegetable oil.

The *Vegetarian Resource Group* has been providing information on food offered at fast food chains for years. Public interest groups such as *Center for Science in the Public Interest* are continually pushing for healthier fast food options. *The North American Vegetarian Society* is presently sponsoring a Vegetarian Express Fast Food Campaign as well. Together we can make a difference!

From "What's In Fast Food", by Sally Clinton, *Vegetarian Journal,* January/February 1992, *Vegetarian Resource Group*, Baltimore, Maryland.

Vegetarian Convenience Foods Choices

New vegetarian foods are also quickly flooding the marketplace as more people go meatless. The fat in some products is surprisingly high. Here is the nutrient information for some products currently available.

Vegetarian "Specialty" Foods

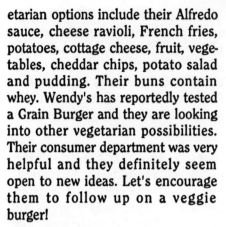

	calories	protein	fat	carbohydrate
LaLoma				
Big Franks	110	11 g	6 g	2 g
Swiss Steak, 3.3 oz.	170	14 g	10 g	7 g
Vege Burger, 3.8 oz.	110	21 g	2 g	3 g
Redi Burger, 2.4 oz.	130	14 g	6 g	5 g
Tender Bits, 4 pc - 2 oz.	80	9	3	5 g
Nuteena, 1/2" slice	160	18 g	12 g	6 g
Meatless fried chicken, 2 pieces	140	9 g	10 g	4 g
Little Links, 2 links	90	9 g	5 g	2 g
Worthington				
Savory Slices, 2 slices	100	8 g	6 g	4 g
Turkee Slices, 2 slices	130	9 g	9 g	3 g
Saucettes, 2 links	150	10 g	11 g	3 g
Vegetable Skallops, 1/2 cup	90	15 g	2 g	5 g

	calories	protein	fat	carbohydrate
Vegetable steaks, 2 1/2 pc	110	17 g	2 g	5
Chili, 2/3 cup	190	10 g	10 g	15 g
Vegetarian Burger, 1/2 cup	150	19 g	1 g	7 g
Grain Burger, 6 Tb.	110	19 g	1 g	7 g

Entree	calories	protein	fat
Angel Hair Pasta with Italian style sauce, zucchini and mushrooms	200	10 g	4 g
Cheese Tortellini	310	14 g	6 g
Cheese Enchiladas Rancheros	260	8 g	10 g
Vegan:			
Michelina's, Spaghetti Marinara	255	11 g	2 g

Source: Manufacturer's labels.

Other Vegetarian Convenience Foods

These are just some of the frozen entrees found in most grocery stores that are either vegetarian (containing cheese or milk) or vegan.

Entree	calories	protein	fat
Healthy Choice Macaroni & Cheese	290	12 g	6 g
Healthy Choice Baked Cheese Ravioli	290	15 g	2 g
Budget Gourmet, Three Cheese Lasagna	390	23 g	17 g
Weight Watcher's			
Cheese Manicotti	260	17 g	8 g
Garden Lasagna	260	19 g	7 g
Fettucini Alfredo with Broccoli	230	15 g	7 g

Questions you May Have:

I just found out I have gestational diabetes; how can I fit vegetarian foods into my meal plan?

Actually a vegetarian diet fits very well into the guidelines of a diabetic diet: high in carbohydrate, high in fiber, and low in fat. Visiting with a registered dietitian would be helpful in planning a vegetarian diet to meet your specific needs. Here are some typical vegetarian foods with their exchanges.

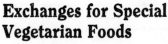

Exchanges for Special Vegetarian Foods

Food	Serving Size	Exchanges
Brewer's yeast	3 Tb.	1 bread
Bulghur, cooked	1/2 cup	1 bread
Carob flour	1/8 cup	1 bread
Kefir	1 cup	1 milk plus 1 fat
Legumes, cooked	1/2 cup	1/2 lean meat + 1 bread
Loma Linda Veggie Links	1 oz.	1 high fat meat
Morningstar Farms Grillers	1 oz.	1 high fat meat
Miso	3 Tb.	1 vegetable
Seaweeds, cooked	1/2 cup	1 vegetable
Soyflour	1/4 cup	1 lean meat + 1/2 brd
Soy grits, raw	1/8 cup	1 lean meat
Soy milk	1 cup	1 milk + 1 fat
Tahini	1 tsp.	1 fat
Tempeh	4 oz.	1 bread + 2 lean meat
Tofu, soft	1/2 cup	1 medium fat meat
Tofu, firm	1/2 cup	2 medium fat meats

Food	Serving Size	Exchanges
Wheat Germ	1 Tb.	1/2 bread (If you use 1/2 cup or more, you need to add 1 fat)

Source: modified from *Vegetarian Journal Reports*, Page 101,

Is a vegetarian diet lower in fat than a diet containing meat?

Generally, yes. However, a vegetarian diet can be as high in fat as a meat containing diet. For example, lacto-ovo vegetarians may eat a lot of cheese, eggs, and lowfat or regular dairy products, which raises the fat content of the diet. A diet that is not well planned can have as much fat and saturated fat as the typical American diet!

A vegan diet can also be high in fat, although most of the fat would be unsaturated (unless coconut products, palm or palm kernel oil were consumed regularly.) For example, nuts, tahini and nut butters, staples for some vegetarians, are very high in fat. Other hidden fats can find their way into the diet through goodies like tofu ice cream and carob.

The important feature for any type of diet is that high fat foods (especially those high in saturated fat), be eaten in moderation.

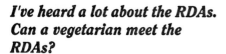

I've heard a lot about the RDAs. Can a vegetarian meet the RDAs?

Many people think that RDA stand for Recommended Daily Allowances, when it really stands for Recommended Dietary Allowances. The RDAs are designed for the maintenance of good nutrition of practically all healthy people in the United States. They have a built in safety margin (11).

Some sources say that the World Health Organization's RDIs are closer to the needs of the vegetarian population. For example, the RDAs for calcium are 1200 mg.; the RDI's for calcium are 1000-1200 mg. (12). Which is correct? Both. The RDAs are based on the typical U.S. diet which contains meat, while the RDIs take into account the needs of other populations that don't eat meat.

How will you know if you are getting enough of all the nutrients? Eat a variety of many foods as outlined in one of the vegetarian meal plans listed previously. Eat as many unrefined foods as possible and enough calories and the rest of your diet will fall into place. Your weight gain and your baby's size (as checked by fundal height and ultrasound) will also show that your diet meets the mark.

I'm worried about being in the hospital and not being able to eat vegetarian...any advice?

First of all, if you pre-register at your hospital, you might be able to request a vegetarian diet then. When you go to the hospital in labor, you will probably be allowed to eat only ice chips or perhaps clear liquid such as apple juice. This is because if you need anesthesia, your stomach should be empty. During this time, you might want to remind your doctor that when you can eat you would like a vegetarian diet. You might even want to write it down before you go to the hospital.

After you have your baby, you will probably be allowed to eat a "real meal." Your meal may depend on what's left in the kitchen-and that depends on what time your baby was born! Babies seem to love to come in off hours, and that may mean "slim pickins" for a very hungry new mom! A simple meal would be just a cheese sandwich, fruit and juice. For vegans, the selection may be very limited if after hours. You may want to bring in some non-perishable snacks from home as options for after delivery.

The Diet Order

The diet, or type of meal that you receive in the hospital must be ordered by your doctor. Make sure he understands that you want a vegetarian meal and specify which type. Many hospitals have options for vegetarians, but they usually aren't vegan.

In addition, a dietary technician or registered dietitian may visit you to see if you have specific likes or dislikes or if you are having any problems eating. Make your preferences known, and also try to select your own menu, if possible. Be polite, but persistent!

For more information about eating after delivery, see page 157, also "Hospital Survival Guide," by

Suzanne Havala M.S., R.D., *Vegetarian Journal Reports, Vegetarian Resource Group.* 1990.

Eating After Surgery

If you have a cesarean section, you may not eat solid food for a day or so, depending on which type of anesthesia you receive. The progression from NPO (nothing by mouth) to a Regular Diet usually starts with clear liquids like clear juices, broth, gelatin, coffee, tea, soda. As your tolerance increases, your diet will progress to a full liquid diet which includes foods like thinned hot cereals, cream soups, and dairy products in addition to clear liquids.

You should be able to omit the non-vegetarian foods and eat double portions of the other foods. Again, make sure that your doctor has left instructions for you to have a vegetarian diet when it's ok to eat solid food.

Special Care for High Risk Pregnancies

What You Will Find In This Chapter:

- Pre-Existing Diabetes
- Gestational Diabetes
- The Diabetic Eating Plan
- High Blood Pressure/Pregnancy Induced Hypertension
- Expecting Twins or More
- Coping with Bedrest
- Age and Pregnancy

And answers to questions you may have:

- What kind of diet should I follow if I have gestational diabetes?
- Should I cut my salt intake if I have high blood pressure of pregnancy?
- How can I eat or prepare healthy meals if I'm on bedrest?
- Are artificial sweeteners safe?
- How much weight should I gain if I'm expecting twins?
- How many calories should I eat if I'm 17?
- Should I eat differently if I'm over 35?
- What are some healthy snacks for a diabetic diet?

When you are pregnant, some conditions may occur that you aren't expecting. It can be scary if you don't know what will happen. This chapter tells you how the condition may affect you and baby, and what you can do. Although there are other complications of pregnancy, this chapter will discuss only the conditions which can affect your nutrient needs or can be affected by your diet. Being informed is the key to taking charge of your health!

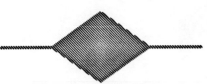

You Are Not Alone

One of the hardest things about having a high risk pregnancy is that you may feel like the only person with your problem. However, there are many women out there who have experienced or are now going through the same challenges you are. Sidelines National Support Network is a network of local support groups for women experiencing high risk pregnancies and their families. Call to find a local support group or a listening ear. Send your own thoughts, poems jokes and anecdotes to share with others.

Sidelines National Support Network, C/O Candace Hurley.; 2805 Park Place, Laguna Beach, CA 92651 714-497-2265

The Confinement Line will find a woman to act as your support-line while your on bedrest 703-941-7183 The Confinement Line Childbirth Education Association., P.O. Box 1609, Springfield VA 2215

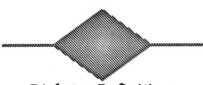

Diabetes Definitions

Glucose: A simple sugar that is the final product of carbohydrate digestion. It is used for energy by every cell in the body.

Insulin: a hormone produced by the pancreas that helps the body use and store glucose produced by carbohydrate digestion.

Pre-Existing Diabetes

If you are currently diabetic, you probably know the long term implications. Before conception and during pregnancy are critical times to control your blood sugar. Before you even think about having a baby, consult your physician. He will want you to be in "tight control" and will want to closely monitor you.

The American Diabetes Association suggests that diabetic moms-to-be keep fasting and pre-meal blood sugars between 60-90 mg., 1 hour after meals blood sugars less than 140 mg. and 2 hours after meal blood sugars under 120 mg. Remember that these are just general guidelines and your doctor may have different guidelines for you (1). Why all the fuss? High blood sugar in the first 6-10 weeks of gestation means a higher risk of birth defects in babies of women who have diabetes. However, moms who maintain acceptable blood sugar control are no more at risk than the general population for having babies with birth defects (2).

The Health Care Team

Before we go further, we should talk about a group of people who are very important to the health of your baby–the health care team. You will need some specialized medical professionals to help in your care. If you

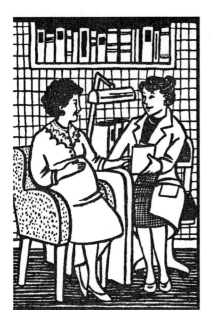

are not already working with these health professionals, you can find them by calling a local medical society, by asking your family physician, calling a local chapter of the American Dietetic Association or the American Diabetes Association.

A diabetologist, endocrinologist, or physician who specializes in care of diabetics is someone you should talk to before you become pregnant to make sure you are in good control.

An obstetrician who specializes in high risk pregnancies, or one who has experience working with pregnant diabetics. A physician who specializes in high risk pregnancies is called a **perinatologist**. Some women consult with a perinatologist before they get pregnant if they have had previous problems in pregnancy.

An endocrinologist is a physician who specializes in caring for people with diabetes and also treats other conditions which involve hormones.

You may be under an endocrinologist's care already or your obstetrician may refer you to one to help manage your diabetes during pregnancy.

A diabetes nurse educator or a nurse practitioner who has special experience dealing with diabetes during pregnancy. The nurse educator or nurse practitioner is a registered nurse who has more education and or experience in a specialized field. She will probably be the person you work closely with for day to day management of your diabetes.

A registered dietitian (R.D.) is someone who will develop an individual eating plan for you. An individual meal plan is important since it can be specifically designed with your activity level, work schedule, lifestyle, and favorite foods in mind. She usually works closely with the nurse educator. Your dietitian can also work with you after you have your baby to help with diet for breastfeeding, and weight loss.

A pediatrician or neonatologist is someone who provides medical care of your baby after it's born. Since babies of diabetics sometimes have problems, a specialist such as a neonatologist might be needed.

You are the most important member of the health care team. You are responsible for the day-to-day management of your diabetes, including contacting other members of the team to let them know how you are doing or when you need help.

What to Expect:

If you are taking insulin, you will probably have to adjust your doses, with the help of your health care team. Some women need to adjust their insulin dosage as often as every five days because of increased need (3). If you were controlled with diet or oral medications (Type II diabetic or non-insulin dependent) before pregnancy, there is a good chance you will be put on insulin during pregnancy. However, after you have your baby, you will most likely return to your prior mode of treatment, especially if you return to your ideal body weight and exercise regularly.

Some women take injections before every meal to keep their sugar in control. Others use a pump. Be prepared to take more shots if needed. Taking more shots will most likely mean checking your blood sugar more often.

Possible Effects on Mom

Pregnant diabetics have a greater chance of having a miscarriage, hypertension, preeclampsia, and excess amniotic fluid (4).

What to watch out for:

Some "normal" conditions of pregnancy can be a real challenge for diabetics. On the other hand, some "normal" conditions for diabetic women are more challenging during pregnancy.

♦ **Insulin resistance:** Insulin needs gradually increase during pregnancy. As pregnancy progresses, especially around the 24-28th week, a hormone produced by the placenta resists insulin. Therefore, much more insulin is needed. Diabetic moms-to-be may need twice the insulin they usually take.

♦ **Ketoacidosis:** Ketones are a by-product of fat breakdown and are a sign that glucose is not available, so the body is breaking down fat stores for energy. As ketones increase in the bloodstream, (usually as a result of high blood sugar from not having an adequate dose of insulin) the pH level of the blood changes and ketoacidosis occurs. Because of changing insulin needs and energy requirements during pregnancy, ketoacidosis can occur more quickly and if not treated can eventually lead to a coma.

♦ **Morning sickness:** If you have this common symptom of pregnancy, it can throw off your usual intake of food. Vomiting can cause dehydration and upset insulin needs. Both can result in low blood sugar. Follow the guidelines in Chapter 1 for morning sickness and guidelines below for "sick day rules."

♦ **Low blood sugar (hypoglycemia):** Low blood sugar can occur because of increased activity, energy demands of baby and from increased insulin dosage. Always have glucose tablets or glucose gel with you or keep in your purse a food that is a quick source of energy like fruit juice or hard candy. Be sure to follow it with a more substantial snack about 1/2 hour later, like half a sandwich or cheese and crackers.

Some doctors recommend having a glucagon kit available for severe hypoglycemic reactions (glucagon is a hormone that increases blood sugar). Make sure that relatives, friends and co-workers know what to do for you if you start having the symptoms of hypoglycemia, including knowing how to use the glucagon kit. Also, be sure to wear a necklace or bracelet that identifies you as diabetic.

♦ **Infections:** Even minor infections can increase blood sugar and change insulin requirements. This can cause a breakdown of fat and lead to ketoacidosis. (See definition above) If you have the symptoms of ketoacidosis, seek medical attention immediately.

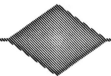

Sick Day Rules

During illness, it is important to follow these rules. If you are sick with a virus or infection, this causes blood sugar to increase, even though you may not be eating much. The following rules are used at the Diabetes Education and Support Center in Colorado Springs:

♦ **Contact a member of your health care team.** This is the first sick day rule during pregnancy, especially if you are vomiting or have diarrhea.

♦ **Continue to take your insulin.** Talk to your physician to see if you should take the same dose. You may actually need more.

♦ **Check blood sugar more frequently.** Your doctor or diabetes educator will let you know how

often. This will prevent any potential problems of high-blood sugar and ketoacidosis. Your doctor may also want you to check your urine for ketones more frequently.

♦ **Prevent dehydration.** Do this by drinking at least 1/2 cup of fluid per hour.

If you can't keep much food down, have 1 serving of a food which contains 10-15 grams of carbohydrate every hour such as:

Fruit Juice or Sweetened Drinks
1/3-1/2 cup apple juice, 1/2 cup orange juice
1/3-1/2 cup soda or fruit punch (not diet)
1/4-1/3 cup lemonade

Solid Foods Easy to Digest
(these foods contain about 10 grams of carbohydrate)
4 saltine crackers
1/4 cup sherbet
about 1/2 popsicle (these vary from brand to brand)
1/4 cup regular jello
10 oz. chicken noodle soup
10 oz. chicken and rice soup
8 oz. cream of mushroom soup (prepared with water)

If you can eat solids, drink plenty of calorie-free drinks to avoid dehydration such as:

Water, broth or bouillon, decaffeinated tea, sugar-free, caffeine-free soda, sugar-free fruit drinks or popsicles, etc.

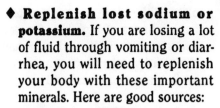

◆ **Replenish lost sodium or potassium.** If you are losing a lot of fluid through vomiting or diarrhea, you will need to replenish your body with these important minerals. Here are good sources:

Sodium: bouillon, canned soups, salted crackers, gatorade (choose regular or sugar free depending on if you are eating other solids)

Potassium: orange juice, melon, papaya, banana, orange-pineapple-banana juice, pineapple juice, tomato juice, vegetable juice, dried fruits.

How Diabetes May Affect Your Baby

Blood sugar crosses the placenta from you to your baby. High blood sugar causes the baby to produce more insulin. The effects of large amounts of sugar and insulin can cause serious risks including a greater chance of stillbirth. However, stillbirth is not common.

Birth defects occur more often in babies of mothers who are diabetic. Fortunately, pre-conception planning, early prenatal care, and keeping blood sugars in a narrow range can dramatically decrease that risk. If possible, seek medical counseling before you consider pregnancy.

Women with diabetes are prone to having bigger babies (macrosomia). High levels of blood glucose in mom, especially during late pregnancy, are thought to be responsible. After 13 weeks gestation, your baby can start producing its own insulin in response to high blood glucose levels. Insulin acts as a growth hormone, causing baby to deposit excess

fat and her increased size may make a C-section necessary.

Babies of diabetics sometimes have hypoglycemia (low blood sugar) immediately after delivery and they must take glucose or sugar water. They are also prone to having higher bilirubin levels, or jaundice, which is easily treated with special lights in the hospital. Babies of diabetic moms can have a higher chance of having respiratory distress syndrome (5).

If your diabetes is advanced and you have some blood vessel damage, you may have restricted blood flow to the placenta, so your baby may have problems growing and may be "small for gestational age."

What you can do to keep your diabetes under good control during pregnancy:

1. **See your doctor before you become pregnant.** You may also want to see a registered dietitian to get a handle on dietary management.

2. **Monitor your blood sugar.** Your physician will give you the blood sugar range he would like you to stay within. The blood sugar range during pregnancy is much stricter than when you are not pregnant. Remember that blood glucose values reflect what has happened in the last 1-3 hours.

3. **Eat regular meals and snacks.** You will want to eat balanced meals at regular intervals. Most women need between 2000-2400 calories, divided between carbohydrate (45-50%), fat (30-35%) and protein (20%). Your calories will be divided between meals and snacks. Especially important is the

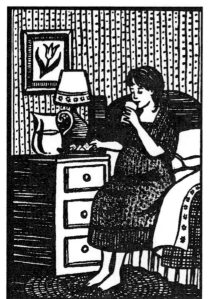

bedtime snack, which should contain carbohydrate, fat and protein. Eating a snack before bedtime (especially one that contains protein) can prevent hypoglycemia in the middle of the night. Some women even need a snack in the middle of the night (such as a glass of milk) to keep their blood sugar up.

4.   Exercise. You should ask your physician about specific guidelines for frequency and duration of exercise and when NOT to exercise (such as when blood sugar is too low or too high). Regular exercise can decrease your need for insulin and also make you feel more energetic! When you exercise, always take glucose gel or tablets, fruit juice or hard candy with you, and eat a snack or meal before you exercise. Never exercise when you know your blood sugar is low or when ketones are present. Also, don't give your insulin injection in an area that you will use immediately in exercise. For exam-

ple, don't give it in the leg if you will take a brisk walk immediately afterwards (See page 116 under Gestational Diabetes for other tips on exercising).

Labor and Delivery

Many doctors will induce labor for pregnant women who are diabetic. With all the high tech equipment available, your physician can tell just when the baby is developed enough to enter our world. About one half of all diabetics will need a cesarean delivery because the baby is too big to fit through the birth canal, or because of other complications (6).

During the first 24-48 hours postpartum, your insulin requirements can drop dramatically. You may need to watch for signs of hypoglycemia. Within a week after delivery, your insulin needs should return to prepregnant levels.

How to Cope

1.   You and your family need to be committed to your pregnancy and unborn child. Everyone should learn how insulin works, the importance of dietary management, and what to do in case of hypo or hyperglycemia. You'll need their emotional support and understanding too.

"It was really tough to put myself first," says Cindy, a woman who has been diabetic for 15 years. "When I was pregnant with my second child, I felt guilty when I had to get myself something to eat because of low blood sugar and my daughter was whining in the background. But I learned that I had to put myself first for the sake of my baby."

2. Remember that the extra time and discomfort you experience now will only last 9 months. When you have your healthy baby, it will all be worth it.

3. Seek out a diabetes support group, preferably one for pregnant women. It has been shown that women who have more social support can follow their dietary and self-monitoring regimens better (7).

4. Keep stress low. Remember that stress can also raise blood sugar. Learn some new techniques to handle your stress like relaxation, visualization and advanced planning. Again, seek cooperation from others to help reduce your stress.

5. Learn to recognize the early warning signs of hypoglycemia, hyperglycemia and ketoacidosis so you can take action.

6. Always be prepared to handle a low blood sugar reaction. See tips below.

Signs of Hypoglycemia:

(Low Blood Sugar)

These signs may develop very quickly

nervousness
shakiness
dizziness
perspiration
cold clammy skin
blurred vision
headache
disorientation, difficulty paying attention
irritability, sudden mood changes
pale skin

How to treat hypoglycemia

1. Take 1-2 glucose tablets or chew 3-4 hard candies or sugar cubes, 1/2 cup juice or non-diet soda (8).

2. Follow with a larger snack such as 1/2 sandwich, peanut butter and crackers or cheese crackers. Milk can be added for a more substantial snack.

3. If you have low blood sugar more than once a week, report this to your health care provider. If you can pinpoint the cause of your low bloodsugar, try to remedy it with the guidance of your health care team. It is often just a matter of eating before exercise, eating a bigger meal or adding a snack, or you may need a different insulin schedule. Many people are surprised to find that they have been giving their injections incorrectly, even though they may have been taking shots for years. This could also affect your blood sugar.

Can hypoglycemia harm my baby?

One animal study indicates hypoglycemia in mom does cause hypoglycemia in baby, and that baby will produce glucose from other sources such as fat for his needs. Continued bouts of hypoglycemia could cause poor growth in the baby (9).

Signs of Hyperglycemia

(High blood sugar)

These signs occur gradually.

hunger
frequent urination
increased thirst

headaches
fatigue

Signs of Ketoacidosis

If you have any of these signs, seek medical attention fast!

(some symptoms are similar to signs of hyperglycemia, but are much more intense)

excessive urination
excessive thirst
fruity, acetone or alcohol breath
listlessness; total lack of energy
nausea
abdominal pains
vomiting
labored breathing

Gestational Diabetes

Almost 3% of all pregnant women will have diabetes of pregnancy or gestational diabetes mellitus (GDM) (10). Diabetes mellitus is a disorder that prevents the body from using a simple sugar called glucose. GDM is a type of diabetes that occurs only during pregnancy and usually disappears after delivery.

Glucose is a simple sugar that is the final breakdown product from foods containing carbohydrate. Carbohydrate is found in all starchy foods like bread, potatoes, and corn, and is also in milk, fruits and vegetables. Forms of simple carbohydrate which enter the bloodstream more quickly are found in candy, jam, syrup, honey and table sugar. Your body can also make glucose from protein and stored carbohydrates.

Insulin is the hormone that allows glucose to enter your body's cells.

During pregnancy, women need 2-3 times more insulin for the body to use glucose. This is due to increased body weight and increased levels of hormones which work against insulin; these hormones peak during the 24th-28th week. When the body cannot produce the insulin it needs, high blood sugar and diabetes are the result.

Effects on Mom

Many women have no signs that they have GDM. Some of the symptoms of GDM are also the typical signs of pregnancy such as fatigue and frequent urination, so you may not be able to tell them apart. Some women have the symptoms of high blood sugar or low blood sugar, listed on page 110. Women with GDM have increased risk of preeclampsia (a type of hypertensive disorder of pregnancy) and urinary tract infections. Symptoms of urinary tract infections include burning during urination and frequent urination (11).

Effects on Baby

The most common problem is delivering a large baby, (macrosomia) which may prove for a difficult delivery, trauma to the baby during delivery, and/or increased need for a C-section.

Less common problems sometimes seen in babies of mothers with GDM include: greater risk of premature delivery, hypoglycemia or low blood sugar at birth, increased bilirubin in the blood (jaundice) and respiratory distress syndrome (12).

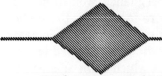

"Who is at risk?"

◆ *For Gestational Diabetes*

Risk factors for gestational diabetes include a history of stillbirth, habitual miscarriages, family history of diabetes, previous delivery of an infant weighing over 9 pounds, previous gestational diabetes, urinary tract infections, hydramnios, sugar in the urine, and overweight. It has also been show that with each subsequent pregnancy, the risk of GDM goes up. As you get older, your risk of having GDM also goes up (13).

◆ *For Adult Onset or Type II Diabetes*

It is estimated that half of all diabetics in the U.S. haven't even been diagnosed. Your chances of becoming diabetic are greater if:

You have a close relative who is diabetic.

You were diagnosed with GDM in a previous pregnancy.

You are overweight.

You have had a baby that weighed 9 pounds or more.

You are African-American, Native-American or Mexican American.

You are over forty.

Testing For Diabetes

When you are between the 24th and 28th weeks or pregnancy, your health care provider will ask you to take a glucose screening test which tests for sugar in the blood. This test is done without special preparation such as fasting or eating certain foods. First you will be asked to drink a very sweet drink called glucose (it tastes like cola syrup before the carbonated water is added). One hour later, your blood will be drawn and the amount of sugar (or glucose) in your blood will be tested. If your blood sugar is over 140 mg., this is considered a positive or "abnormal" test. You may be asked to:

◆ see a registered dietitian (R.D.) for meal planning guidance
OR

◆ take a glucose tolerance test which is similar to the procedure above but lasts 3 hours. You will need to follow a special high carbohydrate diet for 3 days prior to the test. Your health care provider will give you the specific instructions. After drinking the glucose, your blood will be drawn every hour for 3 hours (14).

Once your physician diagnoses you with GDM, you may be referred to a specialist such as an endocrinologist or a perinatologist who probably works with a staff of diabetes educators. However, your physician may decide to treat the diabetes aspect of your pregnancy himself by working closely with an R.D. who will give you a diabetic meal plan and a Nurse Educator, who will teach you about monitoring your blood sugar. (If you aren't referred to an R.D., you should request a referral!)

The Diabetic Eating Plan

Many people think that going on a diabetic diet means they must give up all their favorite foods! This is just not true!

The diabetic eating plan is simply a way of eating that includes balanced amounts of carbohydrate, fat and protein at each meal. All foods are allowed except simple sugars like table sugar, (sucrose), honey, jam or syrup and foods which contain a lot of sugar like cakes, pies, cookies, and candy. However, foods with a small amount of sugar are allowed in moderation, when "counted" into your meal plan. For example, graham crackers, animal crackers and angel food cake are foods allowed in moderation when your blood sugar is in good control.

The goal in managing your diabetes is to keep your blood sugar within a certain range. General guidelines are listed on page 104 under Pre-Existing Diabetes. However, your doctor or nurse educator may have individual recommendations for you. Controlling your blood sugar is done by not eating too many carbohydrates at one time and "balancing" your meals with protein and fat. The protein and fat slow digestion and cause a slow, gradual rise in blood sugar instead of a fast rise that would occur if you ate a carbohydrate food by itself.

Carbohydrate is found in starchy foods such as bread, crackers, cookies, rice, potatoes, corn, milk, yogurt, dried beans, fruit and fruit juice. Carbohydrate is found in smaller amounts in non-starchy vegetables such as green beans, carrots, and squash. Of course, any food containing concentrated sugars also provide concentrated sources of carbohydrate.

Your meal plan will be arranged with your current eating pattern, individual lifestyle and activity level in mind. The calories, carbohydrate, protein and fat that you need in a day will be calculated and then divided between your meals and snacks. Snacks are important because they allow you to eat smaller meals, and prevent your blood sugar from dropping too low. (see page 117 for snack ideas) Following up with the dietitian is important because it is difficult to assess the energy needs and eating patterns of a person in just one visit. Your meal plan may need adjusting as your activity level increases or decreases.

Your Meal Plan

Although many practitioners are using a standard diabetic diet with carbohydrate evenly divided between meals, one trend seems to be to limit carbohydrate before noon. It is common for some women to have high blood sugar in the morning. This is due to hormones from the placenta, which cause your body to be resistant to insulin. A reduced-carbohydrate, higher fat morning meal has successfully controlled the higher blood sugar for some women.

Bev Spears R.D., of The Diabetes Center of New Mexico starts their gestational diabetic patients with just one serving of a starchy food (such as 1 piece of toast) at breakfast. If the blood sugar testing shows that the amount is well tolerated, the carbohydrate will be increased. The preliminary diet also doesn't include milk or juice, because many women's blood sugar are sensitive to the simple carbohydrates found in those foods. Milk may be added back into the diet as tolerated (15). It is generally advised that juice be avoided or drunk sparingly since it can increase blood sugar at any time.

An example of a meal plan that your dietitian might develop for you follows. On the left you will see food groups noted such as starch, protein, fat, milk, vegetable and fruit. Your diet will be probably be based on the Exchange Lists for Meal Planning 1989 from the American Diabetes Association and The American Dietetic Association. It is a plan of eating that uses a combination of foods from seven food groups. Each food in a group has approximately the same number of calories and other nutrients, so they can be "exchanged" for each other. For example, one serving of starch has 80 calories and 15 grams of carbohydrate. You won't have to worry about all those numbers, but do get to know the serving sizes:

1 starch =	1 piece bread
	6 crackers
	1/2 cup pasta
	3/4 cup flake cereal
1 fruit =	1 medium fresh fruit
	1/2 banana
	1/2 cup canned unsweetened fruit
1 milk =	1 cup milk or plain yogurt

1 protein =	1 oz. fish, poultry, cheese, or beef
	1/4 cup cottage cheese
	1 egg
1 fat =	1 tsp. margarine, oil, mayonnaise or butter
	2 tsp. diet margarine
	1 Tb. salad dressing or 2 Tb. diet dressing
	1/8 of an avocado
	20 small peanuts

Source: Exchange Lists for Meal Planning, The American Diabetes Association and The American Dietetic Association, 1989.

Your dietitian will give you a complete list of exchanges from the American Diabetes Association.

The following meal plan has about 2200 calories. Your calorie needs will vary depending on your size, your ideal body weight, and your activity level. An individualized diet developed just for you is very important. The sample below is an example only and is not intended to replace individual counseling by a diabetes educator.

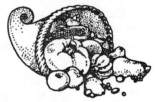

Breakfast:

1 protein	1 egg
2 starch	1 toast, 1/2 cup oatmeal
1 fat	1 tsp. margarine
1 milk	8 oz. sugar free or plain yogurt

Snack

1 starch	6 saltines
1 fruit	1 small apple
1 protein	1 Tb. peanut butter

Lunch

3 starch	2 whole wheat bread, 1 oz. pretzels
2 protein	1 oz. ham, 1 oz. swiss cheese
2 vegetable	1 sliced tomato, raw veggies, romaine lettuce
1 fat	lowfat dip
1 milk	1 cup 1% milk

Snack

2 starch	10 whole grain crackers
1 fruit	1 orange
1 protein	1 oz. turkey

Dinner

3 protein	3 oz. grilled tenderloin steak
2 vegetable	broccoli, carrots
2 starch/ 2 fat	1 small baked potato with margarine/sour cream, 1 whole wheat roll
1 milk	1 cup 1% milk
1 fruit	1/2 frozen banana

Snack

1 starch	1/2 wheat bagel
1 protein	1 oz. fat-free cream cheese
1 fruit	1 1/4 cup berries

After you start a diabetic diet:

♦ Don't be alarmed if you have a small weight loss after you start a diet to control your blood sugar. This is fairly common, especially if you are now eating fewer carbohydrate foods than you did previously. Just remember that it should be temporary-lasting no more than about 5 days. If it continues, talk to your doctor or dietitian.

♦ You may be asked to do self blood glucose monitoring to find out how much sugar is in your blood. On the other hand, some physicians will just test your blood sugar at random during your office visits.

♦ Blood sugar monitoring involves pricking your finger and letting a drop of blood fall on a "test strip." The test strip will be placed in a tiny machine that will "read" your blood glucose level and display it on a panel. Your blood sugar and ketone testing records are good tools to see if you are eating enough food. Go over these records with your health care team.

♦ If you find that your blood sugars are consistently low at certain times of the day, try to figure out why. Some possibilities:

-Not enough food at the previous meal or snack.

-Need to add a snack 2 hours or so before your sugar is low.

-Not the right kind of snack (look below for good snack ideas)

-You are more active or exercise close to this time, and so need more food.

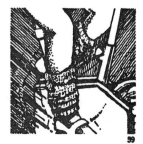

Exercise–A "Shot in the Arm" for Women with Diabetes

Imagine that there was something that would make you feel more energetic and relaxed. This "something" made your legs muscular instead of flabby, allowed you to eat more without gaining too much weight and reduced your long term risk of heart disease. "It" also you avoid taking insulin or reduce your dose. Would you go out and buy "it" by the bucket-full? "It" turns out to be exercise, and it is strongly recommended for women who have gestational diabetes.

It is generally recommended that you exercise 20-30 minutes daily, and at least 3 times per week; some health care providers suggest a daily walk. However, you should talk to your health care provider to see what specific guidelines she has for you. Regular exercise improves the efficiency of your own insulin. It can also help control blood sugar levels so that you don't need insulin.

A study done at the Sansum Medical Research Foundation in Santa Barbara found that regular exercise normalized fasting and post-prandial (after meal) glucose levels, which prevented the use of insulin. The women worked out on arm ergometers (stationery bicycles which use the arms to peddle) 3 times per week for 6 weeks (16).

There is no doubt that we would all "like" to exercise regularly, but it may be a problem to fit it into a busy schedule. The solution is learning to make it a priority and finding the time for it regularly. See Chapter 11, "Fitting Fitness In" to learn how to exercise without thinking about it. Also found in Chapter 11 are exercise guidelines for pregnancy, which are different than before pregnancy.

If you start exercise when your blood sugar level is normal, you could have low blood sugar when you finish. Here are some tips for avoiding low-blood sugar during exercise:

♦ Delay exercise until you have had a meal or snack if you know your blood sugar is low.

♦ Eat one serving of fruit before a 30 minute activity if your blood sugar is within normal range.

♦ Eat one serving of starch and one serving of fruit before an activity that lasts an hour or more if your blood sugar is within normal range.

♦ If your activity is more strenuous, you may need to increase the amount of food at your snack

♦ If your activity is longer than 2 hours, such as a hike, eat before you go and also bring snacks to eat along the way.

♦ Always carry hard candy or glucose tablets with you in case you have low blood sugar or an insulin reaction. Packaged peanut butter or cheese crackers are also good to keep in your purse. See page 110 for how to treat hypoglycemia.

Source: Adapted from Guidelines for Making Food Adjustments for Exercise for People, *Nutrition Guide for Professionals; Diabetic Education and Meal Planning*, MargaretPowers, Ed., The American Dietetic Association and American Diabetes Association, 1988, p. 41.)

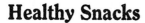

Healthy Snacks

A diabetic snack should contain some carbohydrate, fat and protein. However, it is O.K. to have just a carbohydrate snack alone, as long as it is not juice. Your own lifestyle, activity level, and weight gain will dictate the type of snacks you need. Again, your individual snack needs should be discussed with your dietitian, diabetes educator or physician.

"Balanced Snacks"

Each snacks equals one starch, one meat, and one fat exchange. To add a milk exchange, add 1 cup of milk or 1 cup plain or sugar-free yogurt.

1 oz. Swiss cheese and 6 rye crackers

1 Tb. peanut butter and 2 popcorn cakes

1 piece banana bread and 1 oz. light cream cheese

1 small bran muffin and 1/4 cup cottage cheese

1/2 ham sandwich with 1 tsp. mayonnaise

1/3 cup refried beans with 1 oz. cheese

1/2 cup Tofu Spread on 1 pc toast (page 334)

9 Wheat Thins and 1 oz. turkey

1 Tb. peanut butter and 1/2 small banana

1 oz. cheese and sliced apple

raw veggies, 1 oz. cheese dip and 6 crackers

Starchy Snacks

Each snack is equal to one serving of starch.

6 saltine Crackers

15 cheese nips

2 rice Cakes

1 slice quick bread (with reduced sugar)

1 "Granola bar" sweetened with fruit (the ones from Health Valley are recommended)

3 graham crackers

4 Triscuit crackers

1/3 cup black beans

"Free" Snacks

These foods have very few calories so they can be eaten as desired when you don't have any "exchanges" left from your meal plan. Do not eat these snacks alone before exercise since they will not affect your blood sugar.

Raw vegetables with 2 Tb. of fat-free dressing

Sugar-free jello (if your doctor allows artificial sweeteners)

Vegetable broth

Lettuce and raw greens

Cucumbers, Celery

Gestational Diabetes in a Nutshell; Keys to Control

1. Eat balanced meals at regular intervals. See a registered dietitian to make a personal meal plan for you (see example above).

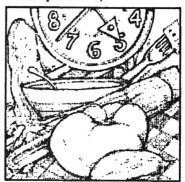

2. Keep your activity level up! Try

to do some activity daily. Talk to your doctor about recommending an exercise program; most approve of walking or swimming. (Note: DON'T exercise if your blood sugar is elevated or if ketones are present in your urine–contact your physician.) See Chapter 11, "Fitting Fitness In" for more information on exercise during pregnancy.

3. Divide the food you eat daily into 3 meals and 2-3 snacks. Especially important is the bedtime snack which should include some starch, protein and fat.

4. Keep a handle on weight gain by making wise food choices. Choose foods that are low in fat.

5. Avoid emotional eating such as eating when sad, angry or stressed out.

6. Avoid concentrated sweets like cookies, candy, pie, sugar, honey and chocolate. Also limit or avoid fruit juices, even unsweetened ones. They contain concentrated amounts of fruit sugar which can raise your blood sugar. Ask your diabetes educator about including juices with meals or snacks.

7. Expect to monitor your blood sugar; your diabetes educator will teach you how to do this. Your blood sugar level will show you how your diet is affecting the amount of glucose in your blood. It will be used to adjust your diet and exercise regimen.

At first your health care provider will ask you to test your blood sugar as much as four to five times a day for the first week. This could include testing in the middle of the night, when blood sugar sometimes drops. When your blood sugar is in good control, you will probably test less often.

8. Keep your diet high in fiber. Fiber helps stabilize blood sugar. So stay away from foods made with white flour as much as possible. Try to eat raw instead of cooked fruits and vegetables. Eat high fiber cereal with milk as a snack. See page 51 Focus on Fiber.

9. Smile! You have a unique opportunity to improve your own and your family's diet! Try to make the changes permanent.

About Artificial Sweeteners

Should you use artificial (non-nutritive) sweeteners while you are pregnant? The answer to that question varies. Many physicians allow their patients to have sweeteners in moderation. Some physicians ask their patients to avoid them totally. The Diabetes Center of New Mexico recommends Nutrasweet® or Sweet One™ instead of saccharin (17). Saccharin has been shown to cause cancer in lab animals, although human population studies have not agreed (18).

Because, saccharin crosses the placenta, the American Diabetes Association discourages use of saccharin during pregnancy (19). It's use has also been discouraged immediately prior to pregnancy (20). The American Academy of Pediatrics Committee on Nutrition concluded that the blood levels of phenylalanine resulting from aspartame ingestion would

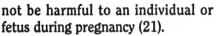

not be harmful to an individual or fetus during pregnancy (21).

The Center for Science in the Public Interest (CSPI, a consumer "watchdog" group) has Saccharin (Sugar Twin, SweeTen, Sweet'n Low), Aspartame (Nutrasweet®, Equal®) and Acesulfame K (Sweet One™, Sunette™) on their "top ten additives to subtract from your diet" list (22). One concern that CSPI has about aspartame is that the breakdown products (aspartic acid, phenylalanine and methanol) could be hazardous to the fetus, particularly if it had phenylketonuria (PKU), a rare genetic disorder in which the amino acid phenylalanine cannot be metabolized and builds up in the body in toxic amounts. Women who have PKU, should not consume any products containing aspartame.

On the other hand, Dr. Richard Black from the University of Toronto, who has done extensive research on sweeteners, says...

> "The amount of breakdown products from drinking diet soda made with Nutrasweet® is negligible compared to the amount of the same products metabolized from eating almost any food." "You'd get more methanol from eating an apple than from drinking a few cans of diet pop. However, like anything, there could be danger to the mother and fetus if she went overboard and drank 2 or 3 liters of diet soda a day, not necessarily from the sweetener, but because of other things found in soda (23)."

With more sweeteners awaiting FDA approval, there's no doubt that soon there will be even more choices of sugar-free sweeteners.

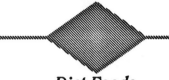

Diet Foods

It's not just sugar and calories that dietetic products may be lacking, some are also missing vitamins and minerals which are so important for you and your baby. One mineral that diet sodas do have is phosphorous, which can be a problem in large amounts. It is thought that a high proportion of phosphorous to calcium in the diet is what causes leg cramps during pregnancy.

If you choose to use artificially sweetened products, moderation is the key. What's moderation? Most professionals consider one to two servings a day moderate–a serving being one diet soda (caffeine free!), one serving diet gelatin, pudding or hot cocoa.

For more information on sweeteners, contact... International Food and Information Council: brochures about artificial sweeteners, additives and food safety; 1100 Connecticut Avenue N. W., Suite 430, Washington D.C., 20036, 202-296-6540

NutraSweet™ Consumer Affairs 1-800-321-7254

Questions You May Have

Will I have to take insulin?

If your blood sugar can't be controlled by diet and exercise alone, you will probably take insulin, which is in the form of a self-administered shot. You may take one, or several insulin shots daily. If you do take insulin, and even if you don't, you will probably be asked to monitor your blood sugar.

Blood glucose monitoring is a great way of seeing how you are doing with your diet. You may be following your meal plan closely, yet seeing high blood sugars. This is because some foods affect your blood glucose quite differently, even though they are similar in carbohydrate value and calories. Also, some women can tolerate carbohydrate better than others.

I've seen diabetic candy sweetened with mannitol. What is that?

Some "diabetic" products contain sugar alcohols. These have names ending with "ol" such as mannitol, sorbitol and xylitol. They are primarily used in candy and chewing gum. They have the same number of calories as table sugar or sucrose, but are broken down in the body differently. They are usually fine if eaten in moderation such as two pieces of hard candy; too much at one time can cause diarrhea.

What else can affect my blood glucose?

Many other factors can affect your blood glucose or blood sugar level:

♦ The combination of foods you eat at a meal (how much protein, fat, carbohydrate, fiber).

♦ How much fiber is in your diet. Fiber slows down digestion and release of glucose into the blood stream is slower.

♦ Your activity level. Exercise uses up extra glucose and causes insulin to work more efficiently, thus decreases how much you need.

♦ Your overall health. Infection and illness can increase blood sugar levels. See page 107 for "Sick Day Rules."

♦ Your stress level. Emotional stress can also increase your blood sugar level.

Will I still have diabetes after I have my baby?

Most women's blood sugar levels go back to normal shortly after delivery. Only a small number of women continue to have glucose intolerance.

However, over half of the women who have gestational diabetes will be diagnosed with Type II or Adult Onset Diabetes 10-15 years after their child is born. Women who have GDM with one pregnancy are very likely to have it with other pregnancies too. The American Diabetes Association recommends having your blood sugar tested 3 months after delivery and then once a year to make sure your blood sugars are normal (24).

Can you avoid it? It's very possible if you maintain your ideal body weight and exercise regularly. Eating a balanced diet is also beneficial.

What about my next pregnancy?

You have a very high chance of having GDM with subsequent pregnancies. Losing excess weight between pregnancies, exercising regularly and eating well can cut your risk.

What if I get sick and can't eat?

If you get ill and don't feel like eating or can't keep food down, you should first contact your health care provider. Women are usually instructed to continue to take insulin (if you are on insulin) because illness can raise blood sugar levels. It is also important to continue drinking fluids, so that you don't become dehydrated. See page 107 for "Sick Day Rules".

Will my baby be diabetic?

Not at birth. The only effect he may experience from your diabetes is low blood sugar which is easily taken care of with a dose of sugar water. However, diabetes tends to run in families. By raising your child with healthy eating and exercise habits, you could possibly prevent your child from having diabetes as an adult. What a nice gift!

The week before I had my blood sugar checked, I was eating a lot of candy and soda. Is that what caused my diabetes?

No. However, you may have craved sweets because of the diabetes. When your blood sugar is high, but you don't have enough insulin to use

the glucose, your body sends out the signal that you need energy.

Sugar does not cause diabetes. However, excess simple sugar and starches in the diet does cause the pancreas to secrete more insulin, and if your body cannot produce the amount of insulin needed, the result is high blood sugar.

High Blood Pressure/Pregnancy Induced Hypertension (PIH)

Sarah was surprised when she went to her doctor's office and found that her blood pressure was elevated. She felt fine! No one in her family had high blood pressure (or hypertension), and she had never had a problem with it herself. Sarah's condition, called Pregnancy Induced Hypertension or PIH, is diagnosed in 10-20% of women expecting their first child.

Sarah was asked to take time to rest. Because she was a salesperson at a local department store, "resting" was virtually impossible while at work. However, she did try to put her feet up for a few minutes when she could and rested a lot in the evenings.

After closely monitoring her blood pressure for several weeks, Sarah's doctor decided she should be on strict bed rest to prevent the blood pressure from getting worse. She took a temporary disability leave which allowed her to keep receiving some income. After 2 months on bed-

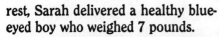

rest, Sarah delivered a healthy blue-eyed boy who weighed 7 pounds.

For Sarah, following the doctor's orders paid off! Keeping her doctor's appointments, and staying in bed kept her blood pressure from going up any more and improved her circulation. The improved circulation allowed adequate blood flow and nutrients to her baby so he could grow adequately.

Had Sarah not taken such good care of herself, the PIH might have escalated into more serious conditions called preeclampsia and eclampsia. PIH, preeclampsia and eclampsia are all forms of *hypertensive disorders of pregnancy*. They are all a progression of the same disease which includes high blood pressure. These disorders are also known as the toxemias of pregnancy, or simply toxemia. Though these are out-dated terms because of new knowledge, they still may be used by some health care personnel.

Following is a list of definitions that will help you to understand high blood pressure during pregnancy (25):

Pregnancy Induced Hypertension (PIH) or Transient Hypertension refers to high blood pressure caused by pregnancy. Women with PIH usually have no symptoms and their blood pressure generally goes back to normal after delivery. They are at risk for developing PIH again in subsequent pregnancies and also may develop chronic hypertension later in life.

Preeclampsia refers to several complications including high blood pressure, protein in the urine, and excessive fluid retention. Kidney and liver damage can occur if untreated.

Eclampsia is a potentially fatal condition in which the mother can go into convulsions or a coma.

Chronic Hypertension is high blood pressure which existed before pregnancy, or that is diagnosed before the 20th week of pregnancy.

Preeclampsia superimposed upon chronic hypertension may occur in women who have high blood pressure before pregnancy who also develop symptoms of preeclampsia.

What Happens to Blood Pressure During Pregnancy

Blood pressure usually drops during the first half of pregnancy and then rises to normal rates. Women with mild hypertension may also experience that drop and may have normal blood pressure by mid-pregnancy. It is not until the third trimester that blood pressure increases to the point where some type of treatment (like bedrest or medication) may be necessary. Once blood pressure increases, it may not drop back down to normal until after delivery.

Though the causes of PIH are not fully understood, poor nutritional status is one risk factor. It appears to occur at a higher rate when a woman has a combination of poor nutritional intake and no prenatal care.

Your overall food intake including adequate calories, protein, and certain minerals appears to be important in preventing high blood pressure. If you don't have enough energy or calories from carbohydrate or fat in your diet, your body will use dietary or tissue protein for energy. This can reduce protein needed for tissue growth and also can limit the protein used in fluid balance. Underweight women who fail to gain weight properly have a higher risk of developing PIH.

You are more likely to develop hypertension during pregnancy if you fall into one or more of these categories (26; 27):

♦ You are pregnant for the first time

♦ You are expecting multiple fetuses

♦ You are diabetic

♦ You have kidney disease

♦ You were overweight before your pregnancy

♦ Your mother had preeclampsia

The information below applies to both women with PIH and also to those with chronic hypertension.

Risk to Mom

The biggest danger of increased blood pressure during pregnancy is the development of preeclampsia. Restricted activity and bedrest are two treatments to ensure that your blood pressure is controlled and your baby has an adequate circulation of blood and nutrients.

Risks to baby

While you may have no symptoms of high blood pressure, it can reduce blood flow–and thus oxygen supply and nutrients to the baby. So your baby may not grow properly and may have IUGR or intra-uterine growth retardation. Your physician will probably monitor your baby's heart rate and his growth with ultrasound tests. Women with hypertension are also more likely to have a miscarriage or still birth. If your blood pressure cannot be controlled, your baby may be delivered prematurely.

What you can do...

If you have high blood pressure before pregnancy:

If you have chronic high blood pressure, see your physician before you become pregnant to establish good blood pressure control and to establish a "baseline" reading of your blood pressure. Losing weight and starting a regular exercise program before pregnancy can help reduce your blood pressure.

When you become pregnant, see your physician as soon as possible to start your prenatal care. Also, be sure to keep your appointments with your health care provider so that you and your baby can be monitored.

What you should do if you are diagnosed with high blood pressure during pregnancy:

♦ Get plenty of rest–at least 8 hours of sleep per night. Also, try to lie down a few hours during the day on your left side to increase blood flow to your baby. When sitting, elevate your legs to above your hips to improve circulation.

♦ Monitor your blood pressure. You may go to your doctor's office more often for a blood pressure check or you may check it at home. Keeping track of it will give you and your physician a better idea of your average blood pressure over time.

♦ Avoid prolonged vigorous exercise including lifting. This is especially important for women with other children at home. Instead of picking up your other children, squat (don't bend over with straight knees!) to their level. Your physician will have more specific exercise guidelines for you.

♦ Because your need for sodium increases during pregnancy it's not necessary to restrict sodium in your diet. However, women who are "salt sensitive" before pregnancy and follow a sodium restricted diet may want to continue to watch their sodium during pregnancy. Ask your physician about your specific sodium needs. Foods with excess sodium include pickles, regular canned soups, smoked and cured meats like bacon, sausage, and ham, and many frozen and ready to eat foods. Sodium information can be found on the nutrition label.

♦ Eat plenty of calcium-rich foods. Research has shown that calcium plays a role in reducing blood pressure and may also reduce the risk of preeclampsia and premature birth (28; 29). Though the evidence isn't conclusive enough to recommend supplementary calcium over the RDA, getting plenty of calcium through diet can only help! Try to have at least 4 servings of calcium rich foods every day. If you are intolerant or allergic to milk, a supplement from your physician may be warranted. If you don't like dairy products, see page 62 for tips on "sneaking" calcium into your diet.

♦ Eat balanced, healthy meals. (Follow The Eating Expectantly Diet!)

♦ Because you will want to restrict your activity or you may be put on bedrest, you'll need super speedy meals. See page 296 for "Meals in Minutes" and page 129 for eating tips for women on bedrest.

♦ Avoiding caffeine, alcohol and cigarettes is even more important for you since those substances can increase blood pressure.

♦ Keep your stress level low. Cut down on commitments and chores. If you're a Type A person, learn to slow down!

♦ Continue drinking plenty of fluids, even if you are retaining fluid.

What can you expect?

There is a possibility that if your blood pressure does increase, you may be asked to restrict your activity, be on bedrest or be hospitalized. Rest has been shown to reduce premature labor, lower blood pressure and help your body get rid of excess water (30).

Even if you aren't given special instructions for rest, you should set aside time every day to be off your feet. Making rest a priority on your own may prevent imposed restricted activity and medications from your doctor! If bedrest or hospitalization becomes necessary, see "Coping With Bedrest" on page 129.

Elevated blood pressure and preeclampsia may warrant an early delivery of your baby, preferably through induced vaginal delivery. However, in cases where a speedy delivery is necessary, a C-section may be done.

In some cases, even if you comply with bedrest or restricted activity orders, this still may not control your blood pressure adequately and you may be hospitalized, be put on medication or deliver prematurely. For women who have chronic high blood pressure before pregnancy, hospitalization is not uncommon.

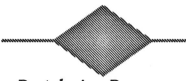

Rest during Pregnancy

Tell the typical woman to "rest" and she'll say "Oh, O.K.," and proceed to take a 15 minute "catnap", but will continue to go about her very busy lifestyle. What most people don't realize is how vital rest is for pregnant women with high blood pressure.

Kathy said her doctor told her to rest and she did lay down for a rest "every so often." She didn't realize what he meant exactly. Eventually, she was put on strict bedrest and when she went into labor, her blood pressure went very high and she had to have an emergency cesarean section. She wished that someone had explained what "rest" meant!

If you're told to rest, this is what you should do:

1. Rest 1-2 hours off your feet in the morning and afternoon every day (ask your doctor for specifics).

2. Arrange with your supervisor to have some type of rest period at work or arrange for a reduced work schedule.

3. Enlist the help of older children to help with household duties, or you may need some extra help with child care.

4. Avoid stressful situations that could increase your blood pressure further.

Questions you may have:

How will I know if I am developing preeclampsia?

These are specific signs and symptoms of preeclampsia:

1. **Swelling of hands, face, feet and legs.** Some water retention during the last months of pregnancy is normal. However, if the swelling moves to the upper part of your body, it may be a sign of preeclampsia.

2. **Sudden increased weight gain.** If weight gain is not explained by temporary increased food or fluid intake and it occurs over a short period of time, this may also be a symptom. If you gain several pounds over a few days or less than a week, check with your physician.

3. **Persistent, violent headache.** If you have a severe headache that just won't go away, contact your physician immediately. This may be a warning sign of a convulsion.

4. **Visual difficulties.** Blurred vision, or partial to complete blindness are signs of preeclampsia. Again, seek medical attention immediately.

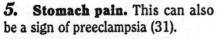

5. Stomach pain. This can also be a sign of preeclampsia (31).

Will I still have high blood pressure after delivery?

Probably not immediately after delivery, unless you have chronic hypertension. Women who have pregnancy induced hypertension are very likely to have high blood pressure later in life. It may be possible to reduce your risk of hypertension by going back to your ideal body weight after pregnancy, exercising regularly, and eating a nutritious diet containing adequate high calcium foods. (For more information on losing weight after delivery see page 164.)

Women with preeclampsia have about the same risk of developing hypertension later in life than those who never had the disease (32).

What about my next pregnancy?

If you have PIH, you have about an 80% chance of developing it again in later pregnancies. If you have preeclampsia along with chronic hypertension, your risk of having the same problem with other pregnancies can be as high as 70% (33).

Looking on the bright side, if you do have the same problem with your next pregnancy, you will be a pro at handling it! You will know how to take it easy and relax, how to monitor your blood pressure, and what will happen during your pregnancy.

For more information on coping with chronic disease during pregnancy, an excellent book is available called *Intensive Caring* by Diane Hales and Timothy Johnson M.D., Crown Books.

Expecting Twins or More

One way to have a ready made family is to have twins, triplets or more! And with suggested weight gain guidelines, you may indeed feel like you are feeding a houseful during your pregnancy.

Weight Gain

The Subcommittee on Nutritional Status and Weight Gain During Pregnancy has concluded that a weight gain of 35-45 pounds produces the most healthy twins (34). A study done in Washington state found a weight gain of about 44 pounds was associated with optimum outcome of pregnancies lasting at least 37 weeks and babies weighing over 5 1/2 pounds (35).   You and your health care provider will probably work out an individual goal for you.

What affects the weight of your twins?

◆ Your diet

◆ Length of gestation

◆ Sex of your babies (same sex vs mixed sex)

◆ Type of twins (identical vs fraternal)

Low birth weight is a concern for any multiple pregnancy. Though twin pregnancies accounted for only 2% of all birth in 1986, 16% of all low birth weight infants were twins (36). Low-birth weight is a problem because it increases the risk of sickness and death in babies. Single babies and twins grow at about the same rate until about the 32nd week, when growth in twin pregnancies appears to slow down. Also, multiple pregnancies are often shorter than the usual 40 weeks. Twin pregnancies average 37 weeks. A pregnancy that is just 3 weeks shorter doesn't seem like it would make much of a difference, but it does. Since babies often increase their weight by up to 1/3 pound per week in the last weeks of pregnancy, three weeks can make a big difference (37)!

There are several factors affecting the weight of your babies, one of them being diet. Besides adding the calories and nutrients that your babies need, diet can actually lower your risk of premature delivery and babies' low-birth rate.

At the Montreal Diet Dispensary, a special program called the Higgins Nutrition Intervention Program was used to try to decrease some of the risks apparent in disadvantaged mothers of twins. The program consists of individualized risk assessment, determination of dietary needs, nutrition education based on clients' eating patterns plus regular follow up. Women not able to afford the prescribed diet were given a supplement of milk and eggs.

The results of the program had previously been proven successful with mothers expecting one baby. The program clearly improved the status of the twins whose moms participated. The twin infants weighed almost 3 ounces more, their rate of low birth weight was 25% less and there were half as many very low birth weight babies, which are the sickest babies who require intensive care. The preterm delivery rate was 30% less.

Some of the specifics of this intervention program include eating 1000 extra calories and 50 extra grams of protein above non-pregnant needs after 20 weeks. Women who are underweight before pregnancy and those with special risk conditions such as poor outcome of prior pregnancy receive further instructions (38).

What can the Higgins program do for you?

One researcher has found that women who have multiple gestations ate about the same as those pregnant with just one fetus (39). That means you probably need to take a close look at what you're eating. Better yet, have your diet analyzed by computer (see form at back of book) and seek the services of a registered dietitian, who can give you individualized dietary advice. Increased calories and protein seem to be a significant factor in preventing low birth weight and prematurity in certain groups of women.

To achieve the 35-45 pound weight gain, you will need to gain about 1 1/2 pounds per week during the second and third trimesters. This may require an additional 500-600 calories per day more than your pre-pregnant weight. Based on the Higgins research, you could need up to 1000 extra calories per day.

How can I possibly eat more food?

You probably feel that you can't really eat much more. The answer is to eat concentrated foods.

First make sure your diet has all the essentials–especially protein, fruits and vegetables. (See "The Eating Expectantly Diet" on page 47.) Then add "extra" foods to boost your calorie intake. The foods most concentrated in calories are fat and sugar– the usual no-nos. However, to get all the calories you need with what seems like an ever shrinking stomach, you must give yourself permission to eat "extras." To insure you are receiving adequate protein, see "Protein Needs" on page 49 about protein.

The easiest extra to add is fat. Add extra margarine to your vegetables, more salad dressing to your salads, etc. It is best to add more vegetable fat than animal fat to your diet. Put avocado and olives in your salads and sandwiches. Another way to add more calories to your diet is through high sugar foods. By that I don't mean you should drink a soda and eat a candy bar every day! There is a category of foods that I call the "good extras". These include milk shakes, puddings, peanut butter cookies and other foods which are high calorie, but also provide nutritional basics to your diet. For snack ideas, see "High Energy Mom-- Snack Ideas" on page 240.

Vitamins and Minerals

Your vitamin and mineral requirements will increase relative to your calorie and protein intake. You may need slightly more of vitamin B6, thiamin, niacin and riboflavin, but the increased amount of food, a well selected diet, and a vitamin-mineral supplement prescribed by your health care provider should take care of that. For examples of foods high in the nutrients above, see page 27.

What about triplet and quadruplet pregnancies?

Since there are fewer triplet and quadruplet births, there is little research pertaining to them. There is also little consensus of advice regarding nutritional needs and weight gain. Triplet and quadruplet pregnancies are usually managed by a specialist, and you will be given very individualized advice according to your prepregnant weight, weight gained so far, and the size of your babies. Here are a few observations...

Triplets

You should expect a preterm delivery, with a baby that weighs less than a baby from twin or single pregnancy. One study showed that on average triplets weighed a little over 3 3/4 pounds. The average hospital stay for triplets was 29 days, and generally more triplets require intensive care than other babies.

The good news is there was no more risk of sickness among moms or serious complications among triplets than among twins. And the odds are on your side if you can follow most of the above information about nutrition for twins (40).

Quadruplets

If you can imagine four babies growing inside you, you probably suspect that your pregnancy will require extra special care! In one study of 70 moms pregnant with quadruplets, bed rest was instituted by about 17 weeks (see the next topic: Coping with Bed Rest!) Tocolytic agents, or drugs which stop the labor contractions, were used in 83% of the women beginning at 25 weeks. The mean age at delivery was 31.4 weeks or at about 7 months gestation. Because of the shortened length of pregnancy, and other factors, the mean weight of the babies was about 3 1/4 pounds.

The average weight gain was only 46 pounds, which is close to the amount of weight gain recommended for twin pregnancies. Complications found in nearly 1/3 of the women were bleeding in the first trimester, pregnancy induce hypertension, (see PIH above) and anemia (41). (See "Focus On Minerals; Calcium and Iron" on page 61.)

Coping With Bedrest

We all dream of just one day in bed, to sleep, watch TV or catch up on our reading. Wishes do come true, but unfortunately, when it rains, it sometimes pours.

Bedrest is prescribed for multiple reasons, including hypertension or preeclampsia, multiple gestation (twins or more,) premature labor, or poor growth of baby (also called intrauterine growth retardation or IUGR). Some women are put on bedrest for several months, which can give a person "cabin fever." The fol-

lowing is a guide to help you make the most of your stay...

Setting up the room:

You will probably want to set up a makeshift bedroom near where your family gathers. A family room off of the kitchen does nicely. Here are the things you'll want to furnish your new room with.

Basic living supplies:

◆ Bed with plenty of pillows (or rent a hospital bed).

◆ Phone that will reach to the bed (think of it as your link to the outside world) and don't forget the phone book.

◆ Ice chest or mini-fridge for bedside

◆ Microwave (not a necessity depending how strict your bedrest is)

◆ Large bedside table (several T.V, trays work well too).

◆ Any medicines you are taking including those you might take rarely for heartburn, constipation, etc.

◆ Large pitcher, filled with fresh water daily and an ice bucket.

◆ Soup cans for doing arm exercises, if your physician approves.

◆ An intercom system. Invest in one for the baby early...this will save your voice and save your family lots of trips back and forth fetching for you.

Bedrest Joke: The best and worst thing about bedrest: You aren't the cook and you aren't the cook! (From Side-lines newsletter, Winter '92.)

Eating

Yes, eating takes on a whole new challenge when your time is spent on a 6 x 4 mattress! Keep in mind that you will need fewer calories than usual since you'll be using very little energy for activity. Here is a guide to "Bedroom Cuisine"

1. Make lists and menus so your husband or friends can shop for you.

2. Keep snacks next to you:

-Fresh fruit, dried fruit like figs and prunes.

-A jar of peanut butter

-Rice cakes

-Raw veggie sticks in plastic container with ice

-Wheat and rye Crackers and graham crackers.

-Cheese food that doesn't need refrigeration.

-Nuts

(Beware that convenience foods needing no refrigeration are often high in fat and salt. Eat accordingly!)

-If you have a microwave next to you:

-Lowfat popcorn

-Decaf tea bags, decaf coffee, hot chocolate mix and mugs

-Cans of hearty single serving soups like split pea, chunky chicken vegetable, bean with ham

-Shelf Stable Meals and Stews (see page 221 for examples)

If you are allowed to get up briefly to make a meal, the following can be prepared in 6-7 minutes.

Frozen microwave dinners (see page 223 for healthy choices)

Refried vegetarian beans, corn tortilla toasted in oven, cheese, lettuce and tomato

Quick leftover meals:

From baked chicken

-Chicken salad with pineapple

-Chicken fajitas, burritos

-Chicken curry over bulgur

-Chicken taco

-Chicken muffin melt

-Chicken sandwich

Pasta

-Pasta with tomato sauce (bottled)

-Pasta salad with tuna

-Pasta Primavera

-Turkey tetrazzini

-Quick tuna casserole

Other ideas

-Chinese takeout or delivery

-Pizza delivery (also delivers sandwiches, pastas, etc.)

-Supermarket deli (ready made meals and snacks)

-Have friends or church take turns making meals for the family.

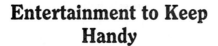

Entertainment to Keep Handy

You may have to be creative with this one!

♦ Have a radio or stereo nearby.

♦ Be within view of a TV and VCR, with remote control in hand (thank goodness for modern technology!) Be sure to have a TV Guide.

♦ Have a mini library set up with magazines, books, stationery, photo albums, etc.

♦ A diary to keep track of your days.

♦ A calender.

♦ A computer to play games on, keep track of finances, write letters on. A modem can really connect you to the rest of the world. The first laptop computer was probably invented by a women on maternity bedrest! You can also borrow your kid's Nintendo or Game Boy!

♦ Large notebook for making all kinds of lists! Things to do, Things for others to do, Things to buy, Things to make, Bills to Pay, What's on sale where, etc.

♦ Puzzles and crossword puzzles.

♦ Crafts like cross stitch, embroidery, knitting etc.

♦ Books on tape for when you get tired of reading.

10 Things to Do to Keep Your Mind Alive

1. Volunteer by phone. Have you always wanted to volunteer, but never had the time? Here's your chance. You could do fund-raising, or check on latchkey kids or elderly shut-ins. Or you could create your own network of other bed-bound moms. A good place to start would be the Red Cross, or check the local paper for volunteer opportunities.

2. Enhance your skills. Take a correspondence course, or a class on TV. Learn a new computer program (desktop publishing seems to be a winner.)

3. Increase your vocabulary. There are several good books on this like "30 Days to a More Powerful Vocabulary." Crossword puzzles and other word games can also help. Keep a dictionary nearby.

4. Learn a language. Parlez vous Français? There are many language courses available by mail. Your new language could be the start of a dream trip to say, Monte Carlo, or Madrid.

5. Shop without dropping! By computer and modem, you can hook into Prodigy, Compuserve, and many other multi-service databases. There are several home shopping networks on TV too. Just be sure to stick to a budget; it could be hazardous to your financial future! If you're worried about getting furniture and clothes for the baby, Sears, Penney's and other department stores still sell through a catalog and can deliver to your door.

6. Have a make-over. You may not feel like putting on makeup, but just for a change, you might have someone come over and give you a new hairstyle or make-up look.

7. Become a financial wizard. Plan your retirement. Send off for information on all those great sounding mutual funds, etc. Keep up with the stock market. Plan how you'll pay for your baby's college.

8. Make a quilt, afghan or rug. Kits can be ordered by mail.

9. Start your christmas shopping, even if it's March. Use TV shopping, catalogs, or start making them with crafts.

10. Master a new cuisine. No kidding! Recently I met a soldier who was in a National Cooking Contest. It turns out he developed his recipe while in Saudi Arabia during Operation Dessert Storm. I was wondering how he ever found access to a kitchen or time to cook. You see, he thought about cooking, wrote down all his ideas for ingredients, etc. When he got back home, he tried a few out and sent them into the contest.

Exercise/Activity

Your activity level is a very individual matter that should be discussed with your doctor. However, you should ask him about doing isometric exercises, and/or arm exercises using light weights or 12 oz. cans. This will help you keep some muscle tone, and avoid feeling sore from lack of movement. Remember that you can always practice your kegels!

Also ask about turning from side to side often during the day. This will help prevent soreness in muscles and skin.

Other Survival Tips

1. Make a "work" schedule of what you'll do during the day. This will make the day seem shorter and less monotonous.

2. Enlist other's help. If you have other children, make a poster of chores for them to do. It may be a good time for them to learn to do laundry, do dishes, even cook, depending on their ages. If you don't have children, you'll need to depend on spouse, significant other, family if they live closeby, or friends. Though it will be tough to ask, make a list of all the little things that need doing and delegate them to different people. Hire a maid service if necessary.

3. Remember it's OK to let the housework go (in this case it's a must!) You have only one priority; for your little one to grow as much as possible for as long as possible. Whether the floor is mopped or the carpet is vacuumed has relatively no importance.

4. Think positively. You might want to invest in a "positive thought for the day" type book. Though the time in bed might be rough, it would be much worse to have a premature or sick baby. Make the most of your time.

5. Find other women in the same boat. Ask your doctor, hospital, or Childbirth Education Association for names of other "at home" moms. Start a support group, or at least find a person that you can chat with. Call the numbers at the beginning of the chapter for more support.

Age and Pregnancy

There once was a time when most women started their families in their early 20's. Now many women are waiting until they are over 35 or into

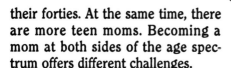

their forties. At the same time, there are more teen moms. Becoming a mom at both sides of the age spectrum offers different challenges.

Women who wait until they are well into 'thirty something' often find that waiting to start a family is the perfect time for them. They are financially more stable, have spent time developing a career and are ready to start on the "Mommy Track!" On the other hand, they may be more set in their ways, may be less physically ready for pregnancy and motherhood, and may be well into a successful career that offers it's own brand of stress. If you are in this group, you are part of a growing group of women, including many celebrities, who want to have it all, but not all at once.

Barbara never really thought about having children until she hit 35. Her biological clock started ticking and suddenly Barbara wanted to join the ranks of moms. She had heard that older mom had a few more risks compared to their younger counterparts, so she visited her physician first to chat about her new goal in life. The doctor assessed that she was in great physical shape. She worked out five times a week, didn't smoke, had no chronic diseases and had already cut out caffeine. She did, however, have the habit of skipping meals, and she often ate on the run.

Her doctor explained that she was on the right track in improving her lifestyle, but that she should work on her diet. He told her that slight nutrient deficits could affect

fertility. She saw a registered dietitian who, after looking at a 3 day food diary, made some suggestions to Barbara about how she could improve her diet. She also started taking a generic brand of multi-vitamins. The dietitian told her about some important studies which showed that a small amount of supplemental folacin (a water soluble vitamin) could decrease neural tube defects by close to 75%. Then they discussed dietary sources of folacin and other nutrients that Barbara was missing in her diet.

Barbara worked a few months on improving her diet, and became pregnant 8 months later. She delivered a healthy baby boy weighing 8 pounds! She was so thrilled with motherhood, that she became pregnant again when Brian was 18 months.

Stories like the above are common, though a few years ago, a pregnant women over 35 sent up a red flag in the minds of health care providers. A recent study done at Cornell University Medical Center revealed that women over 35 had no more important maternal complications than women 20-34 years old. Their babies also had lower rates of perinatal death (death during pregnancy or the first 28 days after delivery) (42).

An even larger study from Mount Sinai School of Medicine found that women between 30 and 34 and over 40 had slightly lower rates of small for gestational age babies and the frequency of fetal and infant death was slightly lower in women over 35. Women over 35 did have a slightly higher risk of having a low-birth weight infant. However, there was no evidence they had more premature deliveries (43). The consensus seems to be that older women can have excellent pregnancy outcomes with early prenatal care and surveillance and commitment to their pregnancy (44).

What can you expect?

Women over 35 can have a higher risk of certain complications of pregnancy such as gestational bleeding, abruptio placentae, and placenta previa. Other problems like gestational diabetes and pregnancy induced hypertension which occur more frequently with older moms, are due to the fact that these problems occur more often in all people as they age.

As women get older, they have higher risks of having a baby with Down's syndrome or other genetic defects. It may also take them longer to become pregnant. Cesarean sections are more common too, though a specific reason is not known. One speculation is that physicians are more vigilant and conservative in their treatment of older women who are pregnant for the first time. Prolonged second stage of labor appears to occur more often in women over 30 (45).

By waiting to start your family, you could end up with an instant family of four! The time frame that women conceive twins peaks from age thirty five to thirty nine. After 40, the odds of having twins go down (46).

Adolescent Pregnancy

Adolescent pregnancy, besides being psychologically stressful to teen and their parents alike, also is a physical stress since the mom-to-be is often still growing herself.

There has been some indication that in young mothers who are still growing, there is a certain amount of competition for nutrients between mother and baby. This is especially true in teens aged 12-15, whose infants are more likely to be born with lower birth weights.

One thing is for sure; whether mom is growing or not, teens are at nutritional risk due to skipping meals, eating away from home, and making poor food choices. In the 1990 Rand Youth Poll (47), 2/3 of those polled ate little or no breakfast. In another study 61% reported snacking on foods high in fat and sugar such as chips, ice cream, candy, and cake (48).

The typical teen diet tends to be low in calcium and iron. As more teens are overweight than in the past, more are turning to unsafe weight loss measures, which further puts them at risk for nutrient deficits.

Add the nutritional challenge of a pregnancy on top of the above factors, and you may have someone who needs a nutrition overhaul.

One study found that 59% of pregnant teens with limited incomes were anemic on their first prenatal visit. The average diet consisted of just 3 servings of milk, 3 servings of meat, 2 servings of fruits and vegetables, and only 5 servings of starch. Those teens weren't meeting their own nutritional needs, much less their baby's (49).

What can you do?

First make sure you are eating 3 meals a day, with a few snacks between. Then, look at what you are eating. Take the food test on page 67. Then compare it to the values below.

Your diet should have AT LEAST the number of servings below:

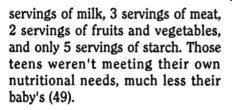

Teen Mom Diet

10 servings of starch/bread

One serving is 1 piece of any type of bread, 1 medium potato (or 1/2 cup), 1/3 cup rice, 1/2 cup pasta, 6 crackers, 1 oz. snack food, 10 french fries.

3 servings of fruits and 2 sevings of vegetables

One serving is 1 fresh fruit, 1/2 cup canned fruit, 1/2 cup fruit or vegetable juice, 1/2 cup cooked or raw vegetables

3 servings protein food

One serving is 3 oz. of beef, chicken, fish or cheese, 2 large eggs, 3/4 cup of cottage cheese, 1 cup dried beans or peas.

5 servings dairy product or high calcium equivalent

One serving is one cup of milk or yogurt, 1 oz. of cheese, 1 1/2 cups soft serve ice cream or frozen yogurt, 1 cup of pudding, 2 cups of soup made with milk. See page 61 for other sources of calcium.

5 servings of fat

One serving is 1 tsp. of margarine, oil or mayonnaise, 1 Tb. salad dressing, 20 peanuts, 1/8 of an avocado.

Ten Eating Tips for The Teen Mom-to-be

1. Eat 3 meals a day.

2. If you eat fast food, have a salad and milk with it. Or have juice to drink. See page 229 for healthy fast food menus.

3. You must gain weight to have a healthy baby.

4. If you have trouble gaining weight, snack on ice cream, milk shakes made with Instant Breakfast mix, and cheese.

5. Calcium in your diet is very important. If you can't tolerate milk, try to eat as much yogurt and cheese as possible. If you don't like milk, see page 62 on "how to sneak calcium into your diet."

6. Snack on fresh or dried fruits, vegetable sticks with dip or a sandwich instead of eating chips or candy.

7. If you don't have time for breakfast try these meals on the go: Tortilla with cheese rolled inside, peanut butter and honey sandwich with banana, granola bars and yogurt or cold pizza. Breakfast doesn't have to be boring! Or participate in a breakfast program at your school if it has one.

8. Easy snacks to take with you to school are cheese or peanut butter crackers, boxes of raisins, fresh fruit, granola bars, string cheese, pretzels, or a sandwich.

9. If it is hard for your family to buy food, you may qualify for the WIC Program (Women, Infants and Children Program), a supplemental food program and nutrition education program for pregnant and nursing women and their children. Contact your local or state health department, or your school nurse for more information.

10. If you are having a hard time coping with the fact that you are pregnant, this can affect your appetite. Find help though programs for pregnant teens, or ask your school nurse for help. Talking to someone will help you deal with the many challenges of teen parenthood.

What Can You Expect?

Teen moms can give birth to healthy normal babies. It depends on you. The amount of weight you gain can directly affect how much your baby weighs and if it is born prematurely. So, don't worry about gaining weight. I've seen teens go almost immediately back to their pre-pregnant weight.

How Much Weight Should You Gain?

The Subcommittee on Nutritional Status and Weight Gain During Pregnancy recommends that you gain 35 pounds if you are considered normal weight for your height. If you were underweight before pregnancy you should gain about 40 pounds. If you were overweight, you should aim for closer to 25 pounds (50). Though this may seem like a lot, remember, you only have one chance to make a healthy baby!

Almost as important as how much you gain is when you put on the weight. Teens who gained little weight in the first six months (less than 10 pounds by the 24th week) had a higher risk of having small babies, even if their weight gain caught up by the end of the pregnancy. Inadequate weight gain also seems to be a factor in preterm birth or birth of a baby that is less than 37 weeks old. Girls who gained less than a pound a week at the end of the pregnancy had more premature deliveries (51).

The problem with "premies" is that the babies usually aren't quite ready for our world yet. Their lungs may not be developed and they can have many other problems. Premies are often kept in the special care unit or intensive care for infants and won't be able to go home for a while. If this necessary, this could cost you and your family a lot of money, since the cost of intensive care can cost tens of thousands of dollars.

Other Nutrient Needs

Concern for calcium in the diet is shared by all women. A low intake of calcium, especially before 30, increases your risk of osteoporosis, or brittle bones. You've perhaps seen older women slumped over-this is probably due to osteoporosis. Or maybe you know a relative who broke their hip and fell. This is probably due to the brittle bone disease too.

How does that affect you now?

Your diet now actually affects how thick your bones will be when you hit age 40. The thicker and stronger your bones are, the lower your risk for osteoporosis.

The Zip of Zinc

Zinc is a nutrient important for cell growth, division and brain development. A study done on teens who didn't have enough zinc in their diets were given zinc supplements. The zinc apparently reduced the rate of prematurity, and caused the pregnancies to last longer than average teens. The babies of teens who were supplemented needed less help in breathing. What zinc may have done is helped the underweight women gain weight, which is vital in preventing premature babies.

What does this mean to you?

While you should never take any supplement that your doctor hasn't given you because some supplements can be poisonous to your baby, you can make sure your diet has plenty of zinc. See page 31 for good foods sources of zinc.

Look back to the Essential Guide to Vitamins and Minerals on page 27 to learn more about the nutrients most important to you and your baby.

9

Considering Breastfeeding

What You Will Find In This Chapter

- ◆ My Experience with Breastfeeding
- ◆ Why You Should Consider Breast-feeding
- ◆ Possible Barriers to Breastfeeding
- ◆ A Note To Dad
- ◆ Nutrition During Breastfeeding
- ◆ Nutrients of Special Concern
- ◆ Drugs and Breastfeeding

And answers to questions you may have:

- ◆ Who can answer my questions about breastfeeding?
- ◆ How will I know if I have enough milk for my baby?
- ◆ What if my husband isn't support-ive of my decision to nurse?
- ◆ Can I drink coffee while breast-feeding? What about alcohol?
- ◆ Should I try to lose weight while nursing?
- ◆ What if my baby is premature-can I still nurse her?
- ◆ What about PCBs in breast milk?

My Experience With Breastfeeding

When my son was born, there was no question which feeding method I would use. In fact, this decision had been made long before I even met my husband! As a health profes-sional who knew all the physical ben-

efits of breastfeeding and also as a registered dietitian who had recom-mended breastfeeding to thousands of women...I had to breastfeed.

The pressure was on! The most diffi-cult week of my life was that first week after Nicolas was born. I had a long labor and a difficult delivery. Nicolas and I didn't catch on to the fine art of breastfeeding right away.

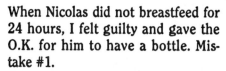

When Nicolas did not breastfeed for 24 hours, I felt guilty and gave the O.K. for him to have a bottle. Mistake #1.

He continued to receive several more bottles in the hospital. At home, our breastfeeding attempts got worse. Finally, in his tries at breastfeeding, he "latched on" and off more times than I could count (or bear) during a feeding. As a last resort, I called our pediatrician who referred me to a lactation specialist. She was our savior.

We had two problems, Nicolas and I. He had "nipple confusion" (sounds like the making of a good joke) and that explained his frequent latching on and off. He had gotten used to a plastic nipple, and so couldn't get the "hang" of mine. And I wasn't positioning him correctly. A week to two after seeing the lactation specialist, we started to learn how this special process worked.

If I hadn't known about the benefits of breastfeeding, and if I hadn't recommended it to so many women, and if there hadn't been that financial pressure (I had quit my job and formula was about $40 a month) I would have surely quit breastfeeding that first week. That's why I feel compassion for all the women who want to breastfeed, but may have a hard time with it at first.

Looking back, I'm so glad that I nursed Nicolas. The time we spent together was wonderful. And Nicolas was never sick while I was nursing him. One of my most memorable nursing sessions took place at a outdoor jazz concert that Frank, Nicolas and I went to when Nicolas was 3 months old. I felt very comfortable feeding him under the privacy of a blanket. Actually, I felt proud, because we were enjoying our own little routine. I didn't feel embarrassed to breastfeed in public like I did at first, and it was nice to feel so self-sufficient; no packing up the bottles, trying to keep them cold or looking for a place to warm a bottle up.

Why You Should Consider Breastfeeding

There is no doubt that breastfeeding is best for mom and baby.

Breastfeeding has been shown to greatly improve a newborn's short term and long term health. These are just a few of the benefits to baby:

♦ Protective against certain respiratory infections and gastrointestinal infections.

♦ Reduced occurrence of middle ear infections.

♦ May be protective against food allergies.

♦ May exert long term protective effects against 3 chronic diseases; Type I diabetes, cancer of the lymph glands, and Crohn's disease (1).

♦ Promotes good jaw and facial development.

Benefits to Mom

♦ A special closeness to your baby and time to get to know him or her.

♦ Uses more calories and helps to get rid of "Mommy Stores" of fat built up during pregnancy. By the way, Mother Nature designed us to gain a certain amount of fat during pregnancy to be used during breastfeeding.

♦ Helps your uterus return to it's normal size more quickly and can also prevent hemorrhage if breastfeeding is started right after delivery (2).

♦ Gives you a special time to rest, recuperate and relax, not to mention catch up on your reading! I remember reading journals from cover to cover during our feeding sessions; something I had never had time to do before.

♦ It's easy. You always have food for your baby with you and at it's always at the right temperature.

Benefits to the Family

♦ Saves money.

♦ May give the family a chance to have "quiet time" together. If you have other children, you can use some of your nursing sessions as a time to read stories to older children.

♦ Your family can do their part in helping with the continuation of breastfeeding-helping around the house, giving expressed milk via a bottle, bringing baby to mom while she is in bed...

Breastfeeding for the Nation

Because breastfeeding has so many health benefits, even the U.S. government recommends it. In Healthy People 2000; National Health Promotion and Disease Prevention Objectives for the Nation, one goal is that 75% of infants would be breastfed at hospital discharge and 50% would be breastfeeding at 6 months of age. As a nation, we're not quite there. In 1988, 54% of infants were breastfed at discharge after birth and 21% were breastfed at 6 months of age. However, individual areas are making more progress; In the Western U.S., over 71% of newborns are breastfed when leaving the hospital and 31% are being nursed at 6 months of age (3).

Possible Barriers to Breastfeeding

There seem to be some specific barriers to breastfeeding, and if you can plan accordingly, you can prevent problems and go around those barriers for a successful nursing experience.

Betty Crase of La Leche League International has nursed 3 out of 4 of her children. She feels the biggest barrier for women in deciding to breastfeed is society. "Society still has a prejudice against breastfeeding. The breast is still viewed as a sex object instead of for nourishing babies. This and lack of support can deter a woman from breastfeeding. Women must have a climate where they can feel comfortable in breastfeeding (4)."

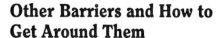

Other Barriers and How to Get Around Them

Family and friends who are not supportive of breastfeeding:

♦ Appeal to the benefit of breastfeeding that would most interest them. For example, spouse might be interested in saving money, or in the scientifically proven benefits. Be assertive in your beliefs.

♦ Find friends or relatives who have breastfed that can support you in bringing your family to your way of thinking! One reason it may be harder to learn to breastfeed is that many of us don't live near extended families who can offer extra support.

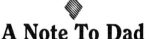

A Note To Dad

**...from Dr. Steven Nafziger,
University Family Medical Center
Pueblo, Colorado**

Until several years ago, I fancied myself as being as much of an expert on breastfeeding as anybody else, and thought that all the advice I gave women on breastfeeding was always adequate and well taken. When my wife made the decision to breastfeed our first child, I quickly learned that simplistic advice such as "just keep trying, it will all come together" fell quite a bit short of adequate. Every day, some very common sense but perplexing questions concerning breastfeeding would arise that made me realize my need to enhance my knowledge about breastfeeding, not only to become more helpful professionally, but as a father.

I'm sure that most fathers recognize at least some of the merits of breastfeeding. Breast milk is by far the best food for your baby. Breast fed babies have fewer allergies and fewer illnesses during the breastfeeding period. Breastfeeding is also economical and convenient.

When moms breastfeed instead of bottle feed, dads do get off the hook for feeding and mixing formula, but there are other helpful and thoughtful things they can do to help out. Breastfeeding requires a lot of a woman's time in which she cannot do other things, especially in the first few weeks. Helping with the housework, laundry, cooking, care of other children, answering doorbells and telephone calls, and bringing baby to mom for feeding, are only a few examples of what a father can do. Bathing or walking the baby, or spending time playing with him or her will not only free up time for mom but can also establish a time commitment to the child, which is the best gift any parent can give.

Of all the things a father can do to facilitate breastfeeding, support is probably the key factor. Many women will make the decision of whether or not to breastfeed on the basis of how their support system feels about it. A woman will be more likely to breastfeed if her partner has an enthusiastic, supportive, and positive attitude toward it rather than an indifferent or negative attitude. Assuring your partner that you are all in favor of her breastfeeding and willing to do whatever you can will help ease any reservations or fears that she may have toward breastfeeding. Breastfeeding for the first time is not only a new experience to the father but also to the mother and requires a commitment from both partners. A father who realizes this has taken the first and most crucial step toward a successful breastfeeding experience (5).

Hospital Staff that are not supportive of breastfeeding.

This appears to be a major problem for women who are still undecided about breastfeeding. If there is just a little bit of doubt and you happen upon a nurse who would rather you bottle feed, the battle may be lost!

First, if possible, find out which hospital is most supportive of breastfeeding. **The most supportive hospitals will have:**

♦ Policies which are conducive to breastfeeding such as rooming in for the baby.

♦ A lactation specialist on staff who can visit you right after delivery to get you started. A lactation specialist is usually a nurse who has extensive knowledge about breastfeeding--they know all the answers! Some hospitals also have a lactation specialist who can visit you in your home to see how things are going. If you receive your prenatal care at a public health department or through an HMO, there is often a nurse who

can visit you after delivery. Check on this while you are pregnant.

♦ Classes about breastfeeding for expectant moms and families. These highly informational classes may "sell" your spouse, significant other, or other family members on breastfeeding as well as give you lots of answers.

♦ Breast pumps for rent. These "industrial" pumps are very efficient and can usually empty both breasts in 15 minutes. This comes in very handy for women who work.

♦ A list of community breastfeeding support groups such as La Leche League, who you can call when you have questions. Their meetings are also open to pregnant women and you may learn quite a lot about nursing just by being around other nursing women.

Pediatrician (or staff) who is not supportive of breastfeeding:

Find a pediatrician (or family physician) who supports breastfeeding before you have your baby. This is probably the person you will call if you have any problems or doubts about breastfeeding. Do some investigative reporting and call the prospective pediatrician's office. Ask to speak to the nurse, since she will probably be the person you will talk to about breastfeeding. Ask her a common breastfeeding question, like: How do I know if I'm producing enough milk? or What do I do if my baby seems hungry all the time? You can ask the doctor about breastfeeding if you plan to interview him ahead of time. Another good way to find a doctor supportive of breastfeeding is to ask other nursing moms; word usually gets around quickly about who the most supportive doctors are.

Having Enough Milk:

Once a mother is breastfeeding her child, her biggest concern may be knowing if she is producing enough milk. You can make enough milk; it's a simple process of supply and demand. The more often you nurse your baby, the more milk your body makes. Here are some tips on what a mother can do to make sure her baby is getting enough breastmilk (6):

♦ Weigh your baby to assure adequate weight gain. Four to seven ounces weight gain per week or 1 pound per month is fine for the breastfed infant.

♦ Monitor wet diapers and bowel movements. These are physical signs that baby is drinking enough milk. There should be 6-8 wet diapers and 3-5 bowel movements per day in the early months.

♦ Make sure you have positioned your baby properly; tummy to tummy. Your baby should be comfortable and have a good grasp of the nipple so that he can empty the milk glands. When the breasts are emptied, more milk is made to fill the demand.

♦ Let baby set the pace for length of the feeding and how often you breastfeed.

♦ Make it a habit to drink a glass of water or other beverage every time you breastfeed.

Betty Crase and other promoters of breastfeeding think an earlier visit to the health care provider may be a real benefit to nursing moms. Betty says, "An earlier visit builds the mother's confidence, and can also be used for problem solving and answering questions (7)." In fact, the Colorado Breastfeeding Task Force is encouraging the American Academy of Pediatrics to make a 5-7 day postpartum visit standard procedure for breastfed babies (8).

Most authorities on breastfeeding agree that the first 2 weeks are crucial for long-term breastfeeding success. If you have trouble those first few weeks, seek help from your health care provider, a lactation specialist or a local La Leche League Leader...fast!

You can reach La Leche League International at 1-800-La Leche.

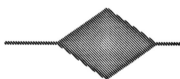

Words of Encouragement From an Experienced Mom

Helene, the mother of five children says: "The bond between mother and child while the child is attached and being nourished in the womb is not over when the umbilical cord is cut. The bond continues and grows as the mother breastfeeds and holds that new miracle of life in her arms. It is not just a nutritional need that is being met for the baby. It is a psychological, emotional and physical need for both as well. There is no sensation that compares with nursing your child. Nothing is as satisfying and fulfilling as nursing. I would tell every new mother that is considering breastfeeding to do it."

Checklist: What Moms Should Do Before They Deliver

_____ 1. Attend a breastfeeding information class, or attend a La Leche League Meeting. Look in the phone book to find a local chapter or call the toll free number above.

_____ 2. Find someone who has breastfed that you can call when you have questions or concerns. This person could be a La Leche League Leader or member.

_____ 3. Find a hospital and a pediatrician that is supportive of breastfeeding.

_____ 4. If returning to work, find out if your company and boss will be supportive of your decision to breastfeed. Do whatever you can now to prepare them.

_____ 5. Prepare yourself for breastfeeding. Though some nipple soreness during nursing is usually a result of incorrect positioning, some may be due to sensitive skin around the nipple. It can be as simple as going braless or topless around the house or not using soap on the nipples. Nipple and breast preparation techniques are no longer recommended because they can cause premature labor. Ask your health care provider for more details.

_____ 6. Have these things on hand: nursing pads (washable cloth pads and disposable cotton pads are avail-

able) and breast pump or access to one (this is useful if you have trouble with engorgement). I found that a battery operated pump worked much better than a hand pump. Some women prefer to rent an electric pump.

Source: modified from the *Colorado Breastfeeding Task Force*

Checklist: What Moms Should Do and Ask For in the Hospital

_____ 1. Tell the doctors and nurses you plan to breastfeed.

_____ 2. Ask to "room in" 24 hours a day with your baby. This enables you to "feed on demand" more easily. However, some moms would rather rest, knowing that their babies are well taken care of and have them brought in frequently to nurse. Ask that your baby receive no any bottles when he is not with you.

_____ 3. Tell them you want to breastfeed as soon as possible after delivery; on the delivery table or recovery room.

_____ 4. Tell them to keep anesthesia and other labor medications to a minimum so you and your baby will be alert during breastfeeding.

_____ 5. Tell them not to give your baby supplemental water, sugar water or formula unless medically necessary.

According to Dr. Nancy Krebs, a Denver Pediatrician,

"Full term babies don't have to drink very much in the first 24 hours or so because most are born relatively well hydrated. Urinating (colorless, dilute urine) and stooling should be watched as indicators of enough intake. Babies who are very small at birth or who may have had a stressful delivery are more vulnerable to dehydration or low blood sugar levels (9)."

Check with your pediatrician or lactation specialist for your own peace of mind if your baby doesn't breastfeed much at first.

_____ 6. Ask a lactation specialist or nurse to help you get started. Contrary to popular belief, breastfeeding doesn't necessarily come naturally. Most of us need to learn and some of us need help in learning.

_____ 7. Nurse your baby as often as the baby wants for as long as the baby wants. Nurse as often as every 1-3 hours. You may need to wake the baby.

Source: *Colorado Breastfeeding Task Force*

These Things Might Happen In The Hospital...

And Here's What You Can Do

1. The nurses or doctors may tell you that you need your rest. Tell them you will not sleep well without your baby and that you need all the nursing practice you can get before you go home and are on your own.

2. The baby may only nuzzle at the first feeding. This is O.K.! It is important for you to get to know each other.

3. The early milk is colostrum. It is thick and yellowish. Even though mature milk will not be in during the first few days, feeding your baby as much colostrum as possible will help protect your baby from illness including jaundice. It also gets you

and your baby started on breastfeeding and helps your baby get enough nutrition and water to begin to grow well, and may help your milk come in sooner.

4. Remember, breastfeeding can be uncomfortable at first, and all of us have different tolerances for comfort. However, it should not hurt. If it does, ask a nurse to help you get your baby properly positioned and latched on.

5. The hospital will probably give you formula or coupons for formula in the discharge packet. This is because formula companies provide it free of charge and does not mean your baby will need it. Your body can make all the milk your baby needs.

6. Before you leave the hospital, be sure to ask for a list of names and phone numbers of people in your area you can call if you have breastfeeding questions or problems.

Source: Modified from the *Colorado Breastfeeding Task Force*

Nutrition During Breastfeeding

The "Best for Baby" Breastfeeding Diet

While breastfeeding, you actually need to eat more than you ate during your pregnancy. And you should continue to "make every bite count!" Below is a meal plan that will allow you to meet your nutrition needs during nursing. Your diet should contain at least the following, which adds up to about 2400 calories.

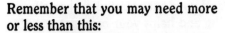

Remember that you may need more or less than this:

12   Servings of starches/grains

One serving is 1 slice of any type bread, 1 flour tortilla, 1/2 cup pasta, 1/3 cup rice or legumes, 6 crackers, 1/2 cup of potato.

4   Servings of fruit

One serving is 1 medium piece of fresh fruit, 1/2 banana, 1/2 cup canned fruit in it's own juice, 1 cup melon or berries, 2 plums or nectarines.

3   Servings of vegetables

One serving is 1/2 cup of any cooked non-starchy vegetable or 1 cup of lettuce.

(Be sure to include at least 1 fruit or vegetable that is a good source of vitamin A and two servings high in vitamin C.)

6   Ounces of protein or equivalent

(Increase your protein intake one ounce for each

serving of milk that you don't drink)

One serving is 1 ounce of lean meat, 1 ounce reduced fat cheese, 1/4 cup cottage cheese, 1/2 cup of tofu, 2 tablespoons peanut butter, 1/2 cup cooked dried beans, 1 egg.

4   Servings of dairy products

One serving is 1 cup of any type milk or yogurt, preferably skim or lowfat.

5   Servings of fat

One serving of fat is 1 teaspoon margarine or butter, or 2 teaspoons reduced fat margarine, 1 teaspoon mayonnaise, or 2 teaspoons reduced fat mayonnaise, 1 slice bacon, 1/2 oz. cream cheese, 1 tablespoon sour cream, 1/8 avocado, 10 peanuts, 5 olives.

And here is an example of a "real" meal plan:

Breakfast:

Corn Bran with berries
Whole wheat bagel with light cream cheese
Milk

Snack:

Vegetable juice
Crackers
Turkey

Lunch:

Grilled cheese sandwich
Raw vegetables with dip
Peach
Sugar cookies
Milk

Snack:

Fibar bar

Dinner:

Grilled chicken
Grilled vegetables
Spinach salad with tomato and mushrooms
Roll
Fresh orange
Milk

Snack:

Peanut butter and graham crackers
Yogurt with dried fruit

Calorie Needs

Your diet should be similar to that during pregnancy, except now you need about 200 more calories over your pregnancy needs (or 500 calories over the amount you ate before you were pregnant). A good way to get the extra calories is through an additional snack or higher calorie snacks. See Chapter 14 for snack ideas.

The suggested calorie intake for lactation takes into consideration the 100-150 calories a day which come from fat stored during pregnancy. For this reason, breastfeeding can help you lose weight; what a wonderful way to do it! The average weight loss for breastfeeding women is 1 to 2 pounds per month, after the first month postpartum. If you breastfeed longer than that, you will probably continue to lose weight, but at a slower rate (10).

Some research shows that the calorie needs for breastfeeding have been overestimated. Therefore, after breastfeeding has been well established, you should evaluate your energy needs based on weight gain during pregnancy, weight loss per week during breastfeeding and your activity level. You may need more or less than 200 calories above pregnant needs, but it's a good place to start (11; 12)!

If you breastfeed more than 6 months, if you didn't gain much during pregnancy, or if you drop below your usual weight, you may need up to 650 calories per day (or even more) over your non-pregnant calorie needs. Also, if you are very active, you will need more calories than the average woman. If you find that you are losing weight too quickly or are having trouble eating the recommended amount of food, you should visit with a registered dietitian for some individualized advice.

Protein needs

Your protein needs also increase during breastfeeding. You'll need 65 grams of protein a day (or 5 grams more than during pregnancy) during the first 6 months of breastfeeding. If you nurse more than 6 months, you will need about 62 grams of protein per day, as baby starts eating solids and drinks less milk (13).

If you can drink or eat the recommended 4 servings of dairy products, you can meet your protein needs by eating just 2 1/2 ounces of protein a day (including the amount of protein in 6 servings of grain products.) This is because each cup of milk contains the same amount of protein as 1 ounce of meat. The Best for Baby Breastfeeding Diet is boosted in protein to assure that you have more of the important nutrients like zinc, iron and vitamin B6, which are found in some protein foods.

If you prefer not to eat much meat, you will need to choose the rest of your diet wisely. See page 61 and page 77 for good food sources of iron and zinc.

Nutrient needs

Most of your nutrient needs stay the same during lactation; some decrease and some increase. You will need slightly more thiamin, riboflavin, vitamin B12, and magnesium. You will need significantly more vitamin C, vitamin E, niacin, zinc, and selenium. You need less folate and iron than during pregnancy. However, many physicians will recommend that you continue to take an iron supplement to help replace iron deficits from pregnancy or blood loss during delivery. For more specifics on vitamins and minerals, see page 51.

Make sure to continue getting plenty of fiber in your diet (See Focus on Fiber on page 51). When I experienced some constipation during the first few weeks of breastfeeding, my doctor explained that the hormones associated with breastfeeding can slow down the digestive process.

Don't forget fluids! Though in the past it was thought that much extra fluid was needed to produce breastmilk, it now appears that drinking to your thirst will provide you with adequate fluid. The exception is the woman who lives in a dry climate or exercises in hot weather; then thirst may lag behind actual fluid needs.

If you were to eat very poorly while breastfeeding, your body would draw from stored pools of nutrients. If you breastfed for 6 months and depended entirely on stored nutrients to feed your baby, you would deplete 19% of protein stores, 4% of calcium stored, 14% of iron stores, 46% of vitamin A stores, and close to 100% of folate stores. Protein is not a problem since most of us get more than enough. But, if your diet is not adequate for calcium, iron, vitamin A and especially folate, your own nutritional status could be in danger. Since pregnancy and breastfeeding are such physically demanding jobs, it's best that your own diet be as good as it can be, so that you will have all the vitality and energy you possibly can (14)!

Nutrients of Special Concern

When looking at average vitamin and mineral intakes of women in the U.S., and comparing them to the needs of breastfeeding women, we find several nutrients that are below the RDAs or Recommended Daily Allowances. When a woman eats 2700 calories per day, only zinc and calcium are likely to be consumed in amounts below the RDA. However, if the diet is less than 2700 calories (and the average nursing woman's probably is), intakes of calcium, magnesium, zinc, vitamin B6, and folate will likely fall well below the RDA.

Improved food choices are better than taking a nutrient supplement for several reasons. Most nutrients are absorbed better from foods than from supplements and there may be unidentified nutrients found in foods not included in supplements. Also, taking a supplement can give you a false sense of security; you may be tempted to make poorer food choices, thinking that your vitamin will make up the difference.

On the other hand, if you do choose to take a supplement, take one that has a broad spectrum of vitamins and minerals that contain no more than 100% of the RDA. Some doctors recommend that you continue taking prenatal vitamins. This is fine except that their high iron content may worsen constipation. Remember that after pregnancy, iron needs generally go down–unless you lost a lot

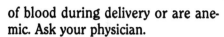

of blood during delivery or are anemic. Ask your physician.

Best Sources of Food for At-Risk Nutrients:

Calcium:

Milk, cheese, yogurt, canned or small fish with edible bones, (salmon, mackerel, sardines), tofu processed with calcium, bok choy, broccoli, kale, collard, mustard and turnip greens, molasses.

Zinc:

Oysters, pork and beef liver, seafood, lean red meats, poultry, eggs, wheat germ, nuts, dried beans and peas, yogurt, whole grains.

Magnesium:

Bran cereal, wheat germ, swiss chard, spinach, nuts, seeds, beans and peas, whole grains, dried fruit, shrimp, scallops.

Vitamin B-6:

Mustard greens, bananas, poultry, meat, fish, potatoes, sweet potatoes, spinach, prunes, watermelon, some legumes, soybeans, lentils, chick peas, pinto beans, fortified cereals and nuts.

Folate:

Spinach, leafy green vegetables, asparagus, liver, black-eyed peas, lentils, kidney beans, fortified cereals, legumes, broccoli, brussel sprouts, orange and grapefruit juice.

Calcium Needs

During pregnancy, women are often reminded about their need for calcium. After delivery, calcium in the diet may not seem that important; it is. The lack of calcium in the diet of a breastfeeding woman promotes loss of calcium from the bone. Osteoporosis is a real threat to American women because of dietary habits and possibly from inadequate amounts of calcium during pregnancy and breastfeeding. The RDA for calcium during breastfeeding is 1200 mg.; the same as during pregnancy (15). See page 61 for calcium contents of your favorite foods. If you cannot obtain the recommended amount of calcium, consult your health care provider about a calcium supplement.

Drugs and Breastfeeding

If you must take a medication during breastfeeding, you don't necessarily have to stop nursing. It depends on the drug and the dosage. For example if you are taking an antibiotic for a breast infection, you are actually encouraged to breastfeed. However, some drugs pose a risk for your baby including antiprotozoal compounds, antineoplastic drugs, some anti-thyroid drugs, and synthetic anticoagulants. Make sure your physician knows you are breastfeeding before he prescribes a medication.

If you must take one of the above drugs, pump your milk temporarily to keep your milk supply up. Discard the pumped milk and resume breastfeeding several days after you stop the medication. Ask your health care provider or pharmacist when the medication will be out of your system so you can start breastfeeding again. If you take a lactation suppression drug to stop breastfeeding, don't give your baby any of your milk while your milk supply is dwindling.

Some over-the-counter drugs should not be taken while you are breastfeeding. For example, acetaminophen (such as Tylenol®) is usually recommended instead of aspirin for pain. Consult your health care provider about which over-the-counter medications she recommends...before the need arises.

Questions You May Have...

I've heard that if I eat gassy foods like broccoli, onions and even milk and chocolate, my baby can get gas. Do I have to stop eating all my favorite foods?

No. Although strongly flavored vegetables and spices may give your milk a different flavor or may cause gas, it is not necessary for everyone to automatically stop eating such foods. After talking to many women, I've learned it seems to be a very individual matter. One friend of mine continued eating plenty of garlic while nursing and her baby had no problem with it. Another friend loved to eat hot peppers and baby apparently liked them too.

Keep in mind that a lot of "gas" can simply be chalked up to an immature digestive system—giving mothers yet another thing to worry about that we might be doing wrong!

If your baby has gas, you might try changing your diet for a several days and see if it makes a difference. The sensitivity to flavor and gas causing properties seems to vary from baby to baby. If there is no problem with gas, I wouldn't worry about any of the above foods in moderate amounts.

We have a lot of food allergies in my family. Can breastfeeding help to prevent them in my baby?

It's possible but not proven conclusively. Some studies suggest that components of food eaten by the mother can pass into the breastmilk and cause allergic reactions in the baby. There has been some success in controlling food and other allergies by eliminating common allergy causing foods from the mother's diet during nursing and even during pregnancy. However, it has not been studied enough to recommend this regimen for everyone.

However, the occurrence of atopic dermatitis, a type of eczema that is sometimes a reaction to a specific food, can be decreased through breastfeeding. As reported in Annals of Allergy, "Among infants at high risk of developing atopic disease because of positive family history, exclusive breastfeeding is associated with a lower incidence and thus a delay in the occurrence of allergic disorders (16)."

Probably the best advice for women who have allergies or family history of allergies is to breastfeed as long as possible and to eat a large variety of foods so that no one food compo-

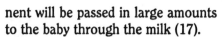

nent will be passed in large amounts to the baby through the milk (17).

Can I start drinking my coffee again?

Your baby will receive about 1% of the caffeine kick that you get in your coffee or other caffeinated beverage. The equivalent of one or two cups of coffee per day is not likely to have a negative effect on baby (18). However, caffeine can accumulate and cause your baby to be irritable and have trouble falling asleep. So again, go easy on the coffee!

I have gone into premature labor. Though I am now on bedrest and medication to stop the labor, I am concerned that I won't be able to breastfeed if my baby comes prematurely. Any advice?

First you should know that the benefits of breastfeeding a premature infant can be even more substantial than nursing a full-term infant. It has been reported that feeding the infection-prone premature infant with colostrum (or first milk) may have even more significant anti-infective factors than in full term infants (19). Another study reports that pre-term infants who were fed breastmilk by a tube in the early weeks of life had significantly higher IQ at 7 1/2 to 8 years of age than did those who received no human milk. The difference was still significant after adjustment for mother's education and social class (20).

If your baby comes very early, he may have to stay in a special area of the nursery where he can be monitored and his environment can be kept at a precise temperature. You may have to express milk so that it can be fed to your baby through a special bottle or tube. In this case you will need to pump your breasts.

It's great that you are thinking ahead; you can arrange to rent a good quality breast pump (Medela is one brand of electric pump) or find out if there is one you can use at the hospital while your baby is there. Taking pictures of your baby and keeping them near you while pumping may help you to be more successful. Not being able to breastfeed your baby may be disappointing, but think of the benefits you are still able to provide for him or her.

My mother says I should drink a beer before I breastfeed to help my milk supply. Will it? And is it safe for my baby?

This old wive's has not been scientifically proven. On the other hand, alcohol is released in the milk, and excessive drinking has caused problems with let-down, high alcohol level in breastmilk and lethargic babies. There has been one report of lowered psychomotor development scores with increased alcohol exposure (21). Since brain development continues to occur during the first year of life, it makes sense to avoid alcohol or drink in limited amounts.

A recent study showed that the smell of alcohol could be detected immediately in the breast milk of moms who had drunk the equivalent of the amount of alcohol in one can of beer. The smell was strongest at 30-60 minutes after the mom imbibed. The babies drank less milk during the feeding, possibly due to the change in taste and smell of the milk. Another theory is that alcohol could decrease the mom's milk supply (22).

If you'd really like to go "out on the town" and have more than one or two drinks, just pump your breastmilk afterwards and discard it. You can give your baby some previously pumped milk. Or if you'd just like an occasional drink, use common sense. Don't drink on an empty stomach as this will speed the flow of alcohol into your bloodstream and to your breastmilk. Ask your health care provider for more information.

I still smoke. Can this somehow affect my milk?

Nicotine and cotinine (another component of cigarette smoke) have been found in breast milk. No symptoms of exposure to the chemicals have been seen in infants though nicotine can affect how much milk you are able to produce. Some researchers advise that if you do smoke (it would be best to quit!), you should not smoke for 2 1/2 hours before nursing and avoid smoking while near your baby (23).

For information on kicking the habit of smoking call 1-800-4CANCER.

Can the HIV virus be transmitted through breast milk?

There have been reported cases of breastmilk infected with the HIV virus (the virus that leads to AIDS). It is doubtful that breastfeeding is a common route for passing on the HIV-1 virus, but in 1985 the Center for Disease Control advised mothers who test positive for HIV-1 not to breastfeed (24). On the other hand, Dr. Frank Oski, professor of pediatrics at John Hopkins School of Medicine reports that there is a substance in breastmilk that can block attachment of the AIDS virus, which may protect a breastfed infant from HIV infection (25).

If I breastfeed, will my baby have a smaller risk of being overweight when he gets older?

Early studies indicated that breastfed babies were much leaner than formula fed babies; later studies show a weaker link. This may be due to different compositions of formula–they are now closer to breastmilk in nutrient and calorie content. Currently, the specific role of breastfeeding in obesity remains unclear (26).

Should I try to lose weight while breastfeeding?

You will probably lose weight without even trying. The priority is to eat all the nutrients you need to supply good quality breast milk for your baby. A diet containing less than 1800 calories usually provides inadequate amounts of some nutrients (27).

However, some research shows that the current energy needs for nursing women are over-estimated. Since individuals burn calories at different rates, it is best to watch your weight loss. If you are overweight, you can lose up to a pound a week while breastfeeding without affecting your milk 28). Any more than that may be a sign that your milk may not contain enough energy. Of course, monitoring the growth and general health of your baby is also a good check point for the quality of your milk.

I want to have another baby right away. Should I still breastfeed if I get pregnant?

It is common in undeveloped countries for mothers to continue breastfeeding well into the second trimester of another pregnancy. However, it can take it's toll on you. Pregnancy and lactation are nutritionally and physically demanding. One study showed that moms who breastfed while pregnant had babies that weighed slightly less.

Much depends on your nutritional status. Not only must you meet the nutritional demands of your growing fetus, but also the nutrition and calorie requirements of your growing baby. This could add up to as much as 900 calories extra a day, depending on the age of your baby! To be sure, you need more calories, protein, vitamins and minerals.

Though it is possible to breastfeed while pregnant, it is best to wait at least a few months after weaning before you conceive again (29).

Does my diet really affect my breast milk?

Yes. In one study, the fat content of the woman's diet directly affected that of the milk. In another study, a very high carbohydrate diet also increased the fat content of the milk. Women on a higher protein diet tended to have higher calorie milk than those on a lower protein diet. In addition, your dietary intake of many vitamins and minerals directly affects their presence in your breast-milk. Every dietary component can

affect breast milk so it's best to continue sticking to a basic, balanced diet that contains a variety of foods (30).

I've heard that women who breastfeed several children for longer than 10 months have a greater risk of developing osteoporosis later in life. Is that true?

Though earlier studies suggested that may be true, it was later hypothesized that women regain bone mineral content after they stop breastfeeding (31). Another study of women who had breastfed from 1-4 children for a long period of time were studied. Their bone mineral mass of the wrist, spine or hip was not significantly different from women who didn't breastfeed. It's important to note here that all of those women consumed the RDA for calcium before and during pregnancy, and while breastfeeding.

Other researchers found that the bone mass of the wrists of women who breastfed was actually higher than those who didn't. A similar study looking at bone mass in the spine found that breastfeeding actually increased bone mass 1.5% for every child that was breastfed (32; 33).

Another study showed that by increasing the calcium content of nursing adolescents' diet to 1600 mg., they prevented a 10% calcium loss from the wrist, as compared with teens consuming only 900 mg. of calcium (34).

Of course there are many other factors involved in osteoporosis. The factors that you can control are calcium intake, regular weight bearing exercising (like walking, aerobics, etc.), moderate intake of protein and regular exposure to sunshine.

I've heard stories about PCB's being found in breast milk. When should you be concerned enough to limit or avoid breast-feeding?

Chemicals such as PCBs and DDT have been found in breast milk of mothers who have consumed minute amounts of these substances over a lifetime. The levels of PCB and DDT in the milk vary with the number of children she has breastfed, the length of time she breastfeeds, where she lives and her occupation.

In addition, alcohol drinkers, smokers and women who eat recreationally caught fish have significantly higher DDE (another pesticide) levels in their breastmilk. Also, as women get older, the levels of both PCB and DDE passed in the milk increases because these chemicals are consumed and stored in a person's body fat over a lifetime.

In the rare event that you have had a direct exposure to a hazardous chemical some time in your life, it would be wise to share this information with your health care provider during your pregnancy so that you can discuss the implications. In one study only about 25% of the women who had direct exposure to hazardous chemicals had higher levels of the chemicals in their milk compared to women who had only a "normal" exposure (35).

Betty Crase, Director of Scientific Information at La Leche League International says,

"Unfortunately, we live in a contaminated world. However, the known and documented benefits of breastfeeding still outweigh the risks of contaminants that may be found in breastmilk. What many don't realize is that artificial infant formula can also contain environmental contaminants, especially if the water used to prepare it contains lead or other chemicals (36)."

During a U.S. Senate Subcommittee on Health and Scientific Research hearing on environmental toxins and breastfeeding in 1977, Dr. Mark Thoman, editor of Veterinary and Human Toxicology said

"On the basis of research to date, no risks to the human infant from contaminants in human milk have been demonstrated and no official group that has studied this matter has recommended the blanket discontinuance of breastfeeding (37)."

The common sense approach is to limit current and future exposure to chemicals in the environment:

♦ Avoid recreationally caught fish not caught by you–fish that is caught by friends or that is sold at a roadside stand. These fish are more likely to come from contaminated water or from water with specific consumption recommendations for breastfeeding women posted by the state health department. A friend that happens to give you the leftovers from their fishing trip may not know you are breastfeeding or didn't pay any attention to the sign at the reservoir that says "pregnant and breastfeeding women should avoid fish A," etc.) If you or your family catch fish yourself, be sure to read any posted signs regarding recommended consumption levels, or call your local health department. For more information on food safety see page 195. Here are a few more tips:

♦ Eat a great variety of foods including fish. The omega-3 fatty acids found in fish are important to your baby's brain development, which still occurs during the first year of life.

♦ Avoid quick weight loss while breastfeeding. Undesirable toxins in the environment are stored in body fat. If you go on an extreme weight loss diet, some of these accumulated chemicals can enter the milk in larger amounts as your body fat is released from storage (38).

♦ Avoid use of pesticides, herbicides and insecticides in your home–even those that claim to be nontoxic.

♦ Avoid eating the skin and fat of poultry, meats and fish.

I just had a case of food poisoning. Can the bacteria that caused my illness be passed to my baby in breast milk?

According to Dr. Steven Nafziger of the University Family Medical Center in Pueblo, Colorado, "The bacteria that cause most common types of food poisoning does not pass through the breast milk. However, some rarer forms of food poisoning involve bacteria which make toxins. These toxins can get through to the baby through the breast milk. I encourage a breastfeeding mom who has flu-like symptoms to come into the office so I can evaluate her condition and make a specific recommendation (39)."

I am a total vegetarian. Is there anything that my milk will be missing?

People who eat no animal protein or dairy products sometimes need another source of vitamin B-12, since it is naturally found only in animal products. You need to consume foods fortified with vitamin B12 or take a daily supplement of 2.6 micrograms (40). See page 85 for more information about vitamin B12.

The calcium requirement for vegetarians is thought be less because their diets are lower in protein than the typical meat-eaters.

If you consume no dairy products, you may need to carefully plan your diet to include high calcium foods, or take a calcium supplement. Zinc and iron are other nutrients that you may have to "work" at getting enough of. See page 76 for vegetarian sources of zinc; page 61 for calcium and iron. If you have concerns about your diet, discuss this further with you or your baby's health care provider or seek a registered dietitian to help you analyze your diet.

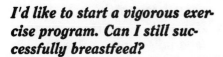

I'd like to start a vigorous exercise program. Can I still successfully breastfeed?

Yes. In one study, women who exercised about 1 1/2 hours per day were found to produce the same amount of milk containing about the same number of calories as sedentary breastfeeding moms. Though these women burned many calories exercising, they also consumed more. These women were very devoted to their exercise; one had previously completed an Iron Man Triathalon and another was a gold medalist in swimming! They were probably equally motivated to eat all the right foods (41).

Can breastfeeding lower my breast cancer risk?

Possibly. Several studies indicate that breastfeeding has a protective effect against breast cancer. However, there are also a few studies that provide conflicting evidence. Since breastfeeding has so many benefits, it would be a pleasant added benefit if it did cut your risk of this dreaded disease (42).

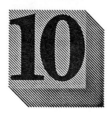

Now That You can See Your Feet Again or...

The First Weeks with Baby

---◆---

What You Will Find In This Chapter:

And Answers to Questions You May Have:

- ♦ When will I be able to eat if I have anesthesia during delivery?
- ♦ How can I possibly eat balanced meals if I'm too tired to cook?
- ♦ What is the difference between breast and bottle feeding?
- ♦ What's a good weight loss diet?
- ♦ How can I tell a good weight loss program from a bad one?
- ♦ How long should I wait before I get pregnant again?

What To Expect After Delivery

The first few days of post-partum life will likely be spent oohing and ahhing over your new arrival as well as recovering from a very tiring event.

You'll need to eat especially well those first few days at the hospital so that you have all the strength possible when you go home.

You may be too tired after delivery to eat a meal–that's normal for some women. You may just feel like drink-

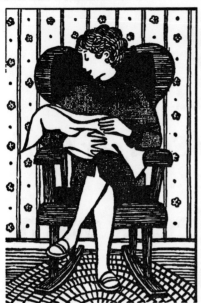

ing some juice or a decaffeinated soda for quick energy. Mary never drank sugared sodas, but after 18 hours in labor, she drank down 18 ounces of 7-Up in just five minutes!

However, some women are so hungry after delivery, that they call out for a pizza!

High Carbohydrate snacks probably available at the hospital include: toasted english muffin, bagel, toast, bran muffins, raisin toast, canned or fresh fruit, graham crackers, milk, yogurt, milkshake, sherbet, angel food cake with fruit, fruit juices and sodas.

When you do feel like eating, these tips will help you get back on your feet:

♦ If you select from a menu in the hospital, pick as many high fiber foods as possible to get your digestive track moving normally. Labor as well as anesthesia slow down your digestion immensely.

Some women have hemorrhoids from pregnancy or from the "pushing" stage of labor. Eating high fiber foods will make your bowel movements softer and easier.

Some high fiber foods you are likely to see on your menu: Raisin Bran cereal, All Bran, 40% Bran Flakes, wheat bread, wheat rolls, fresh apple, orange, banana, strawberries, prunes, raw vegetables, salad, baked potato, legumes, peas, corn, sliced tomato. Also, make sure to drink plenty of liquids when eating high fiber foods.

♦ Those first few days, eat as much as you feel like eating, and especially drink plenty. If you had a long labor, you probably didn't drink much and need to rehydrate. If you are planning to breastfeed, you'll need to continue drinking 8-10 cups of fluids per day-or drink to thirst!

♦ Concentrate on getting your strength back and taking care of the baby those first few weeks. Hopefully, you cooked some meals ahead of time and froze them. Now's the time to start using them! If not, let Dad, or other family members cook. Or, send them out for fast or convenience foods. See Chapter 13 for healthy fast and convenience food menus.

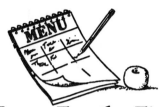

Menus For the First Week With Baby

Those first few days will most likely be too hectic to plan menus. Here are a week's worth of quick meals– some from take-out, and some made quickly at home.

Day 1

Chinese take out night!
Chicken and Snow Peas, Moo Shoo Shrimp or Cashew Chicken, Steamed rice, fresh fruit, milk

Day 2

Canadian Bacon Pizza on whole wheat crust, tossed salad, raspberry sorbet

Day 3

Tuna casserole, Kid's Carrots (page 318), wheat rolls, frozen yogurt

Day 4

Minute Steaks, mixed vegetables, Easy Microwave Potatoes (page 314), canteloupe or canned peaches

Day 5

Crustless Quiche (page x), sourdough rolls, sliced tomatoes with basil, Tropical Pudding (page 312)

Day 6

Bean Tostadas, mexican rice, avocado and tomato salad, frozen bananas

Day 7

Spinach Tortellini with Quick Alfredo Sauce (page 248), garlic bread, mixed green salad, fig bars

The Feeding Decision – Breast or Bottle?

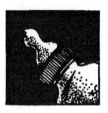

You may have been thinking about this since the day your pregnancy was confirmed. Or because of personal observations, you may have had your mind made up long ago about how you'll feed your baby. Chances are, people will try to persuade you one way or another and you may find yourself searching for an objective opinion.

Breastfeeding is a very personal decision. Whatever method you decide to use, make it a decision YOU feel good about. Don't make your decision based on guilt, others' opinions or anything else.

For a complete discussion of breastfeeding, see Chapter 9 Considering Breastfeeding.

Infant Formula

Today, infant formula enjoys a very high standard of quality. It's nutrient composition is patterned after breastmilk. Here are a few basic facts about infant formula:

◆ Formula is basically the same, can after can. However, breast milk varies over the feeding and between feedings and also varies depending on the diet of mom.

◆ Formula feeding can easily be taken over by other family members, which can help give mom a little extra time off.

◆ Formula has no anti-infective properties. Breastmilk, particularly the colostrum (milk produced the first few days of nursing) contains specific antibodies that protect your baby from infection. Some research shows that this protection could have long-term benefits.

◆ Breastmilk is designed specifically for the human infant, while formula is primarily made from cow's milk. There may be subtle differences in milk that haven't been discovered yet–or copied yet by formula manufacturers.

◆ If your baby is allergic to cow's milk formula, there are special soy formulas and even meat-based formulas that you can try. Ask your pediatrician for advice.

◆ If you feed your baby formula, iron-fortified formula is best for your baby and the American Academy of Pediatrics recommends it (1). Normally, cow's milk is low in iron, so the formula must be fortified with it. Since formula is your baby's sole source of nutrition for 4-6 months, feeding her the iron-fortified formula can prevent iron deficiency anemia.

◆ If you use concentrated formula and the water in your area doesn't contain adequate fluoride, your baby may need a supplement. Ask your baby's health care provider.

◆ If you feed your baby formula, or decide on a combination or breast-feeding and formula, you should not switch to cow's milk until your baby turns one year old. The American Academy of Pediatrics then recommends you start your child on whole milk until he is over 2 years of age when low-fat or skim milk can be used (2).

◆ If you use concentrated formula, make sure that your water doesn't contain too much lead. Three common preparation practices that can increase lead in formula are (3):

–Using the water that is first drawn from the faucet in the morning. Water sitting in the pipes for several hours has the highest amount of lead, if there is lead in your pipes.

–Excessive boiling. This concentrates the amount of lead up to three times in just 5 minutes of boiling.

–Using a lead based kettle for boiling.

For more information on lead see page 39.

Whatever method of feeding you decide on, feeding your baby will be enjoyable but it can also be stressful. Since babies can't tell you what they want, it is sometimes difficult to figure out what they need. Some great advice about infant feeding can be found in: *Child of Mine, Feeding with Love and Good Sense*, by Ellyn Satter, R.D., M.S. (Bull Publishing)

Ms. Satter is a dietitian and a social worker who gives advice about eating and tips on how to encourage a positive relationship with your child.

About Bonding

Bonding is a term often used when breastfeeding is described. However, bonding is touching, cuddling and holding and it can be done regardless of the feeding method. The long-term effects of bonding are very positive and are thought to affect a child's self-esteem as well as the mother's attitude towards the child.

Unlike a formula feeding mom, a breastfeeding mom must be with the baby, unless expressed milk is given in a bottle. Bottle fed babies can also bond with their mom, dad or whoever is giving them the bottle. However, some parents learn that the bottle can be propped by a blanket, etc. so that they can go about doing other things. This is not recommended because of choking hazard and also because this practice does not promote bonding or a close relationship with the baby. Also, if milk sits on the teeth (which happens for example if baby falls asleep with bottle in his mouth), it can cause decay.

Going Back to Work

Most women go back to work when their babies are 6 weeks old. Whether because of economic necessity or for personal fulfillment, this is the situation for many. Going back to work can affect your feeding decision.

During my counseling sessions with pregnant women, I often found that if a woman knew she was going back to work, she threw the idea of breastfeeding right out the window. Fortunately, the two are not mutually exclusive. Here are three examples of how working women handled their feeding decisions:

♦ Barb was determined to breastfeed Joshua. Her company was supportive of breastfeeding. She rented a breast-pump from the hospital and pumped at work. She used the Medela pump with the attachment which emptied both breasts at the same time, which allowed her to use her hands to read, eat a snack, etc. During her lunch break, she came home and fed Josh. Barb found that breastfeeding Josh was just the contact she needed after being away most of the day. I admired Barb for her determination. She carried on this routine for 9 months, until she started day-care in her home where she continued to nurse.

♦ Sarah had a high stress job. Her boss and company policies were not too supportive of motherhood. Yet Sarah wanted to breastfeed. She learned that breastfeeding didn't necessarily mean breastfeeding "full-time." She established a good milk supply while she was home with Erin, then gradually she worked out the routine that worked best for her family. She nursed Erin in the morning, her day care provider gave her two bottles of formula, then Sarah nursed her in the late afternoon while her husband was preparing dinner, and also nursed Erin one more time before she went to bed. Sarah's milk supply adjusted according to Erin's feeding schedule. On the weekend, Erin's Dad helped out with the mid-day bottles, giving Sarah a little break.

♦ Nicole was a little overwhelmed by her pregnancy. She kept changing her mind... breast or bottle? Finally she decided on formula feeding. She was finally glad that she made the decision. After Chris was born and they found their own routine, she knew she had made the right decision. Chris grew appropriately and was healthy.

If you will be returning to work, your environment at work will influence your feeding decision. Try to look into these things ahead of time:

♦ *Parental leave time* – If your company allows an extended maternity leave, this will give you more time to be with your baby. And if you decide to breastfeed, a longer time off will allow better establishment of your milk supply. Even if you decide to breastfeed for just a month, your baby will still receive the colostrum which contains the important disease fighting agents.

♦ *Required travel* – if your job requires you to be out of town a lot, you might want to cut it down to the minimum, whether you breastfeed or not. However, if you decide to nurse, it's not impossible, but will require diligent planning to make it work. Kristen arranged day care with a national franchise so when she traveled she could take Sean with her and the day care center in the other city took care of him. It was a commitment which not many people could do, but shows how creative one can be if needed!

♦ *Flex-hours* – Many companies offer flexible hours. This is useful for the two career couple so that more time can be spent with children. For example, some people work four-10 hour days and have an extra day off. If both partners can arrange this type of schedule, day care would only be required three days a week, giving Mom and Dad extra time with baby. Flex-hours can also help a breastfeeding mom. For example if you can take a long lunch and work a little later to make up for it, you might be able to go to your child and feed him lunch. (On site daycare makes this even easier!)

♦ *Supportive Boss and Co-workers* – It may be emotionally hard to go back to work with an infant at home. Seek out supportive co-workers; perhaps those who also have children. A supportive boss will understand if you need to take breaks to pump your breasts or take a little extra time off to go feed your baby.

Your Body Is Changing!

The "fourth trimester" is the 12 weeks after you have your baby. This period is often neglected, but it is still important to understand. You are now adjusting from being preg-

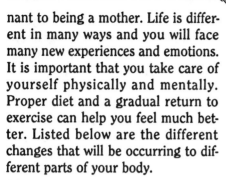

nant to being a mother. Life is different in many ways and you will face many new experiences and emotions. It is important that you take care of yourself physically and mentally. Proper diet and a gradual return to exercise can help you feel much better. Listed below are the different changes that will be occurring to different parts of your body.

Uterus

Immediately after birth your uterus weighs about 2 pounds and is the size of a grapefruit. In the next 6 weeks, it will shrink down to normal; around 3 inches long and 2 ounces in weight. Nursing your baby will help your uterus contract and reduce it's size. You may feel these contractions for 2-3 days, especially if this is your second or third baby.

Lochia

Lochia is the vaginal discharge that occurs the first few weeks after delivery. It is the body's way of getting rid of leftover debris from pregnancy and is a combination of blood cells, skin cells, mucus, white blood cells, bacteria and occasionally some of your baby's stool or hair.

Your blood flow will be red and plentiful for the first few days following delivery. Remember that your body generated a greater volume of blood during your pregnancy and much of that is being reduced at this time. Blood flow is individual, yet within two to three weeks, many women have returned to a whitish discharge.

If you revert back to bright red bleeding, you are being too active...slow down and enjoy these simple days of newborn life. If your flow remains bright red or has a foul odor please contact your physician. Remember that ovulation can occur within weeks after delivery...even if you are breastfeeding. However, ovulation may not occur in the breastfeeding mom until after weaning. The first period may be heavy and irregular for several months. Discuss contraception with your doctor if you want to resume sex within three to four weeks after delivery.

Vagina and Perineum

The area between your vagina and rectum is called the perineum. This area will feel sore due to the tremendous stretching it has undergone, even if you did not have an episiotomy. Ice will be applied in the first 12 hours after delivery to reduce swelling. After this time, heat will promote healing to the area. Many women take sitz baths (sitting for a short time in warm water).

Kegel exercises will help to tone muscles in the perineum area. You should have learned how to do kegels in your childbirth education class or prenatal exercise class. If not, ask your health care provider.

If you had an episiotomy, your stitches will dissolve by themselves. Your vagina will have decreased mucus until ovulation returns to normal, thus intercourse might need additional lubrication. Please note that if you are nursing, ovulation may be delayed for a while, and so you will continue to have reduced mucus.

Abdomen

After the birth of a baby your abdomen still looks very much pregnant yet flabby. This may be one of the biggest disappointments after delivery, unless you are prepared for it. You can start doing exercises to help tighten your abdominal muscles again. Remember that good muscle tone will take time and discipline; diet, good posture and exercise are important. If you have no energy or time to think about exercise at the beginning, think of tightening your perineum (do a kegel) and abdomen, every time you turn on a water faucet!

Losing That Baby Fat - Sensibly!

Ready to get rid of the extra pounds you put on during pregnancy? Not so fast! Remember that it took 9 months to gain the weight, it's not going to come off in a week or two! The key to long term weight loss is a balanced, reduced calorie diet in combination with exercise.

However, it's best not to exercise vigorously the first 6 weeks due to hormonal changes. (Personally, I didn't have to worry about doing anything vigorous the first 6 weeks, I was too tired!) Remember those hormones that were discussed in the third trimester that cause your joints and pelvis to become more elastic? Well, they aren't quite back to normal yet, so you should take exercise easy for a while or you could damage some joints or ligaments. A simple walking regimen should be fine. It's also a great way to show off your new baby to the neighbors or meet other new moms at the mall.

Chances are that if you were at your ideal weight before your pregnancy, you won't need any "diet" at all. If you are nursing, you shouldn't reduce your calorie intake below 1800 calories. (See page 145 for more information. You may just need to consciously cut back on the "extras" and fat you eat, and increase your activity level. The weight will gradually come off.

However, many women want a "program" to follow, even if they have just 10 pounds to lose. Some women were overweight when they became pregnant; they may want something more structured. Later, we will go through steps to help you evaluate a weight loss program.

Regardless of your situation, my advice is to lose as much of your excess weight as possible before you become pregnant again (that is if you are planning to have another child). Many of the women I see for weight loss are in their 50's and explain that they never lost all their weight between pregnancies or after their last baby. By the time they see me they are forced to lose weight because of a medical reason; diabetes, high blood pressure or heart disease. Avoid any of those problems by doing something sensible about losing weight now.

I believe that the reason so many people's weight "yo-yos' is that they are in a hurry to lose weight. I've seen it with many people in my weight loss classes. For example, "Mary" has been overweight for 15 years, but now she has a class reunion to go to and all of a sudden she wants to lose her weight NOW.

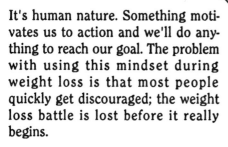

It's human nature. Something motivates us to action and we'll do anything to reach our goal. The problem with using this mindset during weight loss is that most people quickly get discouraged; the weight loss battle is lost before it really begins.

Some experts say it takes close to six months to truly change our habits. Yet, Mary expects to do a major overhaul on her diet and lifestyle in two weeks or less!

When people change their diet drastically they lose quickly at first, much of it being water. When their weight loss tapers down to a pound or less a week, they feel they are unsuccessful and give up. **What they forget is that a pound a week adds up to 52 pounds a year! That's a lot of pounds!**

The key to losing weight is determining which diet or lifestyle habits need changing, gradually altering your eating habits, setting realistic goals and adopting an exercise program that you can stick with for life. Remember–any temporary changes will probably result in only temporary weight loss. I have listed below some of the characteristics I've observed in people who are the most successful in losing weight. Most of my observations are also backed up by research as noted.

1. They exercise regularly (4).

2. They set realistic goals. When they don't meet their goals, they learn from the experience instead of considering themselves a failure and giving up.

3. They have social support from either family, friends, co-workers or support groups (5).

4. They work on liking themselves (or they already do).

5. They are motivated to lose weight for an internal reason instead of an external reason (6). For example, Judy used to lose weight to fit into her old Size 6 Calvin Klein Jeans. Now she loses weight to improve her health.

6. They concentrate not on the bathroom scale, but on some positive outcome, such as lowered cholesterol, or the ability to walk farther without becoming tired.

7. They have conquered emotional eating (7), (or are working on it).

8. They have learned to deal with eating out, eating at parties, while traveling, etc.

Diet Programs

There are many diets programs and diet books out there. Beware. Many promote quick weight loss, which is unhealthy. Others may recommend unbalanced diets which leave out one or more foods or food groups. Some can be downright dangerous. Virtually all diets work–for the short term. However, many diets fail over the long term. Continued dieting with regain of weight, often called "weight cycling" or "yo-yo" dieting can be harmful to the body and devastating to the dieter's self-esteem.

Below are steps to help you evaluate a weight loss program.

Evaluating Weight Loss Programs

1. Does the program promote a balanced diet, allowing most all foods in moderation? Does it omit certain foods or food groups?

A balanced program should allow everything, even so-called "bad" foods as an option at some point in the program.

2. Does the program have an exercise plan or regimen included?

Since exercise is so important for long term success, any program that doesn't address exercise or recommend a specific activity program should be avoided.

3. Is behavior modification (looking at changing current behaviors) included?

For long term weight loss, it is important to find out what your problem behaviors are so that you can change them. The tools used for behavior modification may include self-monitoring, like keeping a diet record, or exercises that promote awareness of eating.

4. Does the program use trained professionals or people who have lost weight as their "counselors?"

Many programs use people who have lost weight, or people who are good salespeople as their counselors. Though they may be very helpful and motivating, they may unintentionally give out inaccurate information.

There are also a number of "quacks" out there, professional and otherwise who are out to make a quick dollar! Beware of anything that sounds too good to be true (it probably is). Look for counselors who are licensed, registered or have a degree from an accredited university.

5. Does the program involve buying special foods or supplements?

Personally, I feel that learning how to eat "real" food is better for long term weight loss. However, some people just don't want to make decisions and would rather buy packaged foods.

6. Does the program provide a foundation for future good eating habits?

Hopefully the program teaches you how to cook more healthfully, plan menus, and learn to eat out in social situations.

The Moderate Approach

The recommended weight loss is about one pound or less per week. You're probably thinking, "One pound a week! I'll never lose this weight!" Consider the importance of long term success, which means keeping the weight off. Those that lose weight slowly seem to keep it off the longest.

To lose a pound a week, you can either cut your food intake by 500 calories a day, use more calories through exercise or do a combination of less food and more exercise.

For example, Colleen walks about 2 miles every evening, which uses 200 calories. She has also cut some extras out of her diet which add up to 300 calories. The diet/exercise approach that Colleen uses works best for long term weight maintenance. Besides being good for muscle tone, cardiovascular health, and endurance, exercise is also good for your mental health! Following is an example of a good fitness program. As you can see, fitness doesn't have to be boring!

Suggested Activity Program for Colleen

Height: 5'4

Weight: 160

Goal Weight: 120

Exercise-Activity Goal: 1 hour six times a week

Monday: 1 hour of light aerobics–burns 217 calories

Tuesday: 1 hour of walking (26 minute mile)–burns 217 calories

Wednesday: 1/2 hour of bicycling at 10 MPH–burns 200 calories

Thursday: 1 hour of walking (26 minute mile)–burns 217 calories

Friday: Day off!

Saturday: 1 hour of lawn mowing – burns 261 calories or 1 hour of hiking–burns 399 calories

Sunday: 1 hour of gardening–burns 232 calories

Source: *Fit III Analysis Program*

Please note that the numbers of calories burned are calculated for Colleen specifically.

Colleen burned over 1700 calories through exercise! To lose one pound per week, she also needs to reduce her diet by 1800 calories per week or about 250 calories per day.

Let's look at the few of the extras Colleen eats that she can easily cut out.

Food	Calories	Action	Calories saved
1 Tb. margarine	100	substitute Butter Buds or Molly McButter	100
1 cola drink	150	substitute diet soda	148
2 chocolate chip cookies	140	substitute 1 peach	100
1 cinnamon roll	230	substitute 1 Quaker Caramel Corn Cake	180
3 cups whole milk	450	substitute 2% milk	90
3 Tb. blue cheese dressing	180	substitute Wish Bone Healthy Sensation Chunky Blue Cheese	120

These changes add up to a reduction of over 700 calories per day! Colleen will only have to make half the changes noted to lose 1 pound per week!

Depending on your weight, height, and activity level, you will probably want to eat from 1200 to 1800 calories per day to lose 1 pound a week. Going below 1200 calories is usually not advised unless you are a very small person. The following menus are for a 1500 calorie program.

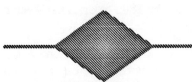

Lose Weight by Leaning Toward Vegetarianism

Cutting down on animal protein is often a way to cut calories and fat–and that leads to weight loss! "leaning towards vegetarian" or even becoming vegetarian might be a goal. If so, see Chapter 7. In addition, here is a good source regarding weight loss for vegetarians: *Vegetarian Weight Loss Guide*, by Suzanne Havala M.S., R.D., in Vegetarian Journal Reports, Vegetarian Resource Group, 1990

1500 Calorie Meal Plan

This meal plan is meant to be a guideline of a healthy weight loss program. It is not meant to take the place of individual counseling with a health professional. If you are breastfeeding, this meal plan does not contain enough calories or nutrients for your current needs.

7   Servings of starches/grains

One serving is 1 slice of any type bread, 1 flour tortilla, 1/2 cup pasta, 1/3 cup rice or legumes, 6 crackers, 1/2 cup of potato.

3   Servings of fruits

One serving is 1 medium piece of fresh fruit, 1/2 banana, 1/2 cup canned fruit in it's own juice, 1 cup melon or berries, 2 plums or nectarines.

2   or more Servings of vegetables

One serving is 1/2 cup of any non-starchy vegetable or 1 cup lettuce.

5   Ounces of protein or equivalent

One serving is 1 ounce of lean meat, 1 ounce reduced fat cheese, 1/4 cup cottage cheese, 1/2 cup of tofu, 2 tablespoons peanut butter, 1/2 cup cooked dried beans, 1 egg.

2-3   Servings of dairy products

One serving is 1 cup of skim or 1% milk or lowfat yogurt.

3   Servings of fat

One serving of fat is 1 teaspoon margarine or butter, or 2 teaspoons reduced fat margarine, 1 teaspoon mayonnaise, or 2 teaspoons reduced fat mayonnaise, 1 slice bacon, 1/2 ounce cream cheese, 1 tablespoon sour cream, 1/8 avocado, 10 peanuts, 5 olives.

For more information about weight loss or healthy eating, see reference section for recommended weight loss books and low-calorie cookbooks.

Questions you May Have:

I've never been much of a breakfast eater, but I've heard that it's good for you. Is it?

You may have heard that "breakfast is the most important meal of the day." It is in many respects. A recent study showed that people who skipped breakfast had trouble working on tasks that required concentration. According to Diane Odland, nutritionist at the U.S. Department of Agriculture Human Nutrition Information Service, "When you consider it's been eight or nine hours since you've had a meal, it's obvious that refueling at breakfast will make you feel and perform better during the day (8)."

Eating breakfast can also help you lose weight. Those that skip the first meal of the day often make up for it later by eating larger meals or tend to snack on high fat, high sugar foods. Whether you stay home with a child, or work outside the home, eating breakfast will definitely improve your energy level.

Will I lose all my pregnancy weight without really trying?

It depends on how much you gained. In one study, women who gained more than 20 pounds retained 5-10 pounds between pregnancies. Those who gained over 40 pounds were an average of 17 pounds heavier at the start of their next pregnancy. Since the current recommendation for weight gain is over 25 pounds, you will probably have to make an active effort to lose weight (9).

How long will it take me to lose my "baby" fat?

Again, it depends on how much you gained, how much you eat and your activity level. A lucky few fit into their "unpregnant" clothes right after delivery (though that wasn't the case for me or any of my friends).

The amount of time it takes to lose the weight and get your "old body" back is probably a big surprise to everyone. It took me close to 9

months to really get back to normal, much to my disappointment. I thought I'd be back to my old self within a few months. When I started aerobics 3 times a week, I saw the biggest change in the way my body looked, and also got rid of those last 5 pounds or so that are so stubborn.

When I surveyed other dietitians about this book, several suggested that I include some realistic expectations for weight loss and body size after pregnancy.

Here are some things you should expect:

*Very few people go back to wearing their "skinny" clothes right after delivery. Expect to wear your maternity clothes for a few more months (even though you probably feel like burning them)!

♦ You may need to buy a few outfits in "the next size" until you get your shape back.

♦ Your body may have re-proportioned itself. Kate weighs the same as she did before pregnancy, but her hips are a few inches wider. Most of us continue to have a little "tummy" unless we diligently practice abdominal exercises. Some find that their ribcages expanded permanently and now they wear a larger bra size. Believe it or not, some women even wear a larger shoe size after pregnancy.

♦ If you are breastfeeding, you may feel like you are "busting" out of your blouses. Judy was depressed because for the first few months of breastfeeding, the only shirts she could wear were her husband's t-shirts and her old maternity shirts.

However, Sandy was rather glad to have an excuse to buy larger tops!

♦ Many women lose the last few pounds after they stop breastfeeding.

♦ Exercise can't be emphasized enough. It will help get rid of baby fat and tone up some of the muscles you haven't used lately.

♦ Overall, be patient. I clearly remember asking my aerobics teacher how fast I could get back in shape after the baby came if I worked out regularly. I wanted real numbers. She said it could be done in 6-8 weeks, but I might need time for recovery. Not me, I thought. I was going to be super-mom! Well, after a tough labor and delivery, and a long adjustment to motherhood, it was months before I had the time and energy to re-start my exercise program. If I had known then what I know now...

Preparing For Your Next Pregnancy

Sometime between when your labor anesthesia has worn off and when you send out birth announcements, someone will ask, "So, when are you going to have another baby?" You may not be ready to answer that question for a long time. However, you may want another baby right away or in the next year. Waiting at least 9 months between pregnancies is a good idea to get your body back in shape and your nutrient stores built up again. When you are ready to think about getting pregnant again, turn to Chapter 2-Contemplating Pregnancy, to learn what you can do for a healthy pregnancy before you conceive.

No matter when you decide to have another baby, or even if you decide not to have another, don't lose the good habits you found during pregnancy. A healthy diet is one of the most important things you can do to insure good health. Giving your children good eating habits is one of the most precious gifts you can give them.

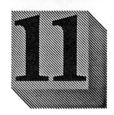

Fitting Fitness In

---◆---

What You Will Find In This Chapter:

◆ Benefits of Exercise

◆ What Every Pregnant Woman Should Know About Exercise

◆ Fitting Fitness Into Your Busy Lifestyle

◆ Exercise After Pregnancy

◆ Tips for Starting a Postpartum Exercise Program

And Answers to Questions You May Have:

◆ What if I don't have time for exercise?

◆ Should I exercise differently while I am pregnant?

◆ How can I relieve back pain?

◆ How does exercise fit in for those on bedrest?

◆ How can I get back in shape after I have the baby?

Benefits of Exercise

Throughout the book, I've mentioned exercise many times.

I'm hoping repetition will bring the message home. Exercise is one of the most important things you can do for your health. It can bring numerous benefits, with just a little time investment.

While you are pregnant, exercise offers even more benefits.

◆ Exercise helps battle the fatigue many women feel during pregnancy.

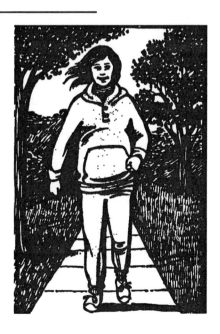

♦ Exercise helps your body get ready for labor by being physically fit.

♦ Exercise helps you feel better mentally about your expanding body size.

♦ Once you've established a fitness routine, it will be easier to resume exercising after you have the baby when you're trying to lose weight.

♦ Regular exercise will help you sleep better; and you may need all the help you can get to sleep during those last few weeks of pregnancy!

♦ You will probably feel better all over, you'll have a better emotional outlook, and you may have improved immunity.

A former "couch potato" says:

"I was never much on exercise, but when I became pregnant, my doctor suggested I get involved in an exercise program for pregnant women at the Y. I went to an aerobics class, mostly for my baby, and I began to really enjoy it, much to my surprise. I started feeling better about my body, which I had always felt negatively about. I shared labor and delivery stories with other Moms-to-be and began a "Mommy Network." Towards the end of my pregnancy, I think it really helped me sleep better. Also I felt much less tired than I did with my first pregnancy. I had more energy and felt vivacious."

If you didn't exercise before you were pregnant, you should ask your health care provider about exercising. He may have some special guide-lines for you, depending on your current situation.

If you had exercised routinely before pregnancy, you can probably continue it with some modifications.

♦

What Every Pregnant Woman Should Know About Exercise

Note: for the most part, these guidelines also apply to the post-partum period (1).

1. **Don't overdo it at first.** Have you ever watched the Olympics and gotten so inspired that you jumped up and decided you're going to run two miles? Don't! Start out slowly, maybe as little as five minutes a day, and don't forget to warm up and cool down.

2. **Be kind to your joints.** The hormones of pregnancy make joints very elastic to prepare them for childbirth. Exercise that requires lots of bouncing, jerky movements, jumping or quick changes in direction could cause joint pain or injury. Also, avoid deep flexing or extending of muscles. Use gentle stretches instead of stretching to the limit to cool down.

3. **Avoid "Iron Man Marathons"** and other rigorous events (unless you are already an athlete and your health care provider has given an O.K.) Competitive sports should also be avoided. Stick to walking, swimming, or low-impact aerobics (preferably classes developed just for pregnant women.)

4. Do kinder, gentler exercise. With the extra weight gain of pregnancy, and the different center of gravity, you should avoid sports which include the potential for falling, including downhill skiing, skating, skateboarding, etc. Exercise should be done on a wooden floor or a tightly carpeted surface to reduce shock and provide a sure footing.

5. Be consistent. It's healthier to exercise regularly, even if it's just for a few minutes. There are thousands of "would be" exercisers with good intentions. Their homes are full of treadmills, stationery bikes, rowing machines, and weight sets. Unfortunately, they serve mostly as dust collectors and clothes racks. Those people would be much better off if they set aside 15 minutes a day to simply go for a walk.

6. Warm up and cool down. Always begin with a 5 minute warm up period of less intense exercise (like slow walking, cycling or water walking for swimmers) to warm up muscles. Strenuous exercise should be no longer than 15 minutes. Follow intense exercise with 5-10 minutes of "cool down"--a gradual slowing down of your workout that ends with gentle stretching.

7. Exercise at least 3 times a week. It is much better for you to exercise just 20 minutes a day, 3 times a week, than to be just a "weekend athlete."

8. Measure your heart rate during exercise. Exercise done at too high an intensity can increase your internal temperature, which can harm the fetus. Measure your pulse at the peak of your activity and before cool down too. To measure your pulse, place your index at your carotid artery on your neck. Keep moving. Count your heart rate either 6 or 10 seconds. Pregnant women's heart rates should not exceed 140 beats per minute. Calculated out, this is 14 beats in 6 seconds or 23 beats in 10 seconds. Check with your health care provider to see if he has an alternate guideline for you.

9. Take your time. Get up slowly and gradually from the floor to avoid dizziness or fainting caused from a drop in blood pressure.

10. Drink, drink drink! Drink water before, during and after exercise to prevent becoming dehydrated. This will also help cool you off. Take a squirt bottle filled with water on your walk or to aerobics.

11. Stay out of the heat. Don't do any vigorous exercise in hot, humid weather, or during an illness when you have fever.

12. Watch out for danger signs. Stop your activity immediately and call your doctor if any of these symptoms occur: pain, bleeding, dizziness, shortness of breath, rapid heartbeat, back pain, pubic pain, difficulty walking.

13. Be kind to YOU! Think of exercise as a special time for YOU. Sometimes it may not feel like it, but it's a way to pamper yourself!

14. Eat enough food. During pregnancy, blood sugar levels are usually lower than non-pregnant levels and carbohydrates are used at a greater rate. So, it's possible to have low blood sugar during strenuous exercise. Make sure you don't exercise on an empty stomach. You may want to eat a piece of fruit, some crackers, dried fruit or juice before your workout for more energy.

If you worked out regularly before pregnancy and continue to have a pretty long workout schedule, keep in mind that you will need to increase your calories accordingly. Your weight gain will let you know if you're eating enough.

Why exercise should be "toned down" or done differently during pregnancy:

♦ Your heart rate at rest is higher than a non-pregnant woman's and rises more quickly during exercise. So, watch the intensity of your exercise.

♦ Your body temperature may rise more rapidly than a non-pregnant woman's. And since your baby is always 1 degree warmer than you are, an elevated body temperature could mean trouble for your baby. Watch out how hard you exercise and how long you exercise.

♦ After your fourth month, your uterus may compress the vena cava, a major vein. This could interfere with blood flow to the fetus. (Don't do any exercise while laying flat on your back after your fourth month.)

♦ Some hormones make joints and connective tissue relax (to get ready for delivery) and can make joints susceptible to injury.

(Treat your joints gently by doing slow stretches daily and don't forget to warm up and cool down!)

♦ Some studies have shown that vigorous activity can cause contractions which may lead to premature labor. One study done with women who had gestational diabetes showed that the safest exercises were those that used mostly the upper body or that put little stress below the waist.

The researchers found that walking on a treadmill was fine, but jogging was more likely to cause contractions. Exercising on a stationary bike caused contractions in half of the women, though exercising on a recumbent bicycle (in which you sit back and legs are in front of you, not under you) caused no contractions. The upper arm ergometer proved to be the safest form of exercise. This is a machine similar to a stationery bicycle except that the arms do all the pedaling (2).

For more specific information about exercise, ask your health care provider or childbirth educator. Always check with your health care provider before starting an exercise program, especially if you haven't exercised recently.

When You Shouldn't Exercise

According to the American College of Obstetricians and Gynecologists, there are several conditions that would totally restrict you from vigorous exercise. If any of these conditions apply to you, ask your health care provider before doing any strenuous exercise.

- History of 3 or more miscarriages
- Ruptured membranes
- Premature labor
- Diagnosed multiple gestation (twins, triplets or more)
- Incompetent cervix
- Bleeding or a diagnosis of placenta previa
- Diagnosed cardiac disease

Some conditions may require you to limit strenuous exercise. If any of these conditions apply to you, be sure to talk to your health care provider before starting an exercise program:

- High blood pressure
- Anemia or other blood disorder
- Thyroid disease
- Diabetes
- Cardiac arrhythmia or palpitations
- History of premature labor
- History of intrauterine growth retardation (slowed growth of fetus)
- History of bleeding during current pregnancy
- Breech position of baby in last trimester
- Excessive obesity
- Extreme underweight
- History of extremely sedentary lifestyle

Reprinted with permission, American College of Obstetricians and Gynecologists. *Exercise During Pregnancy and the Postnatal Period.* ACOG Home Exercise Programs, Washington, DC: ©1985.

Fitting Fitness Into Your Busy Lifestyle

Here is where the "fitting fitness in" comes in. Some people don't exercise regularly because they don't have time. It's true, we live in a very fast paced society. Yet, most of us have 15 minutes a day that we probably waste. Here are a few ideas for fitting fitness into your lifestyle:

- Take a walk every morning before work. If you happen to have a treadmill, you can walk while watching the morning news.
- Make more trips up and down the stairs. One suggestion is to unplug the downstairs phone so that every time the phone rings, you go up and down the stairs once. Although this will give you more activity, this uses only short bursts of energy, and won't improve your overall fitness much.
- Use 1/2 of your lunch hour to take a walk. I did this on the days I didn't go to aerobics. The funny part of it was that I had to turn down so many rides. Everyone must have felt sorry for this big pregnant woman walking down the street!
- Write your exercise "date" down on your calender and keep it!
- Exercise with your spouse or a friend.
- Walk the dog; she'll love you for it!
- Sign up for an exercise class just for pregnant women. Sometimes if

you pay for a class, it becomes more of a priority to go.

♦ On the weekend, take a drive out to the country where you can walk with a scenic view.

♦ Get the whole family into exercising! Take walks or hikes together.

♦ Rent or purchase an exercise video just for pregnant women. *The American College of Obstetricians and Gynecologists have approved a series of exercise videos; Pregnancy Exercise Video and Postnatal Exercise Video ($14.95 each). They can be ordered by calling 1-800-423-0102.*

Your Personal Exercise Schedule

Now take just a moment and write down your plan for exercising.

My goal is to exercise _____times per week, for _____minutes each time.

My exercise schedule:

Monday at (time)_____
Tuesday _____
Wednesday _____
Thursday _____
Friday _____
Saturday _____
Sunday _____

Ten Ways to Exercise Without Thinking About It

Not everyone truly enjoys exercising! If you fit into that category, you'll like the following list which will increase your physical activity level without really working at it!

1. Walk the dog

2. "Shop 'til you drop" – do once around the mall just window shopping.

3. Go dancing–ballroom, country and western, even square dancing will do.

4. Take a stroll around a scenic place, a lake, down a tree lined avenue, or forest trail.

5. Go canoeing or paddle-boating.

6. Fire the maid and do the vacuuming yourself!

7. Go to the pool and just walk from side to side. Bring a friend. With conversation, you don't notice the time passing.

8. Aerobic lawn mowing! Supposedly the latest trend is to cut your grass with a push mower. Start a fad in your neighborhood!

9. Plant a garden. Gardening can increase your activity and you get to enjoy the fruits of your labor!

10. Set a walking date with a neighbor or co-worker. Once you get to talking, you'll hardly notice the time or the exercise.

Exercise After Pregnancy

Women often face weight problems, especially after having children. Those last 5 pounds just don't seem to come off, and then you keep another 5 from the next pregnancy, and before you know it you're 15 or 20 pounds overweight. So what does exercise have to do with weight?

Research has shown that people who exercise regularly lose more weight and have the best odds of keeping the weight off, which is the part that's often the problem. The other benefits of exercising include improved cardiovascular fitness, lowered heart rate, lowered blood pressure, decreased blood lipids, decreased blood sugar, toned muscles, less body fat, improved immunity and more!

Directly after you have the baby, it may take a while for you to get motivated to exercise. That's O.K. You have just gone though one of life's biggest events. It may take you time to get used to a new baby in the house and to set up a new routine. (It took me four months to adjust!) Remember those hormones that made your joints more elastic so that your pelvis could stretch for birth? It takes weeks for those hormones to drop to their normal levels. Most physicians give their O.K. for an exercise program after the 6 week check up. Before that it's generally OK to walk.

A New Mom says:

> "I was one of those people who thought I would be out of the house and back to exercising within days after delivery. Surprise, surprise! After a week, I still had trouble walking! My neighbor had a C-section and she was taking her baby on a walk in the stroller when he was just 4 days old! I was jealous!"

Women have very individual labor experiences. Some breeze through in a few hours. Other's may last a day and a half. If you have a long labor, it may take a lot out of you. If you have stitches, hemorrhoids, or a combination, it may take a long time to feel OK when walking and sitting. Be prepared for the best or worst situation, but remember that this too shall pass.

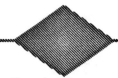

You Don't Have to be a Race Walker to Lose Weight!

Women who walked five days a week for 24 weeks lost 6% body fat. These women walked at a pace of 1 mile in 20 minutes and lost more body fat than faster walkers (3). To use stored fat during exercise, it is best to walk slower, but longer.

Tips For Starting a Post Partum Exercise Program

- ◆ Start at your own pace, no matter how slow it seems!

- ◆ Stretching will be important, even if you don't feel like exercising.

- ◆ Join a fitness class that is for moms and babies; you won't feel like the only one out of shape, you can meet other moms, and you can take your baby along! (Check the YMCA)

- ◆ While you are at home those 6 weeks, the days seem to drift by. Make a little schedule for yourself, including activity. It will give you more of a purpose.

♦ Find activities you enjoy, and if possible, include other family members too.

♦ When you have time between baby's naps, pop in an exercise video. Try one of these considered to be the Ten Best Exercise Videos by American Health Magazine. Numbers 1-3 are considered beginner or intermediate, and may be best if you weren't very active during your pregnancy. Numbers 4-8 are intermediate/advanced and may be appropriate for those who kept up a regular fitness routine during pregnancy. Numbers 9 and 10 are advanced and may be best to step up to after your level of fitness has increased.

1.　Richard Simmons: Sweatin' to the Oldies

2.　Basic Stepping with Walk Aerobics

3.　Jane Fonda's Complete Workout

4.　Victoria's Power Shaping Workout

5.　Kathy Smith's Instant Workout

6.　Kathy Smith's Weight Loss Workout

7.　Jody Watley: Dance to Fitness

8.　The Firm; Aerobic Workout with Weights Volume I

9.　The Firm; Aerobic Workout with Weights Volume II

10.　Technifunk 2000

Source: *American Health Magazine*, March 1992

Probably the most important thing about exercising is the fact that you're doing it.　Do what you have to do to get started, but as the sports shoe commercial says, JUST

DO IT!

For references on fitness, see the resource section.

Questions you may have about fitness:

Doesn't exercise make you more tired?

At first you may feel a little more tired after exercising while pregnant. This is because of the extra weight you are carrying, and the extra blood that must be pumped through your heart. (During the first trimester hormonal changes can cause fatigue) However, since exercise increases endurance, you will gradually feel less tired once your body gets accustomed to exercise. Of course, if you are already used to exercising, you shouldn't feel as tired. If you do, it may be because you are not eating enough foods or the right foods.

How will I know if I'm eating enough to support the exercise during pregnancy?

The rule of thumb here is eat to your hunger, and watch your weight gain. If you're not gaining enough, you need to eat more. If you have a vigorous schedule, and just can't seem to eat enough, you may need to slow down. See page 241 for Snack Ideas for High Energy Moms.

I'm on bed rest. How can I prevent my body from turning into flab?

Pregnancy often causes us to make changes in our lifestyle and habits. Bed rest takes this to the extreme. You will lose your level of fitness while on bedrest. However, by stretching and doing isometric exercises, (if OK'd by your health care provider) you can retain some of your muscle tone. Ask your health care provider for a list of suggested exercises to keep yourself limber. Also remember that after you have the baby, your endurance for exercise will be very low. You'll need to start out slowly! Your body will bounce back and you can become fit again, so think of your situation as temporary.

My back hurts all the time lately, what can I do?

I can sympathize with you. During the last two months of my pregnancy, I couldn't sweep and mop the kitchen floor in the same afternoon, because of back pain. I finally had to give that job to my husband (one of the <u>unexpected</u> benefits of pregnancy!)

Your back undergoes a great deal of stress during pregnancy. Most traditional back strengthening exercises are not recommended during pregnancy because they are done while lying on your back. One that is recommended is the pelvic tilt. If you are attending an exercise class for pregnant women, you probably already know this one.

How To Do a Pelvic Tilt

1.   Stand with feet shoulder width apart and knees bent slightly.

2.   Contract the muscles of the buttocks and abdomen and gently thrust your pelvis forward, rotating the pubic bone upward. Hold this position for 10 seconds and release.

3.   The pelvic tilt can be done while lying or while squatting on hands and knees.

Reprinted with permission from American College of Obstetricians and Gynecologists. *ACOG Guide to Planning for Pregnancy, Birth and Beyond.* Washington DC: ACOG ©1990.

You should try to do the pelvic tilt as often as possible during the day. Keep in mind that after delivery, back pain can still be a problem with all the lifting and carrying of the baby. Continue doing pelvic tilts and other back strengthening exercises to improve back health. Keeping stomach muscles strong supports back muscles and prevents back strain. Stomach crunches (or half sit-ups) where you just lift your shoulders off the ground keeping knees bent is a great tummy exercise for postpartum.

For more information on exercise, an excellent book is "Essential Exercises for the Child Bearing Year" by Elizabeth Noble.

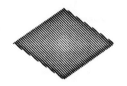

Section II
Shopping, Cooking And Eating Out For A Healthy Pregnancy

Stocking the Pregnant Kitchen

What You Will Find In This Chapter:

♦ A Peak Inside my Pantry

♦ What's on a Food Label

♦ Eating on a Budget

♦ Stocking the Kitchen Tool Box

♦ Cooking and Storing to Keep the Vitamins

♦ Food Safety in a Nutshell for Pregnant Women

♦ The Essential Guide to Food Safety

And Answers to Questions You May Have:

♦ How can I start shopping more healthfully?

♦ What do "lite", and "lowfat" mean on a food label?

♦ Is it safe to drink homemade eggnog?

♦ Are there any fish I should avoid?

♦ Why is a variety of foods so important?

♦ How can I eat well if I have a limited food budget?

♦ How can I avoid food poisoning?

So, now you're motivated to eat well! If your diet is already good, you may not need much help. But, if you're "turning over a new leaf" nutritionally, you may be thinking "where do I begin?"

The best place to start improving your diet is, not surprisingly, your own kitchen. First, you need to find out what your shopping and eating patterns are so you can change them if you need to.

Looking Inside Your Pantry...

1. What takes up the bulk of room in your freezer? Frozen vegetables? Ice cream? Frozen juice? Fish, Chicken, Meat? Fish Sticks? Frozen dinners? Frozen pies or cheesecakes? Pizza?

2. Does the top shelf of your fridge hold milk or soda?

3. Are your produce drawers bulging with fresh fruits and veggies or are there just a few lonely, shriveled carrots?

4. Does your pantry hold many convenience and ready to make foods? Canned vegetables? Canned fruits? Potato Chips? Candy?

5. Do you have a mix of grains such as brown rice, pasta, bulgur, quinoa, whole wheat flour, wheat germ, oats and barley or just white flour, rice and pasta?

6. Do you keep a variety of vegetables in the house, or do you regularly eat your favorite 2 vegetables and fruits?

A Peek Inside My Pantry

As a registered dietitian, people are always curious as to how I eat at home. Sometimes I think they envision me and my family eating "perfectly" all the time. What they don't realize is we are just like any other family; we have our habits, our likes and our dislikes. But to show you how my family eats and shops, I'll let you take a look into my kitchen.

This is what you'll usually find in my Pantry:

Various canned tomatoes, tomato sauce and tomato paste

Jarred spaghetti sauce without meat

Corn, peas, sweet potatoes, pumpkin

Canned black beans, vegetarian refried beans, kidney beans

Assorted dried beans

Canned tuna, Salmon

White, whole wheat flour, skim evaporated milk,

Yeast, sugar, brown sugar, molasses, honey

White rice, brown rice, bulgur, barley, pasta, pasta and more pasta!

Sun dried tomatoes

Raisin Bran, All Bran, Old Fashioned Oatmeal (super-economy size!), Cream of Wheat, grits, Product 19, Multi-Bran Chex, lowfat granola

Raisins, mixed dried fruit

Canola oil, olive oil, soy sauce, many miscellaneous spices

Apple cider vinegar, red wine vinegar, tarragon wine vinegar

Tortilla shells, Boboli Bread

Graham crackers, popcorn cakes, pretzels, fig newtons

Tobler or Cadbury Chocolate (My motto: buy the best but eat one square at a time!)

Potato chips/tortilla chips, or Guiltless Gourmet Oil Free Tortilla Chips (For the occasional batch of guacamole)

Freezer:

Miscellaneous frozen juices

Nutri-Grain Waffles

Healthy Treasures Fish Sticks/regular fish sticks

Trout/Salmon/Sole/Shrimp

Chicken/turkey breast

Top/bottom round/ground buffalo

Mashed bananas (to use later for banana bread or pancakes)

Chopped spinach/broccoli, mixed vegetables, peas

Miscellaneous combination vegetables

Budget Gourmet Light/Lean Pockets/Michelino's Frozen Entrees

Refrigerator:

1% milk, eggs, Kraft Free cheese, regular American cheese,

part-skim Mozzarella or Farmer's cheese, regular or reduced-fat Cheddar, grated Parmesan cheese,

Juice, Diet Coke, decaffeinated iced tea,

Miscellaneous meat, fish or chicken thawing

Turkey polish sausage

Plain nonfat yogurt, plain lowfat yogurt, Yoplait flavored yogurt

Lowfat cottage cheese, ham/turkey breast lunch meat

Promise Light/ I Can't Believe It's Not Butter, Light or Regular

Natural style peanut butter

Mayonnaise, fat-free mayonnaise, Bernstein's regular or Light Fantastic Dressing, homemade vinaigrette dressing, Fat-free Italian Dressing, Light Blue Cheese dressing, Barbecue sauce, Teriyaki marinade, Ketchup, Hoisin sauce, Grated ginger, Dijon mustard, Capers, Horseradish, Lemon juice, Wheat germ (to prevent rancidity)

Various leftovers

In the Produce drawers:

Summer: all kinds of berries, canteloupe, watermelon, apricots, nectarines, peaches, mangos, bananas, pineapple, lemons, tomatoes, carrots, romaine, leaf or boston lettuce, cucumber, broccoli, cauliflower

Winter: apples, bananas, pineapple, pears, grapes, oranges, eggplant, acorn squash, butternut squash, carrots, leeks, cabbage, , broccoli, cauliflower, tomato, lettuce, cucumber

What's On A Food Label

Chances are you are more concerned than you were just a few months ago about what you (and your baby) are eating. Your favorite new pastime may be studying food labels. Why should you read labels? It's the perfect way to put nutrition knowledge into practice by helping you make informed food buying choices.

What can be learned from a label?

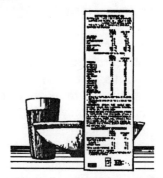

The label contains a virtual goldmine of information. For example, by looking on my box of Raisin Bran, I can see how many calories, how many grams of fiber and how much sugar or sodium a serving contains. I can also find how much protein and fat it has and how my cereal compares to the U.S. RDAs for nutrients like calcium, vitamin A and thiamine.   The U.S. RDA is the highest level of Recommended Dietary Allowances

(RDA) for that nutrient (excluding values for pregnant and nursing women). For example, the requirement for iron is higher in women, so the U.S. RDA for iron is the same as the female RDA.

Suppose I'm allergic to milk protein. I can look on the list of ingredients to see if it's listed there.

Introducing The New and Improved Food Label...

In 1990 Congress passed the Nutrition Labeling and Education Act, and in 1991, the Food and Drug Administration proposed label revisions in accordance with the new law. According to Dr. David Kessler, Commissioner of the Food and Drug Administration,

> "This game of "food label roulette" is a costly game and places the consumer at a disadvantage. It is time to take the guesswork– and the element of chance–out of food labeling."

As this book went to press, the following were proposed to be listed on the new food labels (1):

Calories

Calories from total fat

Total fat

Saturated fat

Total carbohydrates (excluding dietary fiber)

Complex carbohydrate

Sugars

Dietary fiber

Protein

Sodium

Vitamin A, C, Calcium, and Iron (listed as "Percent of Daily Value", which will replace the currently used U.S. RDAs)

Nutrient information should be listed in customary serving sizes and in household measures.

You'll also find that terms that were "loosely" defined will have standard meanings (2):

Fat-free: less than 1/2 gram of fat per serving and no added fat.

Lowfat: contains 3 grams of fat or less per 3.5 ounce serving.

Light: has at least 1/3 fewer calories than a comparable product.

Reduced fat: has reduced fat content by 50% or more, with a minimum reduction of more than 3 grams.

Low in saturated fat: may be used to describe a food that contains 1 gram or less of saturated fat per serving.

Cholesterol free: contains less than 2 mg. of cholesterol per serving and 2 grams or less saturated fat per serving.

Low in cholesterol: 20 mg. or less per 3.5 ounce serving and 2 grams or less of saturated fat per serving.

Percent fat-free: can only be used on products that meet lowfat definition.

Low sodium: less than 140 mg. per 3.5 ounce serving.

Very low sodium: less than 35 mg. per 3.5 ounce serving.

Calorie free: fewer than 5 calories per serving.

Sugar free: less than 1/2 gram per serving

Nutrition and Health Claims

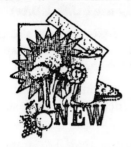

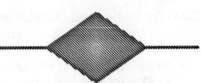

Currently, banners of nutrition and health claims on food labels practically scream at consumers, "buy me!" However, the claims aren't necessarily backed by any scientific study or defined legally. The new labeling law proposes that health claims about diet and disease must be backed by scientific evidence and the FDA will decide which claims it will allow on labels. Those proposed are:

Calcium and osteoporosis

Sodium and hypertension

Fat and cardiovascular disease

Fat and cancer

Claims made using "fresh" "high" or "source of" as in "this product is a good source of fiber" must also meet certain standards.

The Ingredient List

Products contain a list of ingredients—in order of predominance by weight. The new labeling law require that even standardized foods like mayonnaise and ice cream will have an ingredient label now. In addition, all FDA certified color additives will be listed by name.

Sugar is Sugar by Many Other Names

Some ingredients have many names, which makes deciphering the food label even trickier.

Corn syrup, high fructose corn syrup, dextrose, glucose, corn sweetener, sucrose, sugar, brown sugar, fructose, maltose, sorbitol, mannitol, honey, and fruit juice concentrate are all types of sweeteners. There are also "artificial" sweeteners which are sometimes called non-nutritive or non-caloric sweeteners. These sweeteners are widely found in diet products: Nutrasweet®, (the sweetener in Equal®) Saccharin, (found in Sweet n' Low™, Sugar Twin®, etc.) and Acesulfame K (found in Sweet One R). Many other non-caloric sweeteners are currently awaiting FDA approval. See page 118 for information on using these products during pregnancy.

Let's find out how looking at a food label can help you make a healthier food choice: To most people, jam is jam. You may look at the price per ounce, and pick up the cheapest. Or you may be partial to a particular brand and don't look twice at the others. After all, jam is jam...right? Let's see.

Jam # 1

Ingredients: High fructose corn syrup, strawberries, pectin, natural flavoring.

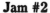

Jam #2

Ingredients: Strawberries, high fructose corn syrup, pectin, natural flavoring.

The better choice would be Jam #2 which, ounce per ounce contains more strawberries than sugar.

Other Ingredients to Look for...

Sugar alcohols, which are often used in diabetic candies, are usually allowed by diabetics because they are metabolized differently than regular sugar. However, they still have the same number of calories as sugar. Their names end in "ol" like sorbitol, mannitol, etc.

Fats are something to keep an eye on because they are higher in calories, and can contribute to risk of chronic diseases. Again, you'll see they have many "alias" names: oil, shortening, lard, partially hydrogenated oil, mono and diglycerides.

Salt or sodium is something many people limit due to high blood pressure or water retention. A certain amount of water retention is considered normal during pregnancy and pregnant women have an increased need for sodium. You shouldn't try to reduce your intake of sodium unless advised by your health care provider.

Other Nutrient Information Proposed for the New and Improved Food Label

Calories: Calories, or the amount of energy a food provides, is an important consideration when making food choices. To determine how many calories are in your typical serving, first look at the serving size listed on the package. For example, a serving size listed for granola is 1/4 cup, and its calories are 130 per serving. Most people look no further and assume that their serving of the food would be 130 calories. But what if you are more likely to eat a 3/4 cup serving? You'd actually be consuming 390 calories instead of 130 and 15 grams of fat instead of 5 grams. That's when "label math" becomes important!

Calories from fat: This helps determine the proportion of calories that are coming from fat, which is important to know if you are watching your fat intake. Ounce per ounce, fat provides more than twice the calories of protein or carbohydrate. Excess fat in the diet has been linked with increased risk heart disease, breast cancer and other cancers.

During pregnancy, too much fat in the diet can put on the pounds; it can also increase heartburn, and the feeling of fullness since fat takes longer to digest. On the other hand, for pregnant women who are not gaining enough weight, increasing the fat in their diet is the easiest way to add calories.

Protein, Vitamin and Mineral content is usually listed as a percentage of the U.S. RDA. However the new label should have values listed as "Percent of Daily Values" which are based on average nutrient needs. These numbers can be used as a "measuring stick" to compare other foods with. Do keep in mind that while pregnant and nursing, your needs will always be higher than the "Daily Values".

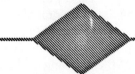

Checking out the Fat

According to the National Consumer's League, 52% of us check the fat content on our food labels.

Fats: Fat is listed in grams and as number of calories from fat   Saturated and unsaturated fat content will also be listed. Saturated fat is hard at room temperature and can lead to increased serum cholesterol. In general, your diet should have as little saturated fat as possible. Large health organizations such as the American Heart Association and the American Dietetic Association recommend that everyone over 2 years old should eat a diet that contains an average of less than 30% of the total calories from fat (2).

Cholesterol: Cholesterol is a fat like substance found only in animal products. The American Heart Association recommends an intake of less than 300 mg. per day for adults (3). A high blood cholesterol level is related to increased heart disease risk. However, a high saturated fat diet is more likely to raise blood cholesterol than dietary cholesterol itself.

Carbohydrates: You may find these on the label:

Total carbohydrates, complex carbohydrates, sugars and fiber. Complex carbohydrates such as bread, potatoes and pasta take longer to digest than sugars. Sugars listed on the label may also include fruit sugar from raisins or other fruit.

Fiber: An intake of 20-35 grams of fiber per day is recommended per day by the National Cancer Institute and other health organizations (4). Fiber is usually listed at the bottom of the label, sometimes with the carbohydrate information. A food is considered a good source of fiber if it has 4 grams or more per serving.

Hey what are all those funny words on the food label?

You may have noticed there are many more things on the ingredient list besides food; these are called food additives. An additive is considered a substance other than a basic foodstuff that is in food as a result of production, processing, storage or packaging.

There has been much in the media regarding food additives; so much so that the word "additive" may bring to mind something negative. In truth, additives often protect our food from spoilage (and therefore keep us from getting sick) and bring clear benefits. For example, many foods are fortified with vitamins and minerals; these are considered additives. Many new fat-free products contain plant gums or seaweed derivatives which have been safely used for centuries. Those are also considered additives.

Listed below are the main categories of additives and what they do:

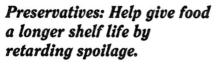

Preservatives: Help give food a longer shelf life by retarding spoilage.

Antimicrobials: Used to prevent food spoilage from bacteria, mold, or fungus. Calcium propionate is used to keep bread from molding.

Antioxidants: Prevent oil-containing foods from going rancid and also delay browing. Vitamin C (ascorbic acid) is commonly used in meats as an antioxidant.

Curing Agents: Used to prevent spoilage in meats. Sodium nitrate is often found in smoked meats.

Flavoring Agents: Directly or indirectly add flavor to a product.

Sweeteners: including natural and artificial. Many new artificial sweeteners are awaiting FDA approval.

Flavor enhancers: Added to food to enhance flavor without leaving a flavor of its own. Monosodium Glutamate or MSG occurs naturally in food and is also added to food to bring out the natural flavors.

Artificial Flavoring: Adds flavor lost in processing or increases natural flavor.

Coloring Agents:

Natural, Nature identical and Synthetic FD&C colorings: Most foods we eat have some added coloring, even cheddar cheese! Color is often added to a product because consumers expect food to be a certain color.

Texturizing Agents

Emulsifiers: Helps to evenly distribute tiny particles of liquid: keeps oil and water mixed as in creamy salad dressings.

Stabilizers or Thickeners: Gives body, or texture. Gums and other thickeners are used in fat-free salad dressings to give them the consistency of regular dressing.

Nutrients:

Vitamins, minerals and fibers are often added to replace nutrients lost in processing or to fortify a food to improve it's nutritional value.

Miscellaneous:

Other types of additives include leavening agents, propellants, pH control agents, humectants, dough conditioners, and anti-caking agents.

Are Food Additives Safe?

Yes; the vast majority of food additives are safe. Some are positively beneficial; others may cause reactions in sensitive individuals. Additives which are questionable continue to undergo evaluation. Keep in mind that overconsumption of any one food or food component can have consequences. Lack of variety in the diet causes an excess of some dietary elements and a deficit of others.

For example, sodium nitrate, which is found in cured meats, can be converted to nitrosamines which may be cancer causing. Vitamin C is often added with nitrates to prevent their conversion to nitrosamine. Sulfites are another type of additive used as an antibrowning agent. They are most often found in dried fruits and in some beer and wine. Up to 10% of the population is sensitive to sulfites; particularly those with asthma. If a food contains sulfite, it is listed on the nutrition label.

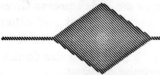

If You Are Concerned about Food Additives

1. Make sure to eat a wide variety of foods

2. Eat as many "whole foods" as possible, limiting mixes and convenience foods.

3. Use fresh meat more often than cured or smoked meats.

4. Eat fresh fruits, vegetables, milk and whole grains for snacks instead of packaged snack foods.

EATING ON A BUDGET

Let's face it, raising children is expensive. If this is your first child, you may have already found that just furnishing the nursery can cost a bundle! You may be looking for ways to cuts costs on food. It is possible to eat a nutritious diet and limit your food costs. But it does take some advanced planning and in some cases, thinking about saving for the long term.

Saving for the Long Term:

Invest in a deep freezer.

Though this represents a great investment, it can allow you to buy in bulk and stock up on things that are on sale.

A grocer in my city often has "buy one, get one free" sales and there is no limit on the number that you buy. Take chicken for example. If you could buy enough chicken for 6 months and get it for half price, that would be quite a bargain. If you live near a cattle ranch, you can invest in a side of beef (or split with a friend) and you'll have tremendous savings as well as very lean cuts of meat.

Buy in Bulk-store or share with a friend.

This only works if you will actually use the food. If half of it spoils before you use it, it's not a bargain anymore! A friend of mine makes homemade granola and lots of other homemade goods. She buys 50 pounds of oatmeal at a time from a health-food store and saves lots of money!

Plant a garden with enough to can or freeze.

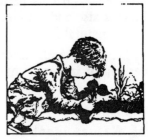

Fresh produce are sometimes the most expensive foods. Having your own garden and canning or freezing what's left for the next winter can save you a "bushel."

Plant fruit trees which will yield fruit in a few years.

Can you imagine stepping out in your back yard and picking a fresh grapefruit? My cousin in Florida does. Or how about some fresh apples to make a fresh apple pie? Check with local specialists to find out which fruit trees grow well in your area.

While Shopping:

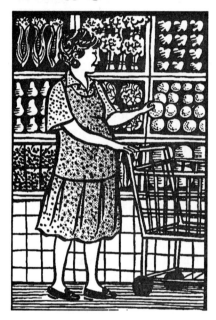

♦ If you have other children, make sure they are not hungry or tired when you shop or try to leave them at home. This will not only give you time to concentrate on reading labels and comparison shopping, it will also prevent you from buying extra treats to keep them happy.

♦ Don't go shopping when tired or hungry. Always shop with a list.

♦ Clip coupons and shop the sales. One saturday I took this a bit too far. I went to 3 stores buying up all the great bargains. It was tiring, but I saved at least 30% on my groceries that week!

♦ Fruit is often cheaper when in 5 pound bags, but produce is not always cheaper when packaged. Mushrooms and tomatoes are good examples of this.

♦ When using coupons, make sure to compare the price of the food with the coupon compared to the store or generic brand. Often I find that even with the coupon, it is still more expensive.

♦ In the summer, farmer's market prices are often cheaper. Again if you can arrange to buy in bulk, you save. For example, we bought a large box of tomatoes for just $5.00 and made homemade tomato sauce, which we froze for future soups and sauces.

♦ Buy your bread at a thrift store. I prefer a brand of bread that is probably the most expensive on the market! However, by buying it at a thrift store, I can also buy fat-free cakes, cookies and ready to make pizza crusts, all at reduced prices. To top it off, if you spend $5 or more, you get one free item!

♦ If you buy staples like beans, cereals, dried fruit, and oats from bulk containers, you not only save money but you reduce packaging which also helps the environment. Ditto for buying a large size of snack food instead of individual packages.

The Cost of Convenience

Americans want their food fast and easy, and we pay for it. When you compare the costs of homemade to various levels of convenience foods, you may be shocked!

♦ Frozen pancakes are 15 cents each, pancakes from a "shake and pour" mix are 10 cents each and those made from a 32 ounce mix are 4 cents each or close to one fourth the price of the frozen.

♦ A popular Italian salad dressing costs $1.65 for an 8 ounce bottle. A mix plus oil and vinegar costs $1.52. By being creative and adding your own herbs and spices, you save the cost of the mix; 8 ounces costs only 55 cents plus pennies for spices.

♦ Instant flavored "ready to eat" oatmeal in individual cups costs 77 cents each. Instant packets of oatmeal costs 30 cents each. Old fashioned oatmeal, which offers the best nutrition value, costs only 7 cents per serving.

♦ Frozen bran muffins cost 75 cents each. Ready to eat muffins from the bakery cost 46 cents each. A Jiffy™ Bran Muffin Mix including added ingredients costs only 5 cents each!

When Menu Planning

♦ Plan your menus with budget in mind. Make less expensive foods like grains, beans and vegetables the main course with more expensive meats "the topping." For ideas on vegetarian meals see page 297.

♦ Plan your menus around what's on sale at the store.

♦ When cooking, use powdered milk. You can double your calcium (which saves money on fresh milk) by using canned evaporated milk.

♦ Fresh fruit may seem more expensive than dessert, but it's usually not!

♦ Plan your menus with leftovers in mind. Think of different menus you can do with one dish (Beef fajitas-night 1, Fiesta Salad with beans and beef strips, night 3) or freeze some in individual containers for future lunches or quick dinners. Most people end up throwing part of their food away, because they forget about it, get tired of eating the same thing night after night or just don't like leftovers! See page 294 for leftover menus.

♦ Are you eating out because of lack of time? Frozen waffles or pancakes, even though expensive, are still cheaper than a meal at a drive-thru. A frozen sandwich like Lean Pockets is still cheaper than a burger meal (though close!) But, if you can plan ahead a bit and arrange for creative leftovers for lunch, you'll probably see the greatest savings on your food budget. The same is true for vending machine snacks, which can "eat" away at your food budget!

Stocking the Kitchen Tool Box

To make great, nutritious meals, you need to have the tools of the trade! I consider the following essential for a cook who wants to eat well but doesn't have lots of time to waste in the kitchen:

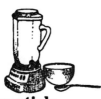

The Essentials

1. **Blender or food processor.** This is essential for making quick soups, lowfat cheese dips, stuffings and "meal on the go" drinks.

2. **Meat thermometer.** To really know if your meat is cooked to the right temperature, a meat thermometer is the most reliable method. If you like your meat rare, it is best to invest in a thermometer to make sure you have cooked your food to the temperature that kills bacteria.

3. **Microwave.** I didn't realize how much I used mine until I started writing down the recipes for this cookbook. Though most people use them just for warming leftovers or heating water, using them for cooking can be a real time saver. Nutrients can also be preserved by cooking in the microwave.

4. **Non-stick pans.** You don't have to add fat when using non-stick cookware. I also like the fact that clean-up is a breeze.

5. **Plastic cutting board.** For food safety reasons, use a plastic or acrylic cutting board instead of a wooden one. (at least for raw meats) Wooden boards are harder to sterilize and can harbor bacteria from uncooked meats.

6. **Microwave safe cookware.** Many people use leftover margarine containers for cooking in the microwave. This is not recommended because some of the chemicals in the plastic (also from plastic wrap) have been shown to migrate into the food. Until further research is done on this, use either pyrex type cookware or containers made especially for the microwave.

7. **Miscellaneous gadgets.** A few good quality knives, nylon spatulas and spoons for non-stick cookware, measuring cups and spoons and a wire whisk should be part of every kitchen. These few tools will make life easier for the cook!

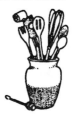

Nice to Have Items

1. **Mini-chopper.** These are mini-food processors which only hold about a cup. They are great for chopping onion, garlic or other vegetables to a fine consistency. This is a great gadget for women who are sensitive to the smells of cooking in the first trimester.

2. **Rotating platter for microwave.** This assures that your food is cooked evenly to the correct temperature. It also saves you from having to stop the microwave every few minutes to rotate 1/2 a turn!

3. **Salad spinner.** I love salad, but I hate washing and drying all those lettuce leaves. We got a salad spinner for a wedding gift and it makes the salad making process much easier.

Really Nice to Have Items

(in other words, your wish list for Christmas after you have a nice college fund going!)

1. **Ice Cream Maker**. Great for making frozen yogurt and sorbets that can satisfy your sweet tooth without a lot of fat.

2. **Bread Maker**. Imagine waking up to fresh bread every morning! Making your own whole grain bread may help you increase the fiber in your diet.

3. **Hand-held blender**. These are the type you see advertised on TV. Some of my clients have told me they really do whip skim milk, they really can grind meat, crush ice and make milkshakes.

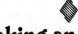

Cooking and Storing to Keep the Vitmins

Which is better, frozen, canned or fresh vegetables?

When it's straight from your garden, nothing beats freshly picked foods. However, frozen vegetable can actually have higher nutrient content than fresh in some cases.

Fresh vegetables may not be so fresh by the time you buy them, and especially if they stay several days (or weeks!) in your refrigerator. The way you cook them can also affect nutrient content. Recently a University of Illinois researcher found that "fresh"

beans from the store which had left the farm 7 days earlier had lost 50% of their vitamin C. After 3 days in a home refrigerator, they had lost 10% more. However, frozen beans had lost only 30% of their vitamin C after 4 months in the freezer. In this case, frozen vegetables were a better choice (5).

Canned vegetables don't hold a candle, nutrient wise, to fresh or frozen. However, some people like the taste of certain canned vegetables, like corn. And it's a good idea to keep some canned veggies in the house for those times when there's "nothing to eat."

Caring for Vegetables Once They're Home.

♦ Store veggies in the crisper in their bags.

♦ To keep lettuce and other greens fresh, wrap in paper towels, then store in their bags.

♦ Don't cut, peel or wash vegetables until it's time to cook or eat them. The only exception to this might be if you like to keep carrot and celery sticks cleaned, cut and ready to eat. Having them ready to eat will increase their chances of being eaten. Eating any vegetables, even with reduced nutrient content is better than eating none at all!

♦ If possible, avoid soaking vegetables to wash them–this will deplete water soluble vitamins.

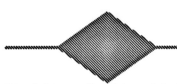

Healthiest Cooking Methods

1. Not cooked

2. Steaming/Microwave cooking

3. Stir-frying

4. Baking

5. Boiling

When foods are "cooked to death", they don't taste good, they have the consistency of baby food, and they also have lost much of their water soluble vitamins like B vitamins and vitamin C.

Tips to cook your vegetables more healthfully:

♦ To cook vegetables in the microwave, add 1-2 Tb. water and cover tightly. Let them stand a few minutes while covered to continue cooking. This is a wonderful way to cooked cubed potatoes. They are so moist they're great without added fat. (See page 314 for variations of this recipe)

♦ When stir frying, put the more dense vegetables in the pan first. For example, start with onion, garlic and spices for flavor, then add carrots, celery, cabbage, broccoli; at the end add softer vegetables like peas, mushrooms and greens.

♦ Steaming over a rack in a pressure cooker is almost too fast! Watch the time carefully to avoid overcooking.

♦ When boiling, use just enough water to prevent scorching. Some

vegetables require covering with water, like potatoes. Cut them in pieces to shorten cooking time.

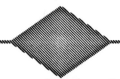

Lowfat, High Fiber Cookies

Those with a sweet tooth will be happy to know that some cookies are now a bit more nutritious. The following cookies are low in fat and are made with whole grain or are high in fiber (6).

Health Valley Fat-Free Fruit Centers

Health Valley Fat-Free

Fat-Free Frookies

Archway Old Fashioned Molasses

Barbara's Bakery Oatmeal

Frookies Animal Crackers

Health Valley Honey Jumbo Peanut Butter

Frookies Fruitins

Since new food products come on the market every day, be sure to check your store for new products that are low in sugar and fat and high in fiber.

Food Safety In A Nutshell For Pregnant Women

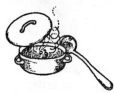

Most of us are so busy cooking all the right foods, exercising and taking other measures for our baby, that we don't stop to think about how we can make our kitchens "safe." By safe I don't mean just making sure the pot handle is not facing out. There are many more dangers lurking in the kitchen and they depend on how you handle your food before, during, and after you cook it, and even how you make your food selections.

Specifically, the concerns in your kitchen usually can't be seen, smelled or tasted. They are hidden in the form of bacteria, fungus and molds. About 9,000 people die of food-borne illness each year in the U.S. Pregnant women have more to risk; fetuses can be severely harmed by some bacteria. A bout of food poisoning could also slow baby's growth from mom's lack of nutrition.

If you don't read the rest of this chapter make sure to read the following summary.

♦ Do choose lowfat fish and meats (Pesticides, chemicals, and metals accumulate in the fat.)

♦ Remove skin and inner organs of fish before making soups and stews.

♦ DO thoroughly reheat leftovers or ready to eat foods such as hot dogs until steaming hot.

♦ Store fish in the coldest area of your refrigerator and cook within a day.

♦ Keep your refrigerator clean and at 35-40° F.

♦ Keep hot foods over 140° F and cold foods at or below 40° F.

♦ Keep hot or cold foods at room temperature as short of time possible.

♦ AVOID raw or unpasteurized milk.

♦ DO eat a variety of foods.

♦ DO keep raw and cooked foods separate. Use separate cutting boards and knives for each to prevent transfer of bacteria.

♦ DON'T eat foods with uncooked or undercooked eggs like eggnog, caesar salads, uncooked souffles and homemade ice creams. (Pasteurized eggnog or that are made with pasteurized eggs are safe.)

♦ DON'T eat any raw fish or shellfish.

♦ When refrigerating large portions of food, divide into smaller containers so they can cool more quickly.

♦ DO cook raw meat to an internal temperature of 160° F, poultry to 180° F and fish to 145° F. Avoid any raw or undercooked animal protein.

♦ If you have cats, don't let them on food preparation areas.

♦ DON'T eat soft cheeses like Mexican style cheese, (Queso Fresca or Queso Blanco), Feta, Brie, Blue cheese and Camembert. These can harbor a bacteria called *Listeria*, which is particularly harmful to fetuses.

♦ If you are pregnant, trying to become pregnant or nursing, eat as little as possible of swordfish, shark, bluefish and salmon from the Great Lakes and Hudson River area. They can be contaminated with heavy metals or chemicals which can harm the fetus (more details on this below.)

♦ DON'T store fruit juice or acidic foods in ceramic containers (especially imported ones), or leaded crystal decanters, because lead can be leached into the food or drink. Also choose seamless cans or welded seam cans instead of soldered seam cans, which may have lead.

♦ Avoid drinking hot liquids like coffee or tea in ceramic mugs which may have leaded glaze. The hot acidic coffee can cause small amounts of lead to leach into your beverage.

♦ If you have lead pipes or lead soldered pipes, let the water run for a few minutes before using. Avoid using warm tap water for drinking or cooking. (See page 39 for more information on lead exposure.)

Source: *Safe Food; Eating Wisely in a Risky World*, Michael Jacobson, Lisa Lefferts, and Anne Witte Garland, Center for Science in the Public Interest, 1991 and Background Paper; *Preventing Foodborne Listeriosis*, USDA, US Department of Health and Human Services and FDA, April 1992.

The Essential Guide to Food Safety

Making Your Kitchen Safe

When you're preparing food:

1. Wash hands in hot soapy water before preparing food and after using the bathroom, blowing your nose, petting the dog, changing a diaper, etc. This is common sense of course, but these are the most common ways in which bacteria are passed through food.

2. Keep raw meats and produce away from each other. Use a separate cutting board for raw meats and uncooked foods. Wash the "meat" board in the dishwasher after use. Use a plastic cutting board instead of a wooden one--the wood can't be cleaned as well and may harbor bacteria. Use paper towels instead of a reusable sponge or rag to wipe away blood from meat, fish or poultry. Wash hands well with soap after handling meat and before handling other foods, especially raw produce.

3. Wash sponges, towels and kitchen rags often; bacteria can survive quite well in them. Replace sponges every few weeks. Between replacing them, try washing them in the washing machine with bleach.

4. Thaw food in the microwave or refrigerator-NOT ON THE KITCHEN COUNTER.

When Eating Out–at Restaurants, Picnics and Friends

1. Don't eat anything that has been sitting out for hours without proper refrigeration or heat. Recently there was an outbreak of *Salmonella* from canteloupe. The canteloupe was cut without the outside being washed and bacteria got onto the edible portion. After sitting out unrefrigerated, the bacteria had a chance to grow to the point that it caused illness.

2. If meat, fish or chicken doesn't look like it is cooked well enough, ask for it to be cooked more thoroughly. Be assertive. (Smoked foods will still look pink, even when done.)

3. If food that should be cold, isn't, don't eat it. Recently, my husband and I ordered a piece of cream pie to share. About half-way through, I realized that it wasn't cold at all and alerted the waitress. She found out that the refrigerator was broken but no one had noticed it!

4. Avoid restaurants that don't practice good sanitation. For example, people that handle food should have a hair covering and should have clean hands. If someone takes your money and then directly touches your food, your food is not very clean! Also, people who work with food must wash their hands after using the restroom, blowing their nose, smoking or eating before they handle food again. If you find workers that don't follow these rules they should be reported to your local health department.

"Is it still good?"

Do you find yourself asking this question often? Here is a guide from the U. S. Department of Agriculture (USDA) about how long you can safely refrigerate and freeze various foods.

Food Storage Guide

Eggs, Meat and Poultry

Food	Suggested storage time in:	
	Refrigerator at 40°F	Freezer at 0°F
Eggs, in shell	3 weeks	Don't freeze
Mayonnaise, commercial, Refrigerate after opening	2 months	Don't freeze
TV dinners, frozen casseroles		3-4 months
Egg, chicken, tuna, ham or macaroni salad (from deli or home-made)	3-5 days	These products don't freeze well.
Pre-stuffed pork & lamb chops, or stuffed chicken breast	1 day	
Store-cooked convenience foods (ready to serve)	1-2 days	
Soups & stews (vegetable or meat based)	3-4 days	2-3 months
Hamburger & stew meats	1-2 days	3-4 months
Ground turkey, veal, pork, or lamb	1-2 days	3-4 months
Hot dogs, opened package	1 week	In freezer wrap, 1-2 months
Hot dogs, unopened package	2 weeks	
Lunch meats, opened	3-5 days	
Lunch meats, unopened	2 weeks	
Bacon	1 week	1 month
Sausage, raw	1-2 days	1-2 months
Smoked sausage	1 week	1-2 months
Hard sausage-pepperoni, etc.	2-3 weeks	1-2 months
Corned beef (in pouch with pickling juices)	5-7 days	Drained, wrapped 1 month
Ham, canned, unopened	6-9 months	Don't freeze
Ham, cooked-whole	7 days	1-2 months
Ham-cooked-half	3-5 days	1-2 months

Food Storage Guide

Food	Suggested storage time in:	
	Refrigerator at 40°F	**Freezer at 0°F**
Ham-cooked, slices	3-4 days	1-2 months
Fresh Meat		
Beef steaks	3-5 days	6-12 months
Pork chops	3-5 days	4-6 months
Lamb chops	3-5 days	6-9 months
Beef roast	3-5 days	6-12 months
Lamb roast	3-5 days	6-9 months
Pork & veal roast	3-5 days	4-6 months
Variety meats-tongue, brain, kidney, liver, heart	1-2 days	3-4 months
Cooked Meat Leftovers		
Cooked meat and meat dishes	3-4 days	2-3 months
Gravy & meat broth	1-2 days	2-3 months
Fresh poultry		
Chicken or turkey, whole	1-2 days	1 year
Chicken or turkey pieces	1-2 days	9 months
Giblets	1-2 days	3-4 months
Cooked, Leftover Poultry		
Fried chicken	3-4 days	4 months
Cooked poultry dishes	3-4 days	4-6 months
Pieces of chicken, plain	3-4 days	4 months
Pieces with broth or gravy	1-2 days	6 months
Chicken nuggets, patties	1-2 days	1-3 months

Food Storage Guide

Seafood Storage Guide

SEAFOOD STORAGE GUIDE

Product	Purchased Commercially Frozen for Freezer Storage	Purchased Fresh & Home Frozen	Thawed; Never Frozen or Previously Frozen & Home Refrigerated
FISH			
FILLETS/STEAKS:			
Lean:			
Cod, Flounder	10-12 months	6-8 months	36 hours
Haddock, Halibut	10-12 months	6-8 months	36 hours
Pollock, Ocean Perch	8-9 months	4 months	36 hours
Sea Trout, Rockfish	8-9 months	4 months	36 hours
Pacific Ocean Perch	8-9 months	4 months	36 hours
Fat:			
Mullet, Smelt	6-8 months	N/A	36 hours
Salmon (cleaned)	7-9 months	N/A	36 hours
SHELLFISH			
Dungeness Crab	6 months	6 months	5 days
Snow Crab	6 months	6 months	5 days
Blue Crabmeat (fresh)	N/A	4 months	5-7 days
Blue Crabmeat (pasteurized)	N/A	N/A	6 months
Cocktail Claws	N/A	4 months	5 days
King Crab	12 months	9 months	7 days
Surimi Seafoods	10-12 months	9 months	2 weeks
Shrimp	9 months	5 months	4 days
Oysters, shucked	N/A	N/A	4-7 days
Clams, shucked	N/A	N/A	5 days
Lobster, live	N/A	N/A	1-2 days
Lobster, tailmeat	8 months	6 months	4-6 days
BREADED SEAFOODS			
Shrimp	12 months	8 months	N/A
Scallops	18 months	10 months	N/A
Fish Sticks	18 months	N/A	N/A
Portions	18 months	N/A	N/A
SMOKED FISH			
Herring	N/A	2 months	3-4 days
Salmon, Whitefish	N/A	2 months	5-8 days

Footnotes:

- N/A - not applicable or not advised.
- These storage guidelines indicate optimal shelf life for seafood products held under proper refrigeration or freezing conditions. Temperature fluctuations in home refrigerators will affect optimal shelf life, as will opening and closing refrigerators and freezers often.
- Although the above storage times ensure a fresh product for maximum refrigeration storage life at 32°F., the consumer should plan on using seafood within 36 hours for optimal quality and freshness of the product.
- To determine approximate storage time for those species not listed, ask your retailer which category (lean, fat, shellfish, breaded or smoked) they fall within and refer to the guide.

National Fisheries Institute, 2000 M Street, NW, Suite 580, Washington, DC 20036

Food Storage Guide

Dairy Products

Food	Suggested Storage Time*	
	Refrigerator at 40°F	Freezer at 0°F
Milk	8-20 days	Not recommended due to reduced quality of product after thawing.
Buttermilk	2-3 weeks	
Sour Cream	3-4 weeks	
Yogurt	3-6 weeks	
Eggnog	1-2 weeks	
Ultra Pasteurized Cream	6-8 weeks	
Parmesan cheese	almost indefinitely	
Swiss and cheddar cheese	1 month	6-8 weeks
Grated cheese in moisture proof packaging, unopened	12 months	6-8 weeks
Process cheese food in jars, unopened	3 months	Not recommended

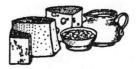

*Refers to the amount of time after processing, not after purchasing.

Source: *Newer Knowledge of Milk*, National Dairy Council, 1988 and *Newer Knowledge of Cheese*, National Dairy Council, 1986.

According to DeeAnn Whitmire a registered dietitian and Communication Specialist with Western Dairy Council, "A good rule of thumb is that you can keep a dairy product one week after the date printed on the package or the "pull" date. Also, when in doubt, throw it out, since how you handle a product can affect it's freshness (7)."

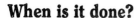

When is it done?

Don't be impatient when cooking meats; it takes time to cook them thoroughly and it takes thorough cooking to kill harmful bacteria.

To check visually if it's done, red meat is done when it's brown or grey inside; poultry is done when juices run clear; and fish is done when it becomes opaque and flakes with a fork.

Cook eggs until the white is firm and yolk is no longer runny. This lessens the chances that the egg is harboring *Salmonella*.

Cook beef, pork and lamb to an internal temperature of 160° F; whole chicken or turkey to 180° F. Cook fish to a temperature of 145° F for at least 5 minutes. In general fish should be cooked 10 minutes per inch of thickness.

Other Hidden Risks in Your Food Supply

O.K., you decide you're going to avoid all those preservatives by simply eating fresh fruits and vegetables, homemade grains, and fresh fish chicken and beef. Now you're totally safe from the undesirable compounds in food, right? Wrong!

Unfortunately, it's hard to get away from all risks in food. The important thing is to keep food safety in perspective. Pesticide use is still common, though reduced use is becoming possible through crop rotation and biotechnology. Organic farming is also gaining popularity.

Although growth hormones have widespread use, their use is looked upon as safe. Polluted waters can cause our fish to be contaminated with heavy metals like mercury and other chemicals. Improper handling of any raw fish, poultry or fish can cause bacterial growth.

Despite the potential dangers in our food, our food supply is one of the safest in the world.

According to Dr. Martha Stone, Professor of Food Science at Colorado State University, "Our food supply is the safest, most wholesome, most abundant in the world. Aren't we fortunate? (8)"

It is important to be "picky" about what you eat and how you prepare foods while pregnant. While exposure to some contaminants is harmless for you, it may be harmful to your baby. Also, eating a variety of many different foods is vital to decrease your exposure to various contaminants as well as to increase your intake of a variety of nutrients.

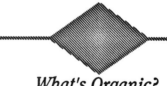

What's Organic?

Organic simply means grown without synthetic pesticides and herbicides; instead farmers use biological methods of pest control such as compost and beneficial insects. There is no national standard for "organic" though states like California, Oregon, Minnesota, Texas, Washington and Colorado have certification programs. However, there are national standards being developed and should be in effect in a year or two. Check with your State Department

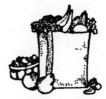

of Agriculture or Department of Health for more information.

Organic doesn't necessarily mean "free of pesticide residues". Some growers take over plots of land that contain enough pesticide residue in the soil to grow perfect looking produce. However, they can still claim "no pesticides used" (9). The only sure way to know you are getting true pesticide free produce is to buy "certified organic." Fortunately, organic farming is becoming more popular and we should be seeing more organic products in the next few years. According to Helen Davis of the Colorado Department of Agriculture, "Organic farming methods do not change the nutritional quality of produce. However, organically grown produce is often fresher, which would slightly improve it's nutrient value 10)."

To Lower Your Risk

The following section will give you tips on selecting and handling foods so that you can have the safest food possible.

Fruits, Vegetables, Grains and Nuts

The biggest risk regarding fruits and vegetables is not consuming enough! The slight risk of illness due to pesticide exposure is minimal compared to the risk of illness from not consuming enough produce.

◆ Grow your own

◆ Buy locally grown produce; it's fresher, picked closer to it's peak ripeness, and probably isn't coated with wax or sprayed with post-harvest pesticides. Usually a local farmer's market or roadside stand is great for this. However, last summer when I asked where the produce came from at my local farmer's market, some of it was from four states away!

◆ Buy domestically grown produce (this is also good for local farmers.) Ironically, pesticides that are banned in the U.S. are still produced for export. Some of those pesticides find their way back into the country on imported foods.

◆ Buy fruits and vegetables in season. If you buy a canteloupe in the dead of winter, you can be sure it was grown pretty far south. That means it had to be picked early, and was probably sprayed with post harvest pestiticides and wax to make sure it showed up at your store looking just picked!

◆ The large national brands of peanut butter probably have the highest quality standards in terms of aflatoxins, a naturally occurring carcinogen. Throw away any moldy, discolored or shriveled peanuts, pecans, walnuts, almonds, Brazil nuts, and pistachios–they can also have aflatoxins.

◆ Store potatoes in a cool, dark place. Trim away any green or damaged marks--they contain a toxin (glycoalkaloids) that can affect the nervous system (10).

♦ Consider certified organic produce. (In Colorado, this means that there have been no pesticides used on the land for 3 years, though pesticide residues may still be present.) However, since the cost is sometimes prohibitive, following the other tips in this chapter may work best for you. If you do buy organic, beware that it won't look perfect. One reason pesticide use is so popular is that Americans demand that perfect looking orange, or flawless lettuce!

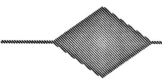

Questions about using pesticides or their safety?

Call the National Telecommunications Network Hotline, funded by the EPA and operated at Texas Tech University: 1-800-858-PEST, 24 hours a day, 365 days a year.

Putting Pesticides in Perspective

According to Dr. Bruce Ames, Chairman of the Biochemistry Department, University of California, Berkeley,

"The man made pesticide residues in the American diet are present in trivial amounts and are not a credible risk factor for causing cancer. The danger has been widely exaggerated by piling worst case assumptions–none of these assumptions are turning out to be true. The FDA and EPA are doing an adequate job of protecting our food supply from carcinogenic contaminants."

Instead of worrying about risks that have very little real danger, we should look at the whole picture of food safety. According to Dr. Sanford Miller of the University of Texas Health Sciences Center in San Antonio, "There simply is no public health problem with pesticide residues. The real risks in the food supply are microbiological hazards;... risk for illness from microbes is 1 in 100, while risk of illness from pesticides is 1 in 1,000,000 (11)."

Although less than 1% of food samples analyzed for pesticides in 1989 exceeded tolerances set by the EPA, the amounts were often just a fraction of EPA tolerances. Nevertheless, it is always a good idea to wash produce to remove any tiny amount of residue that may be present.

Guide to Peeling and Washing Produce

To peel or not to peel? It's a toss up: peeling does completely remove all surface pesticides (whereas washing might not remove them all), but peeling can also mean losing valuable fiber and nutrients. As a general rule, peel produce if your diet is otherwise rich in fiber–especially produce that is obviously waxed, to remove the wax and any pesticides that might have been applied with it.

Always wash produce. Adding a few drops of dish soap to a pint of water is more effective than plain water at removing many pesticides. Just choose a soap brand that isn't loaded with dyes and perfumes. Don't use salt water or vinegar-they won't help, and salt is something we get more than enough of anyway. And there's no evidence that those specially formulated pesticide and wax removing washes are more effective than regular dish detergent-and they cost up to eight times as much! Use a vegetable brush, and be sure to rinse completely.

Here are some tips for handling specific types of produce (instead of buying organic food):

♦ For leafy vegetables like lettuce and cabbage, discard outer leaves and wash the inner leaves.

♦ Wash celery after trimming off the leaves and tops.

♦ For recipes that call for grated peel, buy organic fruit if possible.

♦ Peel carrots (you won't be losing out on fiber, since it is found throughout. Peel cucumbers if they're waxed. Peel apples, peaches and pears if you get plenty of fiber from other sources, since these are apt to contain risky residues.

♦ Wash eggplants, peppers, tomatoes, potatoes, green beans, cherries, grapes, and strawberries. Cut up cauliflower, broccoli, and spinach before you wash them, since pesticides may be hard to wash off otherwise.

Copyright 1991, Reprinted from *Safe Food*, which is available from CSPI, 1875 Conn. Ave., N.W., #300, Washington DC, 20009 for $9.95.

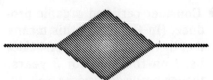

Food Safety Issues–Who to Believe?

In 1989, two stories about food safety hit the headlines and people all over the country lingered at their plates, wondering if anything was safe to eat. First the Alar scare came, which Washington apple growers are just now recovering from. Soon after, a story about two cyanide infected grapes made the news. As a result, the purchase of all imported foods from Chile dropped off, causing economic hardship there.

Food safety issues often appeal to our emotions, since the safety of our children is often cited. However, when we react with our hearts instead of our minds, our opinions and decisions are likely to be based on feelings, not facts.

Many activist groups are involved in food safety issues and for the most part, their claims are valid. However, when scientific information is taken out of context and blown out of proportion to it's real effect on our health, people are needlessly misled, confused and frightened.

Depending on which side of an issue you are on, there is probably a scientific study to back you up. Therefore, it is hard to know what the answers are. Frankly, we don't know all the answers about nutrition and health, which is why you may hear one story today and hear a completely different story tomorrow. When an issue

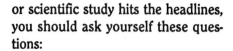

or scientific study hits the headlines, you should ask yourself these questions:

1. Who is reporting the information? It is a neutral group or someone with something to gain from the results? For example, someone who is selling vitamin supplements may recite this or that study. Though the points made may be valid, it's important to separate facts from opinion, especially when a person's opinions may be biased.

On the other hand, it's common for many large companies to fund research by well respected universities. However, this doesn't mean the research is biased or of lower quality. Let's face it, who would want to put up millions of dollars for research on oatmeal–besides the producers of the food?

2. If it is a scientific study, was it done on animals or humans? Though many effects are the same in animals and humans, it can't always be assumed that the results can be equally compared.

3. How large was the sample size? Research using a group of 10 people won't be as reliable as research on a group of 1000.

4. How many studies have been done on the subject? It takes many studies to prove anything conclusively. One study shouldn't cause you to change dietary habits drastically, unless the evidence is very strong.

Dairy Products

The biggest potential risk from eating dairy products are from drinking raw or unpasteurized milk, and from bacterial contamination due to improper handling.

Like all perishable foods, dairy products are very safe foods, if handled properly. One issue that has gotten some recent attention is the use of BST on dairy cows.

You may have heard of cows being given a hormone called Bovine Somatotropine (BST). This is a naturally occurring hormone produced by dairy cows. Scientists have found a way to produce the hormone synthetically, and when given to cows it can increase their milk production by 10-30%.

The National Institutes of Health (NIH) has concluded that milk from BST treated cows is safe for humans (12). The use of supplemental BST is generally regarded as safe by the medical community (13).

So what's all the fuss? Actually, much of the controversy surrounding this issue is based on social or economic grounds. Some people feel that an increased milk supply may take away jobs from dairy farmers and some people are concerned that injections of BST may adversely affect dairy cows. Others are just opposed to biotechnology in general.

Tips for eating and storing dairy products:

♦ Buy only pasteurized milk and milk products. Avoid any raw milk, including goat's milk.

♦ Avoid cheeses that have been known to be contaminated with the dangerous *Listeria* bacteria; Brie, Camembert, Feta, Blue Cheese and Mexican Style soft cheese (Queso Blanco and Queso Fresca).

♦ Keep your refrigerator at or below 40° F. and keep milk refrigerated. If you like to put milk on the table for meals, don't keep it out long. Milk left out at room temperature just briefly can allow bacteria growth and speed spoilage. Never return unused milk to its original container after it has been sitting out for a while.

♦ See chart on page 202 for storage times for dairy products.

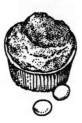

Eggs

The number one food safety problem with eggs is with *Salmonella* bacteria, which are often passed on from the hen before the egg is formed. Though rare, *Salmonella* poisoning can be fatal, especially if someone with a weakened immune system is affected. Unfortunately, *Salmonella* poisoning is on the rise, especially in the Northeast. Luckily, there is no need to avoid eggs; the protein in eggs is of very high quality! Here are some tips for keeping your eggs safe.

Buying and Storing:

♦ Buy only eggs that have been refrigerated.

♦ Store them in their own container, to keep them from getting microscopic cracks.

♦ Don't wash the eggs; they are usually washed, sanitized and a coating of mineral oil has been put on to keep out bacteria.

♦ Buy eggs that aren't cracked–bacteria can seep through. You have a better chance of getting uncracked eggs if you buy AA or A eggs, which are required to be clean and uncracked.

Eating:

♦ Avoid any food containing raw egg, or egg white. According to Dr. Pat Kendall, Food Science Specialist with Colorado State University, most of the *Salmonella* bacteria is found in the egg yolk (15). When you eat out, question "health shakes," Caesar salad dressing, and cold mousse desserts or souffles, which may contain raw eggs. Also avoid unpasteurized eggnog and homemade ice cream or eggnog that is made with raw eggs.

♦ Cook your eggs well. If you prefer your eggs runny, you might opt for an egg substitute, which contains pasteurized eggs. Eggs with the shell should have the yolk and white cooked until firm.

♦ Avoid the temptation of licking the spoon of cake batter or cookie dough containing raw eggs.

Beef and Pork

The potential food safety risk from eating beef or pork is from bacterial contamination due to improper handling during processing, or more often, by the consumer. Eating raw or undercooked beef can increase your chances of toxoplasmosis, an illness caused by a parasite, which can be harmful to the fetus.

The danger from trichinosis in pork is much reduced from past generations. Trichinosis is an illness caused by eating raw or undercooked pork that is infected with a type of worm. It is completely destroyed at 138° F (15).

The Facts about Drugs and Hormones

One of the main concerns one reads about regarding safety of animal meat is that of drug residues. About 40 years ago it was discovered that small, preventive doses of certain antibiotics improved growth in livestock. The National Cattlemen's Association recommends against the routine use of antibiotic in feed for cattle and it is thought that most beef producers are following their recommendation. When antibiotics are used to treat illness in cows, there is a standard weaning period before the cow goes to the market.

Hormones

"Growth hormones have been used safely and successfully for almost 30 years to increase lean production and feed efficiency," says Lowell L. Wilson, Animal Science Department, Pennsylvania State University (16).

Hormones improve animal growth. For example, beef cattle that have a tiny amount of growth hormone implanted in the ear grow faster, go to market sooner and are leaner. According to the Beef Industry, if hormone implants were not used, the supply of beef would be smaller and prices that consumers pay would be higher.

A Texas A & M report concluded that it is now agreed in the scientific community that the proper use of certain hormones is harmless to the consumer and may enhance animal growth performance by as much as 20% (17). The University of California Wellness Letter, March 1989 reported "At the prescribed dosages used in feed lots, these hormones have been certified safe by numerous scientific studies."

Surprisingly, hormones are present in nearly all the plant and animal foods we eat. In fact, many common foods exceed the level of estrogen found in beef given a supplemental dose of the hormone.

Estrogen Levels in Food

Food	Serving Size	Estrogen (in nano-grams)
Beef, from a cow implanted with estrogen	3 oz.	1.85
Beef, from a cow not given estrogen	3 oz.	1.01
Egg	1	1, 750
Cabbage	3 oz.	2,016

(one nano gram is one billionth of a gram; compared to a gram, a nanogram is equal to one blade of grass on a football field

Source: Inter-American Institute for Cooperation of Agriculture, *Report on Use of Hormonal Substances in Animals*, December 1986.

Men, women and children also produce estrogen in their bodies at levels thousands and millions of times that are found in beef. In the third trimester of pregnancy, your body will produce 37 million times the amount of estrogen found in a 3 ounce serving of beef.

From what I know about the Beef Cattle Industry and it's membership organizations, beef is probably the safest animal meat around. They follow voluntary bans on antibiotic use, and they are dedicated to production practices which will meet the consumer's demands for a safe and wholesome product. Karen Baker, Director of Consumer Affairs for Colorado Beef Council says, "Beef producers take the safety and wholesomeness of the food that they produce to heart. When the food you produce not only feeds the world, but your own family as well, there is an inherent commitment to food safety (18)."

Poultry

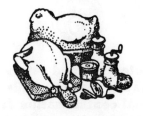

The two greatest potential risks from eating poultry are illness from two food borne bacteria, *Salmonella* and *Campylobacter*. They can be reduced or destroyed by proper cooking and handling.

Chicken is the most popular meat among my clients. It can be low in fat and prepared quickly. However, poultry can have two traveling companions that can make you sick; *Salmonella* and *Campylobacter jejuni*. *Salmonella* is a bacteria which is in the feces of chicken and spreads to other parts of the chicken during processing. Improper handling in your own kitchen adds to the risk of food poisoning from *Salmonella*.

Probably the best defense against it is sanitary kitchen procedures, as noted previously in this chapter. *Salmonella* can multiply at room temperature--a good reason to thaw poultry in the refrigerator or in the microwave instead of on the counter-top. It's also why you should keep things in a cooler or on ice when having a picnic or buffet dinner. Keeping hot foods hot (above 140° F) and cold foods cold (below 40° F) keeps *Salmonella* at bay.

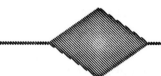

Campylobacter is another bacteria that chicken are often contaminated with. It is thought to be a very common, but under-reported ailment that sickens 2-6 million people a year. Since the symptoms (cramps, diarrhea and fever) are flu-like and can occur up to five days after eating the affected food, only one in 100 cases is thought to be reported.

Like *Salmonella*, *Campylobacter* is also a "bug" that is passed between chickens during processing. Luckily, you can control it's growth with good kitchen techniques. Here are a few tips that apply:

♦ *Campylobacter* can live in your refrigerator for weeks! Make sure to clean any juices that spill from a defrosting chicken. If juice falls on a food that will be eaten raw, (like lettuce, fruit or cheese), throw it away.

♦ Because microwave ovens cook unevenly, they may not completely kill *Campylobacter* (or *Salmonella*), so traditional methods like baking, broiling or boiling are preferred.

♦ Research shows that most of the cases of *Campylobacter* reported occur during barbecue season; a sign that perhaps people are under-cooking their grilled chickens! A combination of microwaving and grilling would ensure thorough cooking as well as a time savings. (An internal temperature of 180° F ensures "doneness.")

♦ Since *Campylobacter* is sensitive to freezing, buy frozen chickens, or freeze for a few days before using.

For more information about poultry, call the toll free USDA Meat and Poultry Hotline: 1-800-535-4555

Fish

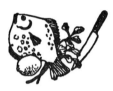

Ben Franklin said "Fish and house guests begin to smell after 3 days." He should have said two days, at least for fish, for it's unwise to keep unfrozen fish longer than that!

The greatest potential risks from eating fish are bacterial food poisoning and consumption of chemicals in fish that come from polluted waters. Proper handling and cooking can reduce or kill bacteria. While you are considering pregnancy, and when you are pregnant or breastfeeding, you should limit tuna consumption to one or two times a week and shark and swordfish intake to once a month.

Americans are eating more fish, up 25% in the last 10 years. The healthfulness of fish is probably the main reason: it's low in fat and calories and high in protein, and all varieties provide omega- 3 fatty acid-a fat component believed to have disease fighting properties.

However, there's a bit of bad news about fish and a recent study done by Consumer Reports Magazine uncovered it. They reportedly found that 30% of the fish they sampled were of poor quality, half the fish were contaminated by bacteria, and some species were contaminated by polychlorinated biphenyls (PCB's) and mercury. Part of the blame can be placed on polluted waters, while some can be put on the handling of the fish; from the fishing boat, to the processor and even in your local store (19).

Critics of the Consumer Reports study thought that the study looked at too few samples and used poor research methods.

However, the study does give us food for thought and reminds us not to take the quality of our food for granted.

Dr. Michael Bolger, a toxicologist with The Center for Food Safety and Applied Nutrition of the Food and Drug Administration disagreed with some findings of the study:

> "The data on PCB's and mercury are uncertain. They didn't do a good job of presenting that fact. They didn't give the benefits of eating fish, making the report unbalanced. Their sample size was inadequate and there was no distinction within salmon samples— they weren't from the Pacific Ocean but the Great Lakes, where only a small amount of commercial fishing is done."

> "There is no question that in certain areas PCB's continue to be a problem, such as Boston Harbor and the Great Lakes. The problem is seen in inland waters such as rivers and lakes. In marine species, there is no evidence that it is a concern except with several inshore species like Bluefish and Striped Bass."

> "The two main sources of salmon from the Great Lakes is from sports fishing and from Native Americans who have exclusive fishing rights. Those who fish in the Great Lakes should check with their local health department for fish advisories (20)."

In a 1991 report on Seafood Safety, the National Academy of Sciences said that "Fish and Shellfish are nutritious foods that constitute desirable components of a healthy diet. Most seafoods available to the U.S. public are wholesome and unlikely to cause illness in the consumer." The FDA agrees with the NAS conclusions and reminds consumers that fish and shellfish are highly perishable products that can spoil or lose quality between harvesting and consumption (21).

Janis Harsila, a registered dietitian from the National Seafood Educators says

> "The Consumer Reports article tells us not to eat any salmon but that study looked at a very small sample. When Alaska analyzed their fish they found virtually no PCB's or other pollutants, so Alaskan salmon is actually one of the safest fish to eat. Some of the purest waters are in Alaska and any

fish caught their are usually safe (22)."

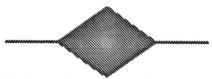

Did you have your Omega-3 Today?

In recent years a type of oil found primarily in fish, omega-3 fatty acid, shows great promise in controlling blood pressure, reducing heart disease, and improving the symptoms of rheumatoid arthritis. Now we know that developing babies need DHA (one of the omega-3's) for building brain tissue, nerve growth, and for development of the retina in the eye. Before birth, your baby gets DHA from you (that is, if you eat your share of fat-rich fish) and after birth from breast milk. Omega-3 fatty acids are so important that some scientists think that lack of the fat could result in delays or deficiencies in nervous tissue development and possibly impaired vision (23).

Good sources of omega-3 include: Anchovy, Atlantic Salmon, Coho Salmon, Herring, Mackerel, Pilchards, Pink Salmon. Sablefish, Sardines, Sockeye Salmon, Spiny Dogfish and Whitefish.

Moderately good sources include: Chum Salmon, Pompano, Rainbow Trout, Shark, Smelt, Spot, Striped Bass, Swordfish, Pacific oysters, Squid

Source: National Fisheries Institute

The Facts on Fish

Fish are among the most perishable of foods. They have a shelflife of 7-12 days once they're out of the water. Some fish stay on the fishing boat for several days, so once it gets to the store it may have little "life" left! If the fish gets warmer than 32 degrees, the shelf life decreases; it can be cut in half if kept at 42 degrees. Fattier fish and cold water fish spoil even faster.

Poor sanitation practices, such as not washing knives and cutting boards often enough, can increase bacterial growth. So can some display procedures. For example, if a fish is kept under a hot light, the fish gets warm and bacteria can multiply at a quick clip. If raw fish is displayed next to cooked fish, the cooked fish can be contaminated. (Fortunately, the bacteria in fish can be killed with proper cooking, see below.)

Other contaminants found in fish include PCB's and methylmercury, which don't pose an immediate threat to most people, but which can be harmful to the fetus. PCB's (a chemical previously used in transformer fluids) were banned in the 1970's though residues remain and will continue to be around for years to come. They accumulate in body tissue, especially fat, so they can be passed up the food chain and back down again when fish eat other fish and when some fish is turned into fish feed.

In the body, too much accumulated PCB is thought to affect neurological behavior and cognitive development in the growing fetus. Methylmercury is thought to have the same effect. There is not much data to support how sensitive the fetus is to these chemicals. One example of methylmercury poisoning was a tragic accident in Japan when fish were highly contaminated with methylmercury. The infants born during this time had severe problems similar to cerebral palsy.

Dr. Bolger of the FDA sees the subject of mercury contamination as a "grey" area; "What we know about lead and mercury is like night and day." He gives food for thought when comparing our fish eating habits with the those of the Japanese. "The Japanese eat five times more seafood than we do. If mercury has the effect that we think it has (on neurological development) you would expect to see the effects in academic achievement and economic success. Why is it then that the Japanese are doing as well as they are? If they consume more mercury than Americans do, why do they always come out on top academically (20)?" Good questions, Dr. Bolger.

Surely someone inspects fish?

Most of us assume that all fish is inspected, but up until now it has been "hit and miss." The National Marine Fisheries Institute has had a voluntary inspection service for years. Fish processors can pay to have the conditions at their plant and store observed and subsequently be given a seal of approval. According to the Consumer Reports Study, about 18% of the fish eaten currently is inspected under this program. Local and state health departments

also do some inspection of seafood, mostly through control of shellfish harvesting.

However, there's good news for fish lovers. A newly created Office of Seafood under the Food and Drug Administration will play an increasing role in seafood's safety. Already the office inspected over 3/4 of all seafood processing facilities in the U.S during it's first year of existence.

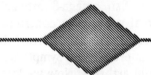

Buyer Beware

Labels which say "USDA Inspected, or US Govt inspected" is sometimes found on fish labels. USDA inspects beef, pork and chicken, but not fish.

Are all fish safe for pregnant and breastfeeding women to eat? Are there any fish that should be limited or avoided?

There are frequently many answers to the same question. Here are the positions of various people in the seafood industry, government, and consumer organizations.

Consumers Union: "For pregnant women or women who expect to become pregnant, there's little choice but to avoid...salmon, swordfish, and lake whitefish... [which] may well contain PCB's which can accumulate in the body to the point where they pose a risk to the developing fetus. Swordfish and tuna too often expose women to mercury,

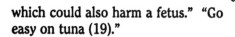

which could also harm a fetus." "Go easy on tuna (19)."

Food and Drug Administration: Dr. Michael Bolger, a toxicologist with the Food and Drug Administration says, "If a woman is concerned about contaminants in fish, the most prudent thing to do is reduce intake, but it is unwarranted to avoid eating fish if you know what the health benefits are. Eating tuna 1-2 times per week and eating shark and swordfish no more than once a month would be consistent with what we now know."

"The tolerance and action levels of PCB's and methylmercury are both being reviewed. It is more likely that the action level for methylmercury will be reduced (20)."

Center for Science in the Public Interest: "Avoid swordfish, shark and marlin. Limit yourself to 1/2 pound per week of tuna (24)."

American College of Obstetrics and Gynecology: ACOG has no specific recommendations about eating seafood. They feel seafood should be part of a varied diet (25).

Colorado Department of Health: Dr. Mike Wilson, Chief of the Environmental Toxicology Section, Colorado Department of Health says, "If you are pregnant or planning a pregnancy in the next year, you may wish to reduce your consumption of predatory fish, such as swordfish and shark to the lowest degree possible. Given the limited existing data on mercury toxicity to the developing nervous system, this is the most cautious approach (26)."

Tom Messenger, Director of the Consumer Protection Division, recommends that pregnant and breastfeeding women avoid shark and swordfish due to their mercury content. He adds that eating young fish, lean fish and fish that are lower on the food chain would help insure the lack of contaminants (27).

Tom Messenger put it all in perspective when he said "You can damage yourself with overconsumption of anything. A variety of food leads to a healthy and nutritious diet."

The bottom line on fish...

With controversy over safe levels of consumption of fish that could contain PCB's, mercury, and other environmental contaminants, I think the conservative approach is best. My advice is to try to eat fish several times a week, but limit tuna to once or twice a week and shark and swordfish to once a month. Variety and moderation are the key.

Remember, you should not AVOID fish during pregnancy or breastfeeding. They contain important nutrients for your baby. Just limit the high risk fish and eat a variety of others.

What You can Do

You can eat fish without worry by taking a few precautions:

Buying Seafood:

♦ From a health risk standpoint, frozen fish is often the best choice. It is usually quick-frozen or frozen right on the boat where it was caught, resulting in a fish that is actually fresher than "fresh." Look for and avoid freezer burn, ice crystals, and broken wrappers. Try to avoid buying fresh salmon, bluefish and catfish and freezing it when you get home. According to Clare Vanderbeek of the National Fisheries Institute, "Fish with a higher fat content deteriorate more quickly than lowfat fish. Consumers should buy those fish already commercially frozen, which will ensure a higher quality product (28)."

◆ If you choose to buy fresh fish, learn how to recognize freshness. Gills should be bright red and moist, not covered with mucus or brown colored. Eyes should be bright, clear and bulging. Avoid fish with cloudy or slime-covered eyes. The skin should have a translucent "varnished" look. Fish with skin that is starting to discolor, that has tears or blemishes should be left at the store.

◆ Watch for troubling display habits: fish stacked in large piles (harder to keep at coldest temperatures), raw fish next to cooked fish, strong "fishy" odor (means more bacteria), or fish displayed under bright, hot lights.

◆ If you can, find out where your fish came from–the further from shore, the better. You can also ask to see a tag for shellfish that tells when it was caught and shipped. Both pieces of information may require some real "fishing" however...

◆ The National Fisheries Institute recommends avoiding recreational fish–those caught by a friend, etc., since fish caught recreationally are more likely to be from contaminated waters or not handled properly. It's probably best to avoid buying shellfish at roadside stands; they can be "bootlegged"– or caught from polluted waters.

◆ Good choices for pregnant women and breastfeeding women include flounder, cod, pollock, orange roughy, squid, clams, rockfish, alaskan salmon, shellfish and sole (19; 22; 24.) Variety is important!

Storing and Handling Seafood:

◆ To keep your fish as fresh as possible:

◆ Before refrigerating, remove the fish from its package, rinse under cold water and pat dry with paper towels. To keep cleaned fin fish more than 24 hours, place the fish on a cake rack in a pan, fill with crushed ice, and cover tightly with plastic wrap or foil. Rinse the fish daily, cleaning the rack and changing the ice.

◆ Keep fish stored at 32-38° F or in the coldest part of your refrigerator and use within one day. Keep frozen fish at 0° F and use within six months.

◆ Store live oysters, clams, and mussels in the refrigerator. Keep damp by covering with a clean, damp cloth or moist paper towel, but do not place on ice or allow fresh water to come in contact with them. Never place in an airtight container because it will kill them.

◆ Keep live lobsters, crawfish and crabs in the refrigerator in moist packages (use seaweed or damp paper strips), but not in airtight containers, fresh water, or salt water. Lobsters should remain alive for about 24 hours.

♦ Keep freshly shucked oysters, scallops or clams in their shells and store in the coldest part of the refrigerator, preferably surrounding the package with ice.

♦ Be sure to discard any fish juices and marinade used for raw fish, and do not re-use sponges, utensils or cutting boards used for raw fish. Also don't forget to wash your hands well after handling raw seafood.

♦ Throw out fish with a strong fishy or ammonia smell.

♦ Discard any shellfish that die during storage.

For more information, see *Consumer Reports Magazine*, February 1992, p 103-120. *FDA Consumer 91-2246*, *Seafood A to Z*, by Janis Harsila R.D. and Evie Hansen, *National Seafood Educators*

Cooking Seafood

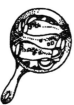

♦ **Avoid raw, and undercooked fish and shellfish at all costs!**

♦ Don't leave raw or cooked seafood out of the refrigerator for more than 2 hours including preparation time and time on the table.

♦ Cooking fish well will destroy most all bacteria present. Fish is done when the flesh is opaque and begins to flake easily when tested

with a fork at the thickest part. You can also check with a thermometer. Fish is ready when it's internal temperature reaches 145° F.

Fin Fish:

Though you don't want to undercook fish, it is also easy to overcook it, making your fish less tasty. Follow these suggestions from National Seafood Educators for perfectly cooked fish every time!

♦ For baking (400-450° F), broiling, grilling, poaching steaming and sauteing: Measure fish at it's thickest part. If it is stuffed, measure after it's stuffed. Then cook 10 minutes per inch, turning halfway through cooking time. Pieces that are less than 1/2 inch thick don't need to be turned.

♦ Add five minutes if fish is cooked in foil or sauce.

♦ Double the cooking time for frozen fish that hasn't been defrosted.

Shellfish:

♦ It takes 3-5 minutes to boil or steam 1 pound of medium shrimp in the shell.

♦ Shucked oysters, clams and mussels become plump and opaque when done. Overcooking causes them to shrink and toughen.

♦ Oysters, clams and mussels in the shell will open when cooked. Remove them one by one as they open.

♦ Sea scallops take 3-4 minutes to cook through; the smaller bay scallops may take as little as 30-60 seconds.

♦ Sauteed or deep fried soft shell crabs take about 3 minutes each. Steamed hard shell crabs or rock crabs take about 25-30 minutes for a large pot of them.

♦ If you poach or steam fish, let liquid come to boil first, then add fish and cook as described above.

To Microwave:

♦ Split-second timing is important when cooking fish in the microwave. Since the food will continue cooking after it is removed from the microwave, take it out before it looks done, when the outer edges are opaque with the center still slightly translucent. Allow the fish to stand, covered for a few minutes before serving.

♦ Use a shallow microwave safe dish.

♦ Arrange filets with the thicker parts pointing outward and the thinner parts toward the center of the dish. Rolled fillets cook more evenly than flat fillets.

♦ Cover the dish with plastic wrap and lift one corner to vent.

♦ Cook 3-6 minutes per pound of boneless fish at 100% power.

♦ Cook thawed, shucked shellfish 2-3 minutes per pound, stirring and rotating 1/2 turn during cooking. Allow to stand for 1/3 of the cooking time.

♦ Place clams, mussels or oysters in the shell in a single layer in a shallow dish. Cover with plastic wrap, venting one corner. Cook for 2-3 minutes on high. Check and remove shellfish as they open.

From: *Seafood, A Collection of Heart Healthy Recipes* by Janis Harsila R.D. and Evie Hansen, *National Seafood Educators*. This book has everything you want to know about seafood including how to buy, store, cook and even how to introduce it to picky eaters. The 180 recipes give new meaning to "fast food" since recipes can be cooked and on the table in 30 minutes or less.

13

Fast Foods–Eating Out and Eating In

◆

What You Will Find In This Chapter:

- ◆ Tips for Choosing Convenience Foods
- ◆ Frozen Convenience Foods; How to Have a Complete Meal
- ◆ Putting it All Together; Healthy Convenience Food Menus
- ◆ Sit Down Restaurants; Making the Best Choices
- ◆ The Most Nutritious Fast Foods
- ◆ Healthiest Fast Food Menus for Pregnancy

- ◆ Last Minute Meals from What's In the Cupboard

And Answers to Questions You May Have

- ◆ What can I add to a frozen entree to make a quick, complete meal?
- ◆ Are there any fast foods that are high in iron?
- ◆ Which fast food restaurants serve grilled chicken?
- ◆ Is it possible to eat out and have a lowfat meal?
- ◆ What can I keep at home in the pantry to put together a quick meal?

We live in a very fast paced society and we often don't have time to cook. Approximately 40 cents of every food dollar is spent on food prepared away from home. You may be wondering...is it possible to eat out or prepare convenience foods and still have a balanced diet? The answer is yes-with a little thought and planning.

Tips For Choosing Convenience Foods

Convenience foods such as frozen dinners, shelf-stable meals and dinners-in-a box are becoming more and more popular. Some are better than others. Consider these points when looking for dinners:

- Are they balanced; containing protein, starch and vegetable and/or fruit?
- How much fat do they contain? A good rule of thumb is to look for no more than 10 grams of fat per 300 calories.
- How is the sodium content? More than 800 mg. per serving could be excessive. However, since you need more sodium during pregnancy, this should not be a concern unless you were following a low sodium diet before pregnancy and your physician has advised you to continue doing so.
- Are they a good value? One often pays for convenience, so cost is something to consider. When considering the total price of a dinner, make sure to consider the cost of ingredients that you add, such as chicken or tuna.
- Is there a long list of additives and preservatives? If you are concerned about this, read the ingredient label.

The following frozen dinners offer convenience and good nutrition. Thousands of new foods enter the grocery store every year. The exclusion of some items on the list does not imply they are bad choices.

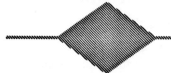

Doing your Math

Remember, the average pregnant woman needs about 2200 calories. (Your calorie needs can range anywhere from a modest 2,000 calories to more than 3,000 calorie depending on your size and activity level.) You can count on about 400 calories for breakfast, 500 calories for lunch and dinner and two 300 calorie snacks or three 200 calorie snacks. Most low-cal dinners have 300 calories. After adding milk, fruit and starch, you have 550 calories and a well balanced meal for you and your baby!

Frozen Convenience Foods; How To Have A Complete Meal

Below you can find out what to add to the different types of frozen convenience foods to make them a balanced meal:

Low-Calorie Entrees

  Budget Gourmet Hot Lunch

  Kraft Eating Right

  Healthy Choice Entrees

  Weight Watchers Ultimate 200 and Entrees

  Lean Cuisine Entrees

  LeMenu Light Style Entrees

Start with one of the entrees above and add:

1 cup milk or yogurt

1 fruit

1 piece of bread, or roll and you have a complete meal!

The reason the "lite" or lower calorie meals are good choices is that they are low in fat. Too much fat could give you heartburn, as well as add too many extra calories. However, the entree type meals don't always include a fruit or vegetable and they can be too low in calories. Adding some foods makes a balanced meal.

Stir fry meals: These offer yet another choice for a quick nutritious meal; they can be cooked in 6 minutes. An added benefit is that if you cook it as little a possible, the vegetables will retain more vitamins. Again, they are made with the dieter in mind, so add some milk or yogurt, fruit and bread or starch. These meals can be prepared in the microwave or on the stovetop.

Chicken pot pies, frozen pizza, fried chicken, chicken nuggets, fish sticks: these foods contain 50% or more of their calories from fat, and they are usually less expensive than other frozen dinners. However, there are many "lite" versions of those foods available now, which are better choices (but more expensive.) If you are having a hard time gaining weight or don't have an appetite, you can choose the "original" versions in moderation. Just watch out for indigestion due to their high fat content.

Frozen turkey roasts: in general, a quick meal that can be used the next day for sandwiches or leftovers.

Low-Calorie Dinners

These dinners offer a complete meal, but still contain only 300 calories.

Healthy Choice Dinners

Budget Gourmet Light and Healthy Dinners

Budget Gourmet Hearty and Healthy Dinners

Budget Gourmet Quick Stirs

LeMenu Healthy Dinners

Tyson Supreme Dinners

Ultra Slim Fast Dinners

Lean Cuisine:
Chicken and Vegetables
Breast of Chicken in Herb Cream Sauce
Turkey Dijon

To have a complete meal add:
milk or yogurt,
some type of starch
and maybe dessert!

Quick extras to add to your meal:

Starches:

bulgur, instant brown rice, whole wheat english muffin or bagel, bran muffin, bread sticks, canned legumes, corn or peas.

Fruit:

Frozen bananas or grapes, frozen melon balls, canned pineapple, instant pudding with bananas, fruit shake, yogurt parfait, fresh fruit.

Vegetables:

Ready to make coleslaw or salad, pre-cut vegetable sticks, shelf stable vegetables, canned or frozen vegetables.

Shelf Stable Foods

Don't have access to a refrigerator? Or are you stuck on bedrest? Pack one of the many shelf stable meals into your bag or (or keep them at your bedside). The variety of shelf stable foods are expanding quickly; you can find whole meals, soups, stews and even vegetable dishes that don't need refrigeration. These foods redefine the meaning of fast food; they can be ready to eat in 1 1/2 to 2 minutes! To top off your shelf stable keep dried fruit or individual

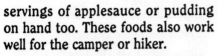

servings of applesauce or pudding on hand too. These foods also work well for the camper or hiker.

Read the labels on the shelf stable products; some of the smaller products are soups or side dishes, not entrees.

Make sure to add milk or yogurt, a fruit and a starch to the entrees so that you have adequate calories and nutrients.

Dinners:

Dinty Moore American Classics (a few are high in fat)

Top Shelf (a few are high in fat)

Hormel Health Selections

Kraft Microwave Entrees

Entrees/Side Dishes

Healthy Choice Soups

Lunch Bucket Light and Healthy (formerly Light Balance)

Lunch Bucket (some are high fat)

Chef Boyardee Main Meals

Hormel Micro Cup

Libby's Diner

Green Giant Shelf Stable Vegetables

Campbell's Microwave Soups

Watching Your Sodium?

The following frozen meals and entrees contain 700 mg. or less of sodium. Remember that your need for sodium during pregnancy goes up. However, your physician may ask you to moderate your salt intake if you had a condition existing before pregnancy such as hypertension or kidney disease.

Sodium content is in parentheses.

Hormel Health Selections

Italian Style Chicken and Vegetables (440)

Beef and Mushrooms (390)

Turkey and Vegetables in Sauce with Rice (420)

Hormel Top Shelf

Sweet and Sour Chicken ((280)

Boneless Beef Ribs (510)

Chicken Cacciatore (680)

Chicken Ala King (690)

Kraft Eating Right

Healthy Choice Entrees and Dinners

Healthy Choice French Bread Pizzas

Healthy Choice Shelf Stable

Budget Gourmet Quick Stirs

Primavera Vegetables with Sirloin of Beef (680)

Primavera Vegetables with Loin of Beef (680)

Milano Vegetables with Shrimp (640)

Ultra Slim Fast

Beef Pepper Steak (690)

Sweet and Sour Chicken (340)

Tyson Premium Dinners

Chicken Supreme (480)

Chicken Picatta (550)

Tyson Chicken Stir Fry Kit (480)

Budget Gourmet Quick Stirs

Rigatoni with Chicken and Tomato Sauce (550)

Herbed Vegetables with Shrimp (640)

Source: Manufacturer's Labels

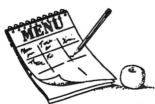

Putting It All Together; Healthy Convenience Food Menus

These menus show how to make a complete balanced meal starting from a frozen dinner.

Mexican/Southwest

Light & Healthy Chicken Fiesta (Shelf Stable)
2 Wheat tortillas
1 oz. reduced fat cheese
Orange

Weight Watchers Chicken Enchiladas Suiza
Guiltless Gourmet Tortilla Chips (or homemade chips)
with Black Bean Dip (page 243)
Avocado and Tomato slices
Milk

Healthy Choice Beef Fajita Entree
Three bean salad with tomato
Yogurt with graham crackers
Vegetable juice

Italian

Weight Watchers Baked Cheese Ravioli
Wheat rolls
Italian green beans
Carrot & raisin salad
Milk

Weight Watchers Italian Cheese Lasagna
Bread sticks
Marinated artichoke hearts with tomato and spinach
Melon
Milk

Lean Cuisine Zucchini Lasagna
Garlic Toast
Tossed salad with cheese
Broiled grapefruit

Budget Gourmet Shrimp and Scallops Marinara Dinner
Minestrone soup or Minute Minestrone (page 280)
Wheat crackers
Peach cobbler

Americana

Weight Watchers Broccoli and Ham
Baked Potato
Tossed Salad with kidney beans
Fresh apple
Vanilla pudding with banana
Milk

Healthy Choice Mesquite Chicken Dinner
Wheat rolls
Mixed fruit salad
Yogurt

Budget Gourmet Stuffed Turkey Breast Dinner
Corn muffins
Fresh mango
Milk

Budget Gourmet Special Recipe Sirloin of Beef Dinner
Grilled tomato halves
Dinner rolls
Fruit sorbet
Milk

Continental

Healthy Choice Chicken A' L'Orange
Entree
Corn
Bran muffin
Fresh Strawberries with yogurt

Healthy Choice Seafood Newburg
Entree
Tossed Salad with carrot and bell
pepper strips
Bagel
Grapefruit half

Healthy Choice Chicken and Pasta
Divan Dinner
Coleslaw
French bread
Milk

Budget Gourmet Primavera Vegeta-
bles with Sirloin of Beef
Cream of tomato soup
Sourdough roll
Tropical fruit salad
Milk

Tyson Beef Champignon
Spinach salad with parmesan cheese
(or carrot salad)
Rye bread
Apple or applesauce

Budget Gourmet Herbed Chicken
Breast with Fettucine
Caesar salad
French bread
Frozen yogurt with raspberries

Kraft Eating Right Shrimp Vegetable
Stir Fry
Bran muffin
Lemon yogurt with peaches
Milk

Chinese

Weight Watchers Sweet 'N Sour
Chicken Tenders
Budget Gourmet Spinach Au Gratin
Side Dish
Cherries
Milk

Budget Gourmet Teriyaki Chicken
Breast Dinner
Carrot sticks and broccoli with dip
Wheat roll
Milk

Lunch on the run...

Banana
Turkey, Broccoli and Cheese Lean
Pocket
Yogurt

Economy Frozen Meals

Swanson Chicken Pot Pie
Fruit cocktail and yogurt
Milk

Fish sticks
Easy Microwave Potatoes (page 314)
Sliced tomatoes
Peach halves
Milk

Jeno's Canadian Bacon Pizza
Tossed salad
Pineapple slices
Milk

Turkey with Stuffing and Mashed
Potatoes
Pumpkin Parfait (page 250)
Milk

Macaroni and Cheese
Carrot and pineapple salad
Tomato juice
Pudding

Tyson Fajita Kit
Refried vegetarian beans
Frozen melon balls and bananas
Milk

Sit Down Restaurants; Making The Best Choices

Dining out offers many many choices; which foods are best for the mom-to-be? If you eat out often, your diet will most likely be higher in fat and lower in other nutrients such as calcium, folacin, and vitamin C, unless you make your choices wisely!

Some specific challenges for the pregnant diner are:

◆ Typically large servings may tempt you to overeat; take half of it home in a doggy bag! Or order a half portion or from the appetizer menu.

◆ Higher fat foods and fried foods may cause heartburn.

◆ Servings of vegetables and fruits are usually minimal–making your meal consist of meat and starch. This is changing though, as more restaurants offer healthier fare!

◆ Milk may not be available--this could be a problem if you dine out regularly.

Salad Bar Savvy

Most people think a salad bar means a healthy meal! It can be–but beware the high fat foods! Here are a few tips for making your trip to the salad bar a healthy one!

◆ Make sure to get enough protein foods: Ham, turkey, cottage cheese, kidney beans, garbanzo beans, cheddar cheese.

◆ Go easy on the hidden fats: sunflower seeds, Chinese noodles, coconut, salad dressing, bacon bits, olives, marinated vegetables, puddings, mousses and salads made with mayonnaise. Also try to stay away from the fried foods on the "super bars" such as fried zucchini and potato skins.

At the Table

◆ Good choices from the menu: By looking for these key words, you should be able to order a healthy entree: Marinara sauce, vegetarian, grilled, baked, poached, steamed, stir-fried, lean, and light.

◆ Try to avoid meals described with these words: Butter, butter sauce, hollandaise, raw (as in seafood), au gratin, alfredo, creamed, cream, sauteed, pan fried, or fried.

◆ Order foods which contain 1 or 2 servings of vegetables. You may want to order ala carte to get what you want. Pasta, potatoes, brown or wild rice are good side dishes. Avoid fried potatoes.

◆ Order any salad dressings or sauces on the side.

What's For Dessert?

Fresh fruit, sorbet and lowfat frozen yogurt are good choices. If you want to indulge in something heavier, split it with your dining partner.

The Most Nutritious Fast Foods

Which fast foods are healthiest? A good question...and the answer depends on what you are looking for...Lowfat content? High vitamin C or A content? High fiber content? Every day the choices available at the drive-thru seem to expand. It's now possible to eat a healthy, balanced diet when you eat fast food regularly. The key is to follow through in making the best choices, (many of us have good intentions!) and to round out your diet by snacking on fruits and vegetables that might not be available when you eat in the fast lane...

Fast Foods Highest in Vitamin C

Company/Product	Percentage of RDA for Pregnancy
Taco Bell Taco Salad with shell	107
Orange juice, 6 fl. oz.	102
Wendy's Chef Salad	94
Grapefruit juice, 6 fl oz.	86
Carl's Jr. Fiesta Potato	86
Taco Bell Bean Burrito with red sauce	75
KFC Apple Shortcake Parfait	71
Wendy's Baked Potato, sour cream and chives	64
Arby's Baked Potato, Broccoli & Cheddar	64

Company/Product	Percentage of RDA for Pregnancy
Taco Bell Beef Tostada with red sauce	64
Wendy's Cauliflower, 1/2 cup	60
Wendy's Baked Potato, Broccoli & Cheddar	51
Wendy's green peppers, 1/4 cup	51
Burger King Garden Salad	49
Taco Bell Mexican Pizza	44
Jack in the Box Chef Salad	39
Taco Bell Combination Burrito	38
Subway Chef Salad or 6 inch sandwich (any choice)	36
KFC Cole Slaw	31
Long John Silver's Seafood Salad	26
Wendy's Honeydew melon, 2 oz.	21
Pizza Hut Traditional Hand-Tossed Pizza, Supreme, medium, 2 slices	17
McDonald's Wheaties, fortified	17

Adapted from *The Completely Revised and Updated Fast Food Guide*, Copyright 1991, CSPI, Available from CSPI, 1875 Conn. Ave. NW, Washington, DC 20009 for $7.95.

Calcium and Fast Food

Calcium is a mineral that is very important to your future bone health, and you can jeopardize that if you don't have enough calcium in your diet while you are pregnant or breastfeeding. However, if you choose a fast food just for it's calcium content, you're likely to get a lot of extra calories in the form of fat and sugar that you probably don't need. For example, if you choose the Pizza Hut Personal Pan Pepperoni Pizza, you'd get 675 calories and 29 grams of fat along with your calcium. Hardee's shakes will give you 41% of the RDA for calcium, along with 9 grams of fat and 10 teaspoons of sugar or more! McDonald's offers a lowfat milkshake providing 30% of the RDA with 8 1/2 teaspoons of sugar and just 1 gram of fat. Sometimes it's worth it to splurge–just not too often!

Fast Foods Highest in Calcium

Company/Product	Percentage of RDA for Pregnancy
Pizza Hut Traditional Hand-Tossed Pizza, Cheese, large, 2 slices	83
Wendy's Taco Salad	66
Pizza Hut Personal Pan Pizza, Pepperoni, whole pizza	61
Pizza Hut Thin n' Crispy Pizza, cheese, medium, 2 slices	55
Jack in the Box Ultimate Cheeseburger	50
Carl's Jr. Shake, large	41
Carl's Jr. Double Western Bacon Cheeseburger	41
Hardee Shakes	41

Company/Product	Percentage of RDA for Pregnancy
Dairy Queen Heath Breeze, regular	41
Carl's Jr. Cheese Potato	37
Domino's Pizza Double Cheese/Pepperoni, 16 inch, 2 slices	32
Wendy's Frosty Dairy Dessert, medium (11 oz.)	32
McDonald's Lowfat Milk Shakes	30
Carl's Jr. Breakfast Burrito	29
Baskin-Robbins Lowfat Frozen Yogurt, large (9 oz.)	28
Taco Bell Taco Salad, with shell	27
Milk, 1%, or 2% lowfat, 8 oz.	25

Adapted from *The Completely Revised and Updated Fast Food Guide*, Copyright 1991, CSPI, Available from CSPI, 1875 Conn. Ave. NW, Washington, DC 20009 for $7.95.

Fast Foods Highest in Zinc

Company/Product	Percentage of RDA for Pregnancy
Wendy's Triple Hamburger	72
Taco Bell Burrito Supreme	39
McDonald's Quarter Pounder with cheese	38
Wendy's Double Hamburger	37
Arby's Beef and Cheese Sandwich	36

Company/Product	Percentage of RDA for Pregnancy
Burger King Whopper	35
McDonald's Quarter Pound Hamburger	34
Wendy's Single Hamburger	32
Jack in the Box Jumbo Jack with Cheese	32
McDonald's Big Mac	31
Taco Bell Regular Taco	26
Arby's Roast Beef Sandwich	22
Fried Drumstick & Thigh	21
Taco Bell Beefy Tostada	21
Taco Bell Bean Burrito	20
Taco Bell Beef Burrito	15

Source: Nutritionist III Analysis Software

Fast Foods Highest in Folate

Company/Product	Percentage of RDA for Pregnancy
Taco Bell Regular Tostada	18
Taco Bell Bean Burrito	18
Arby's Ham and Cheese Sandwich	18
McDonald's Egg McMuffin	11
Taco Bell Burrito Supreme	11
Arby's Beef and Cheese Sandwich	10
McDonald's Large French Fries	10

Company/Product	Percentage of RDA for Pregnancy
Arby's Roast Beef Sandwich	10
McDonald's Egg Sausage Biscuit	10
Wendy's Single Hamburger	9
Burger King Egg-Cheese Croissant	9

Source: Nutritionist III Analysis Software

Fast Foods Highest in Vitamin B6

Company/Product	Percentage of RDA for Pregnancy
Wendy's Triple Hamburger	28
KFC Fried chicken breast & wing	26
Wendy's Double Hamburger	25
Arby's Beef and Cheese Sandwich	15
Wendy's Single Hamburger	15
KFC Fried chicken-leg and thigh	15
McDonald's Large French Fry	14
Burger King Whopper	14
Jack in the Box Jumbo Jack	14
Taco Bell Burrito Supreme	12
Arby's Roast Beef Sandwich	12
McDonald's Big Mac	12

Company/Product	Percentage of RDA for Pregnancy
Burger King Egg-Cheese-Ham Croissant	10

Source: Nutritionist III Analysis Software

Tips for Making your Fast Food Meal the Healthiest

♦ Choose lowfat or skim milk, hot cocoa or fruit juice as a beverage.

♦ Try to bring along fresh fruit or vegetables to go with your meal or order a side salad. Some McDonald's now carry packets of fresh carrot sticks.

♦ If you have trouble with heartburn avoid fries, burgers, fried pies and other fried foods, which are high in fat and will aggravate your heartburn. (The exception is reduced fat burgers such as the McLean Deluxe.)

♦ If you are trying to keep your weight gain down, choose lower calorie fare such as grilled chicken, fajitas or bean burritos. Skip the additional toppings such as cheese, sour cream and guacamole. Choose low-calorie or fat-free salad dressings.

♦ If you eat at the salad bar, choose raw vegetables such as tomato, broccoli, cauliflower and carrot sticks and fresh fruits. Have cottage cheese, beans, ham or chopped eggs for a protein source. Go sparingly on the mayonnaise based salads, puddings, olives, etc. Be sure to have a source of starch such as bread sticks or crackers.

♦ Cut the fat on sandwiches by asking for no mayonnaise or sauce. You can also ask for any sauces on the side. Cutting the cheese will also cut the fat; unless cheese is your primary calcium source.

♦ Remember that having a food high in vitamin C with your meal will increase the amount of iron your body absorbs. This can be done by drinking orange juice, having a salad with tomatoes, or having fresh fruit or other vegetables from the salad bar.

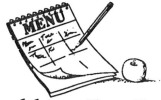

Healthiest Fast Food Menus For Pregnancy

The menus below have been chosen because of their lower fat content as well as higher values for some nutrients. All foods listed have less than 50% of their calories coming from fat. The main dishes marked with an (*) have 30% or fewer of their calories coming from fat. Most meals average 500 calories.

Breakfast Fast Food Menus

McDonald's

*Apple Bran Muffin
(Contains no fat.)
*Cheerios or Wheaties
2% milk
Orange juice

Egg McMuffin
2% milk
Grapefruit juice

Sunday Brunch at McDonald's
*Hot Cakes with margarine
and syrup
Scrambled eggs
Orange juice
2% milk

Burger King

Potato, Egg, and Cheese Burrito
2% milk
Orange Juice

Breakfast Bagel Sandwich
2% Milk

Arby's

*Blueberry muffin
2% milk
Orange juice

Ham and Cheese Croissant
Orange juice
2% Milk

Carl's Jr.

*Bran muffin
Orange juice
1% milk

Hot Cakes
Orange juice
1% milk

Light breakfast/mid-morning snack

*English muffin with margarine
1% milk

Dunkin Donuts

*Bran Muffin with raisins
Milk
Juice

*Egg Bagel
Milk
Juice

Hardee's

*Pancakes
Orange juice
2% Milk

Ham and Egg Biscuit
Orange juice
2% milk

Jack in the Box

Scrambled Egg Pocket
Orange juice
2% milk

Breakfast Jack
Orange juice
2% milk

Lunch and Dinner Fast Food Menus

Arby's

*Light Roast Beef Deluxe Sandwich
Lumberjack Mixed Vegetable Soup
Milk

*Chicken Fajita Pita
Garden Salad
Orange juice

*Light Roast Turkey
Deluxe Sandwich
*Tomato Florentine Soup
2% Milk

Broccoli and Cheddar Baked Potato
Beef with Vegetables and Barley
Soup
2% milk

French Dip 'n Swiss Sandwich
Garden Salad
2% milk

Burger King

*BK Broiler
Side Salad
Orange juice

*Chunky Chicken Salad
Lite Italian dressing
Crackers
2% milk

Cheeseburger
Garden Salad
2% Milk

Ocean Catch Fish Filet
Orange juice or water
Breyer's Chocolate Frozen Yogurt

Carl's Jr.

*Santa Fe Chicken Sandwich
Garden Salad
Reduced-Calorie French Dressing
1% milk

*Charbroiler BBQ Chicken
Sandwich
Small vanilla shake

Fiesta Baked Potato
Small Orange Juice

Dairy Queen

*BBQ Beef Sandwich
Side Salad
Yogurt Cone

*Grilled Chicken Fillet Sandwich
Side Salad
Milk

Fish Fillet Sandwich
Side Salad
Milk

Single Hamburger
Small French Fries
Orange Juice

Domino's Pizza

*2 slices 16 inch Ham pizza
Tossed Salad
Mixed fruit salad (from salad bar)
Milk

2 Slices Sausage Mushroom pizza
Salad Bar
Milk

Hardee's

*Roast Beef Sandwich
Side salad
2% milk

*Real Lean Deluxe
Side Salad
Orange Juice

*Grilled Chicken Sandwich
Crackers
Side Salad
2% Milk

Chicken Fiesta Salad
Chocolate Frozen Yogurt Cone
2% Milk

Jack in the Box

*Chicken Fajita Pita
Guacamole
Side Salad
2% milk

Hamburger
Small French Fries
Orange Juice

Chef Salad
Crackers
2% Milk

Grilled Chicken Fillet Sandwich
Side Salad
2% Milk

KFC

Breast Center (original)
Mashed potatoes with Gravy
Coleslaw
Milk

Thigh (original)
Coleslaw
Corn on the cob
Milk

Meatless meal at KFC

*Baked beans
*Corn on the cob
*Coleslaw
*Milk

McDonald's

*McLean Deluxe
Garden Salad

*Chunky Chicken Salad
Crackers
Strawberry Frozen Yogurt Sundae

For a Hungry Appetite!

Quarter Pounder
Orange Juice
Lowfat Frozen Yogurt Cone

Hamburger
Carrot sticks
1% Milk
Orange Sorbet Ice Cone

Pizza Hut

2 slices Canadian Bacon Pizza
Salad Bar
Lemonade

2 slices Cheese Thin n' Crispy Pizza
Salad Bar
Water or milk

1/2 Personal Pan Pizza Supreme
Salad Bar
Milk

Skipper's

Baked Alaska Fish
Baked Potato
Coleslaw
Milk

Shrimp and Seafood Salad
Cup Clam Chowder
1/2 serving Fries
Milk

Subway Sandwiches

*Subway Club- 6 inch
Large garden salad
Milk

*Seafood and Crab Sandwich
Broccoli-Cheese Soup
Orange Juice

*Ham Sandwich
Small chef salad
Milk

Taco Bell

*Bean Burrito with red sauce
Milk

*Soft Chicken Taco
Pintos n' Cheese
Orange Juice

Regular taco
Tostada with extra tomatoes
Milk

Chicken Salad
Fiesta Tostada
Milk

2 Beef Fajitas
Guacamole
Milk

Wendy's

Single Cheeseburger
Salad bar with fruit
2% Milk

Hot Stuffed Chili and
Cheese Baked Potato
Side Salad
2% Milk

Grilled Chicken Salad
Breadstick
2% milk

Salad Bar
Breadsticks
2% Milk

Luscious Snacks and Desserts

When you feel like splurging on dessert, these are low in fat, but delicious.

*Arby's Jamoca Shake

*Baskin Robbin's Nonfat Frozen
Yogurt

*Burger King's Breyer's Frozen
Yogurt

*Dairy Queen Small Strawberry
(yogurt) Breeze

*I Can't Believe It's Not Yogurt's
Nonfat Frozen Yogurt

*McDonald's or Dairy Queen's Frozen Yogurt Cone

*Taco John's Apple Grande

*TCBY's Nonfat Frozen Yogurt

Wendy's Frosty Dairy Dessert

(Also available is sugar-free yogurt at TCBY and I Can't Believe It's Not Yogurt)

Source of nutrient information: Manufacturer's nutrient analysis.

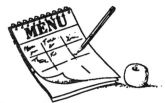

Last Minute Meals From The Cupboard

To avoid spending too much of your food budget on convenience foods, you can keep a supply of staple ingredients on hand for quick meals at home.

With the ingredients on the left, you can make all the foods on the right; some of them gourmet!

Ingredients	Meals
Pasta	Spaghetti with marinara sauce
Spaghetti sauce, Boboli Pizza,	Pizza with artichoke hearts
english muffin or pita bread	Chicken with mushrooms and
Canned Chicken	capers over pasta with Italian sauce
Canned mushrooms	
Capers	Quick Calzone
Artichoke hearts	Chicken Tetrazinni
Canned biscuits	
Mozzarella Cheese	Fettuccine Alfredo
Cottage Cheese	with tuna or with peas
Tuna	Tuna casserole
Salmon	Linguini, salmon,
Evaporated skim milk	and parmesan cheese toss,
Pasta	Macaroni and cheese
Parmesan cheese	
Olives	
Canned peas	
Mushroom soup (reduced salt and fat)	
Refried beans	Bean tostadas,
Taco shells	Chicken tacos,
Pineapple tidbits	Chicken salad with pineapple
Tostada shells	Spanish rice with chicken
Instant brown rice	Baked potatoes with chicken topping
Canned chicken	
Mixed vegetables	
Canned tomatoes	Black bean and chicken soup
Black Beans	Black bean tostadas
Corn	Black bean and Corn salad (recipe page 243)
Tostadas/Corn Tortillas	with tortilla chips
Fat-Free Dressing	
Baked beans	Black bean soup
Cornbread mix	Cornbread and Bean Bake
Kidney Beans	Hoppin' John (page 317)

Menus and Recipes for the First Trimester

About the Eating Expectantly Menus

The menus were planned especially for the cooking moods and eating challenges of pregnancy. Beverages are not necessarily included in the menus, though it is assumed that milk will be your choice of beverage at least 2 times per day! Other good choices for drinks include vegetable and tomato juice, fruit juices, and club soda mixed with fruit juice. Of course, you should try to drink plenty of water throughout the day too!

The recipes included in the menus are usually located immediately after, though some recipes will be located in other sections if the book. All recipes are listed alphabetically.

About the Eating Expectantly Recipes

When it comes to food, I have my likes and dislikes like anyone else. And the recipes in this book reveal my own food biases. For example,

you won't find any recipes that contain mustard greens or liver since these are not among my favorites! You will also find a French influence, since my husband is French, and a few southern recipes since I am originally from Texas. The Eating Expectantly Recipes were developed and chosen for their taste, nutritional value and ease of preparation. Most recipes call for ingredients that are readily available; the majority will be found in your own pantry.

Nutritional Analysis

All recipes were analyzed using Nutritionist III™ Software Version 7.2 from N-Squared Computing. All numbers are rounded off. When more than one ingredient or more than one serving amount is listed, the first number listed is the one used for analysis.

Protein is listed so that you can have an idea of how a recipe compares to your total goal for protein intake. Fat is included because most people are interested in fat content these days; women who have heartburn will be interested in choosing the lowest fat recipes. Carbohydrate is listed for the benefit of diabetics and health professionals, so they can plan special diets using them. The fiber listed is dietary fiber. If fiber is not listed, it is because the recipe contains less than 1 gram per serving.

Key Nutrients

Recipes were compared to the RDA's for pregnancy and are listed as a percentage of the RDA's. By looking at the key nutrients, you can pick foods high in a variety of nutrients; you can also learn what types of foods are most nutritious.

Diabetic Exchanges

Diabetic exchanges are included to assist in meal planning for women who have diabetes or gestational diabetes. They are calculated according to the Exchange Lists for Meal Planning developed by the American Diabetes Association and the American Dietetic Association. Exchanges are also rounded off as needed. Women who have diabetes should consult with a registered dietitian for an individualized meal plan based on their weight and activity level.

The diabetic exchanges are based on principles of good nutrition, so women who are not diabetic can also use them for keeping track of how many servings of food from the different food groups they are eating.

Diabetic Variations

A few of the recipes contain a significant amount of sugar; a sugar-free variation follows the recipe. These variations contain Equal. (See page 118 about use of artificial sweeteners during pregnancy.) Use Equal only with your physician's approval. When a Diabetic Variation is listed, the exchanges which follow it are for the diabetic variation.

Menus You Will Find in This Section

Don't Feel Like Eating Menus

Don't Feel Like Cooking Menus

Don't Feel Like Cooking or Eating Menu

Feel Like Staying in Bed But Can't Menu

Feel Great Menu

Blender Breakfasts (or Snacks to Go)

Snack Ideas

High Energy Mom Snack Ideas

First Trimester Recipes

Plain pasta
Applesauce

Creamy Asparagus Soup (page 246)
Wheat crackers

Tofu Spread (page 334) or cream
cheese on bagel
Pears

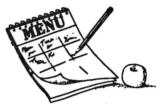

Menus FOR THE
FIRST TRIMESTER

Keep in mind that during the first trimester, the priority is not weight
gain–it should be to make your diet
as high quality as possible and to
improve other life-style habits. Don't
worry if because of nausea, you
don't eat much at all for a little
while. It should only become a concern if you begin losing weight.

Don't Feel Like
Cooking Menus

Tomato stuffed with Pea salad and
cheese (page 249)
Fresh apple

Black Bean and Corn Salad with
Homemade Tortilla Chips (page 243)
Sorbet

Tostadas with refried black beans
(page 268) beans, cheese, lettuce,
avocado and tomato
Milk
Frozen banana

Quick and Easy Lunch for Friends:

Salmon pate on crusty bread
Shrimp stuffed avocado with ranch
dressing
Fresh pineapple slices

Tuna and Pasta Salad
with artichoke hearts
Rye crackers
Canteloupe slices

Cold Sesame Beef (page 330) served
warm over mixed greens
Marinated vegetables
Tropical Pudding (page 261)

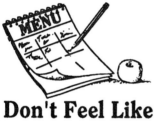

Don't Feel Like
Eating Menus

Many women find that drinking their
liquids between instead of with
meals helps with nausea.

Cream of mushroom soup
Wheat toast
Peach slices

Chicken noodle soup
Saltine crackers
Frozen yogurt with peaches

Jello with pears
Cottage cheese
Toast

Lowfat yogurt and banana shake
Graham crackers

Egg custard
Graham crackers

Melted goat cheese on toast rounds
over mixed greens and vegetables
Wheat roll
Yogurt Fruit Parfait (page 262)

Rigatoni Combination (page 328)
Carrot-apple salad
Wheat roll
Watermelon

Canned Black Bean Soup
Cornbread Toaster Biscuit
(Enteman's)
Grilled grapefruit

Tabouli salad with cheese
French bread
Fresh fruit salad

Fresh Tortellini with Quick Alfredo
Sauce and Peas (page 248)
Tossed salad
Wheat rolls
Sunshine Sorbet (page 333)

Lite Lunch:

Thrive on Five Bread (page 260)
with fat-free cream cheese
Apple Pie ala Mode Shake
(page 253)

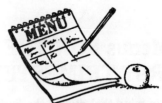

Don't Feel Like Cooking or Eating Menu

Breakfast

Dry toast
Fruit spread or jam
Milk or juice (later)

Snack

Crackers
Milk

Lunch

Fresh fruit with cottage cheese
Vanilla wafers

Snack

1/2 ham sandwich
Jello

Dinner

Spinach quiche or poached egg
Tomato soup
Wheat toast
Milk

Snack

Cinnamon toast
Milk

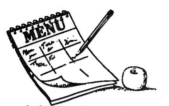

Feel like Staying in Bed, But Can't Menu

Before arising

Saltine crackers
gingerale (later)

Snack

Jello with peaches
Graham crackers

Lunch

Pasta
Mozzarella cheese
Sliced tomatoes

Snack

Frozen fruit juice bar

Dinner

Chicken or tuna salad
Wheat crackers
Apple slices

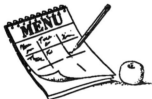

Feel Great Menu

If you are one of the lucky ones, you will feel close to normal and will want to eat "as usual". Here's an example of a good day's diet.

Breakfast

Raisin bran
Banana
Milk

Snack

Dried figs or prunes

Lunch

Ham and cheese sandwich
Fresh or canned peach
Raw broccoli and carrots with dip
Milk

Snack

Vegetable juice
Popcorn

Dinner

Broiled salmon steak
Roasted New Potatoes (page 329)
Carrots Antibes (page 245)

Snack

Tangy Salad (page 288)

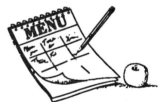

Blender Breakfasts (or Snacks to Go):

Banana Ginger Shake (page 254)
Cinnamon Graham Crackers

Pina Colada Frappe (page 256)
Oat bran toast

Very Berry Shake (page 258)
Health Valley Apple Bake

Peanut Butter Chocolate Shake (page 255)

Raspberry Surprise Shake
(page 257)
Bran Muffin

Apple Pie ala Mode Shake
(page 253)
Peanut butter on crackers

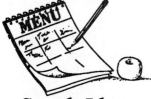

Snack Ideas

Here are snack ideas for the first, second and third trimesters, so that you won't run out of ideas for something different!

First Trimester

Rye crisp and pimento cheese

Melba toast and reduced-fat Laughing Cow Cheese

Cinnamon rice cakes and yogurt

Rice pudding

Bran flakes and granola, milk

Jello with peaches

Health Valley Date Bake Bar

Graham crackers and milk

Stewed prunes

Favorite Snack Cake (page 315)

Second and Third Trimesters

Toasted cheese and tomato sandwich

Neufchatel cheese,
raisins and cinnamon spread on
toasted English muffin

Deviled eggs and rye crackers

Pear and cottage cheese

Apple and colby cheese

Thin sliced lunch meat rolled around lite cream cheese with flavored crackers

McDonalds Low Fat Frozen Yogurt Cone

Banana and peanut butter

Peach Yogurt Parfait (page 262)

Popcorn cakes with string cheese

1/2 pita bread stuffed with salad, Farmer's cheese and vinaigrette

Quaker Caramel Corn Cakes, milk

Tuna salad with apple, crackers

Apple Date Bran Muffin (page 242) and milk

Harvest Crisp wheat crackers with spinach cottage cheese dip

Popcorn, milk

Figs stuffed with light cream cheese

Crustless Quiche (page 312)

Frozen yogurt with fresh strawberries and blueberries

Toasted wheat berry english muffin, yogurt

Fibar bar, milk

Leftover pizza, vegetable juice

"Guiltless Gourmet" Nachos

Raw vegetables, ranch dressing, crackers

Orange juice with club soda, yogurt with Grape Nuts and raisins

Strawberry Bread (page 259), milk

Hot Apple Cider, Thrive on Five Bread (page 260)

Ham and cheese in wheat tortilla

Chicken salad on 1/2 bagel or bagel crisps (baked)

Corn muffin with Monterey Jack Cheese, tomato juice

Orange, Pimento Cheese on celery, carrots and cucumbers

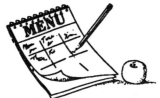

High Energy Mom Snack Ideas

Peanut Butter Chocolate Shake (page 255)

Fig Newtons

Egg custard, Ginger Snaps

Rocky Mountain Quesadilla (page 251)

Oven Baked Potato Chips with parmesan cheese and Italian seasoning (page 329)

Delightful Spinach (page 247) in a flour tortilla, milk

"Macho Nachos" (Corn tortilla toasted and served with melted cheddar, refried vegetarian beans, bell pepper strips, lettuce, tomato and light sour cream, and avocado

Egg and olive salad on rye, tomato juice

Wendy's Frosty, Graham crackers

Tortellini Pasta salad with ham

Peanut Butter cookies, frozen vanilla yogurt

English muffin with melted part-skim mozzarella cheese, sun-dried tomatoes and marinated artichoke hearts

Fat-free chocolate frozen yogurt with strawberry and granola topping

Old fashioned banana pudding with vanilla wafers

Ole' Version of Pita Pizza (page 325), pineapple juice

Raspberry Surprise Shake (page 257), granola bar

Refried Beans with cheese, vegetable juice

Cheesecake with raspberries

Pound Cake with peaches and Caramel Creme Sauce (page 308), milk

Pumpkin Parfait (page 250), milk

Favorite Snack Cake (page 315) with cream cheese

Avocado and shrimp salad, hard rolls

Tropical Pudding, Vanilla wafers (page 261)

First Trimester Recipes

The following recipes are found in the menus above.

Apple Date Bran Muffins

This recipe was developed by Deborah Compton who loves to cook as a hobby. You can bake the muffins now or keep them in the refrigerator for up to one week!

24 Muffins

1 cup oat flake cereal

2 cups 100% bran cereal

1 cup low-fat buttermilk, scalded or 1 cup plain non-fat yogurt, heated

2 large eggs or 1/2 cup egg substitute

1/2 cup margarine, at room temperature

1 1/2 packed brown sugar

1 cup low-fat buttermilk or 1 cup plain non-fat yogurt

1 cup unsweetened applesauce (choose one with vitamin C)

2 cups all-purpose flour

1/2 cup whole wheat flour

2 1/2 teaspoons baking soda

1/4 teaspoon salt

1 cup dates, chopped

1. Preheat oven to 400° F. In a large bowl, combine oat and bran cereals; pour scalding buttermilk over and stir. Add eggs, margarine, sugar, the other cup of buttermilk and applesauce; mix to blend.

2. Stir dry ingredients into cereal mixture until just moistened. Fold in dates.

3. To bake now, grease muffin tins, spray with non-stick spray or paper liner. Fill muffin tins 2/3 full. Bake 20-25 minutes.

Nutrient Analysis per Serving:
    147 calories
    3 g protein
    27 g carbohydrate
    4 g fat
    2 g fiber
Key Nutrients:
    Small amounts of all nutrients
Diabetic Variation:
    Reduce brown sugar to 1/2 cup; add 1/2 thawed apple juice concentrate.

Nutrient Analysis per Serving:
    134 calories
    3 g protein
    24 g carbohydrate
    4 g fat
    2 g fiber
Diabetic Exchanges:
    1 Starch, 1 Fat

Black Bean and Corn Salad with Homemade Tortilla Chips

This dish is chock-full of important nutrients for you and your baby!

4 Servings

1-16 ounce can black beans, drained

1 cup corn, drained

1/2 cup fat-free Italian dressing

6 corn tortillas

4 oz reduced fat cheddar or monterey jack cheese

1/2 cup plain non-fat yogurt

1/2 teaspoon cumin

1/8 teaspoon garlic powder

2 tomatoes

4 cups romaine or leaf lettuce leaves, torn

1. Mix corn, beans and dressing. Marinate in refrigerator at least 30 minutes.

2. Spoon corn and bean mixture over lettuce. Sprinkle 1 ounce of cheese on each serving. Garnish with 2 tomato quarters.

3. Mix yogurt with cumin and garlic powder.

Serve with tortilla chips and yogurt sauce.

Homemade Tortilla Chips

Preheat oven to 350 F. Cut each tortilla into 6 pieces and bake on cookie sheet for 20 to 30 minutes, turning once.

Nutrient Analysis per Serving:
367 calories

22 g protein

8 g fat

10 g fiber

Key Nutrients:
(percentage of RDA for pregnancy)
Folate-63%
Potassium-43%
Magnesium-38%
Calcium-28%
Zinc-20%

Diabetic Exchanges:
3 1/2 Starches, 1 1/2 Medium-fat Meat, 1 Vegetable

Bridget's Garden Salad

I often create meals from what's in the fridge, or in this case, in the garden. With a little luck, many of my creations work (though my husband can attest that some don't). This salad was created one week when green beans seemed like the only thing our garden was producing.

4 Servings

4 cups torn leaf or romaine lettuce

2 cups cooked green beans or a mixture of green and wax beans

1/2 cup shredded purple cabbage

4 large mushrooms, sliced

2 tomatoes, coarsely chopped

4 ounces smoked turkey, cubed

1/2 cup kidney beans, drained

2 ounces grated reduced-fat cheese

1/2 cup fat-free Italian dressing

2 tablespoon lowfat sour cream

Sesame or sunflower seeds, optional

1. Toss all ingredients except cheese, dressing and sour cream. Mix sour cream and dressing in small bowl.

2. Toss salad with dressing. Sprinkle cheese on top. Garnish with toasted sesame seeds or sunflower seeds if desired.

Variation:

Substitute 4 cups of pasta (twists or shells work well) for lettuce. Increase the fiber by using whole wheat pasta.

Nutrient Analysis per Serving:
  177 calories
  17 g protein
  16 g carbohydrate
  6 g fat
  5 g fiber
Key Nutrients:
  Vitamin C-50%
  Vitamin A-26%
  Vitamin B6-19%
  Zinc-10%

Diabetic Exchanges:
1/2 Starch, 2 Lean Meat, 1 1/2 Vegetables

Carrots Antibes

While visiting my husband's family in France, I ate this dish at a restaurant on the coast of the Mediterranean. Pureed vegetables are popular with Europeans; once you try Carrots Antibes, you'll know why! This is my version of the dish, which many two year-olds absolutely love!

---

4 Servings

**8 carrots, peeled and sliced
(about 1 pound)**

1/2 cup water

1 egg

1/2 teaspoon sugar

1/4 teaspoon nutmeg

1. Place carrots and water in microwave safe dish. Cover and cook 10 minutes in microwave on High, turning once half-way during cooking. Drain.

2. Place in blender or food processor with egg and spices. Blend until well pureed.

3. Return to microwave dish. Cook 4 minutes, rotating once.

Nutrient Analysis per Serving:
 82 calories
 3 g protein
 15 g carbohydrate
 2 g fat
 5 g fiber

Key Nutrients:
 Vitamin A-509%
 Potassium-24%
 Vitamin C-19%

Diabetic Exchanges:
 3 Vegetables

Creamy Asparagus Soup

Cooking the asparagus minimally in the microwave saves the important B-vitamin folacin from being destroyed.

4 Servings

1-10 ounce package frozen asparagus

1-12 ounce can skim evaporated milk

1/2 cup water

1 chicken bouillon cube or 1 heaping teaspoon broth mix

1/4 cup each finely chopped onion and celery

1 1/2 tablespoons cornstarch

2 tablespoons cold water

2 teaspoons margarine

1/2 teaspoon salt

1/4 teaspoon garlic powder, or to taste

1/8 teaspoon pepper, or to taste

1. Cook asparagus in covered microwave safe dish on High in microwave 2 minutes. Rearrange spears and cook 3 minutes more, or until tender. Leave covered several minutes to cool and cut into 1 inch pieces.

2. Meanwhile, mix 1 bouillon cube (or enough to make 1 cup broth) in 1/2 cup water. Bring to boil. Add celery and onion. Simmer until tender.

3. Add evaporated skim milk to pan. Mix cornstarch with 2 tablespoons cold water and stir into milk mixture. Cook until slightly thickened. Stir in margarine.

4. Pour milk mixture into blender; add asparagus. Blend briefly until desired consistency is reached, about 30 seconds.

5. Serve warm with Bridget's Garden Salad and bran muffins.

Variation:

Substitute 1-10 ounce package broccoli for asparagus. Add 2 ounces of grated reduced-fat cheddar cheese and let melt before blending.

Nutrient Analysis per Serving:

132 calories
10 g protein
18 g carbohydrates
3 g fat
1 g fiber

Key Nutrients:

Folate-26%
Vitamin C-27%
Calcium and Vitamin A-22%

Diabetic Exchanges:

1/2 Starch, 1 Vegetable, 1/2 Skim Milk, 1/2 Fat

Nutrient Analysis per Serving for Broccoli Soup

168 calories
14 g protein
18 g carbohydrate
5 g fat
3 g fiber

Diabetic Exchanges

1/2 Starch, 1/2 Medium-fat Meat, 1 Vegetable, 1/2 Skim Milk

Delightful Spinach

Do you groan at the thought of greens? This simple recipe will make you go back for seconds! The creamy sauce boosts it's calcium and protein content.

3 Servings

1-10 ounce package frozen chopped spinach

4 ounces fat-free cream cheese or yogurt cheese

1/2 teaspoon mixed herbs

Salt and pepper to taste

2 drops tabasco sauce, optional

1. Cook spinach (or thaw completely) and squeeze out all the water.

2. Add cream cheese and spices and stir until well blended. Serve.

Variations:

You can use this recipe for swiss chard, mustard greens or any green including cooked lettuce.

Nutrient Analysis per Serving:
41 calories
6 g protein
3 g carbohydrate
<1 g fat
1 g fiber

Key Nutrients:
Vitamin A-61%
Folate-23%
Magnesium-16%
Vitamin B12-10%
Diabetic Exchanges:
1/2 Lean Meat, 1 Vegetable

Pasta with Quick Alfredo Sauce

Love alfredo sauce, but hate how rich (and expensive) it is to make? Try this delicious, more healthful version.

4 Servings

1 cup low-fat cottage cheese

4 tablespoons parmesan cheese, preferably freshly grated

1/4 teaspoon garlic powder

1/4 cup skim milk

2 dashes nutmeg

1 cup frozen peas, thawed or lightly cooked

4 cups cooked pasta

1. Puree all ingredients except peas and pasta in food processor or blender.

2. Pour into microwave safe container and cook on Medium-High for 2 minutes. Or place in saucepan and cook gently until warm.

3. Toss pasta with peas.

4. Pour sauce over pasta. Garnish with more parmesan.

Variation:

Use canned mushroom pieces instead of peas.

Nutrient Analysis per Serving:

313 calories

20 g protein

46 g carbohydrate

5 g fat

Key Nutrients:

Vitamin B12-24%

Calcium-16%

Folate-10%

Diabetic Exchanges:

3 Starch, 1 1/2 Lean Meat

Pea Salad

I developed this recipe for those days when you just want something light; it's high in protein and calcium. It tastes best when eaten the say day it's prepared.

4 Servings

2/3 cup cottage cheese

1 tablespoon mayonnaise

1/4 teaspoon salt; pepper to taste

Dash of dill and garlic powder

1-17 ounce can peas or

  2 cups frozen peas, thawed or cooked

1/2 cup finely chopped celery

4 ounces reduced-fat cheddar cheese, cubed

1 tomato, sliced or 4 hollowed out tomatoes

1. Puree cottage cheese with mayonnaise and spices in blender or food processor until it is creamy and no longer has lumps. Set aside.

2. Mix together cheddar cheese, celery and peas. Add cottage cheese mixture. Stir until just mixed.

3. Serve with tomato slices or in hollowed out tomato.

Variation:

Add 1/4 cup of water chestnuts.

Nutrient Analysis per Serving:
  178 calories
  16 g protein
  14 g carbohydrate
  7 g fat
  3 g fiber

Key Nutrients:
  Vitamin C-25%
  Vitamin A-18%
  Zinc-11%

Diabetic Exchanges:
  1 Starch, 2 Lean meat

Pumpkin Parfait

6 Servings

1-16 ounce can pumpkin

1/3 cup brown sugar, packed

1/3 cup apple juice concentrate, thawed

2 teaspoons pumpkin pie spice

1 1/2 cups non-fat vanilla yogurt

1 cup light whipped topping, divided

1/4 cup fat-free granola (I like Health Valley)

1. Mix first four ingredients with 1/2 cup of whipped topping.

2. Layer pumpkin mixture and yogurt alternately in a round casserole dish or in 6 individual parfait or wine glasses.

3. Top with reserved 1/2 cup of whipped topping and granola.

Nutrient Analysis per Serving:
   186 calories
   4 g protein
   37 g carbohydrate
   4 g fat
   2 g fiber
Key Nutrients:
   Vitamin A-210%
   Calcium-10%
   Riboflavin-10%

Diabetic Variation:

Omit brown sugar and substitute Equal--equivalent of 4 tablespoons of sugar. Use plain or sugar-free non-fat yogurt instead of vanilla yogurt.

Nutrient Analysis:
   113 calories
   5 g protein
   20 g carbohydrate
   3 g fat
   2 g fiber
Diabetic Exchanges:
   1/2 Starch, 1 Vegetable, 1/3 Fruit, 1/2 Fat

Rocky Mountain Quesadillas

This can be a snack, an appetizer or a light meal. The figs gives it a real nutritional boost!

1 Serving

1 small whole-wheat flour tortilla

1 ounce Farmer's cheese, grated or sliced

4 figs

1. Cut figs in half. Arrange on one half of flour tortilla.

2. Top with cheese. Broil until cheese is just melted. Fold over.

OR, fold over tortilla and cook in microwave on Medium-High for 45 seconds to 1 minute.

Nutrient Analysis per Serving:
268 calories
10 g protein
44 g carbohydrate
7 g fat
4 g fiber

Key Nutrients:
Calcium-23%
Potassium-15%
Magnesium-11%

Diabetic Exchanges:
1 Starch, 1 Lean Meat, 2 Fruit

Salmon Pate

This creamy spread can be used as a dip or a sandwich filling. It tastes so good you won't believe the low-fat content!

20 Servings

- 1- 15 1/2-ounce can salmon with skin removed
- 2 1/2 tablespoons grated onion
- 2 teaspoon white horseradish
- 2 1/2 tablespoons lemon juice
- 1 teaspoon dry dill or 1 tablespoon fresh dill
- 2 teaspoons dry parsley or 2 tablespoons chopped fresh parsley
- 8-ounces fat-free cream cheese or 8 ounces low-fat cottage cheese

1. Place cheese in food processor. Process until smooth.

2. Add remaining ingredients and process until smooth. When you taste it you shouldn't feel any bones.

Serve with rye crackers, toasted pita bread or on a sandwich with thinly sliced cucumbers. As an appetizer, stuff cherry tomatoes, spread on crackers with a carrot curl for garnish, or stuff mushroom caps.

Nutrient Analysis per Serving:
- 41 calories
- 6 g protein
- <1 g carbohydrate
- 1 g fat

Key Nutrients:
- Vitamin B12-48%
- Selenium-22%
- Calcium-4%

Diabetic Exchanges:
- 1 Lean Meat

Shakes

These shakes can be made with plain yogurt or milk. Yogurt adds a little tanginess.

Apple Pie ala Mode Shake

2 Servings

1/2 cup applesauce, frozen

2 tablespoons brown sugar

1 cup skim milk or plain non-fat
   yogurt

1/2 teaspoon each cinnamon and
   vanilla extract

ice as needed

1. Blend all and serve.

Nutrient Analysis per Serving:

   133 calories

   7 g protein

   0 g fat

   1 gram fiber

Key Nutrients:

   Vitamin B12-21%

   Potassium-15%

   Calcium-13%

Diabetic Variation:

   Substitute 1 packet of Equal for brown sugar.

Nutrient Analysis:

   86 calories

   4 g protein

   17 g carbohydrate

   1 g fiber

Diabetic Exchanges:

   2/3 Fruit, 1/2 Milk

Banana Ginger Shake

2 Servings

1 cup skim milk or plain non-fat
  yogurt

1 frozen banana

1/2 teaspoon ginger

2 teaspoons brown sugar

1 tablespoon molasses

1 teaspoon vanilla

1. Blend all and serve. Add ice as needed.

Nutrient Analysis per Serving:

169 calories

5 g protein

38 g carbohydrate

0 g fat

1 g fiber

Key Nutrients:

Potassium-40%

Vitamin B12-31%

Calcium-24%

B6-19%

Magnesium-11%

Diabetic Variation:

Substitute Equal for sugar and
molasses.

Nutrient Analysis:

99 calories

5 g protein

17 g carbohydrate

0 g fat

1 g fiber

Diabetic Exchanges:

2/3 Fruit, 1/2 Skim Milk

Peanut Butter-Chocolate shake

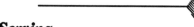

This shake is filling; drink it when you're hungry, not gaining enough weight, or when you don't feel like eating a meal.

1 Serving

1 cup plain non-fat yogurt or skim milk

1 package chocolate instant breakfast mix

2 tablespoons smooth peanut butter

ice

1. Blend all and serve.

Nutrient Analysis per Serving:
351 calories
24 g protein
43 g carbohydrate
9 g fat

Key Nutrients:
Vitamin B12-90%
Vitamin A-66%
Potassium-55%
Calcium-46%
Magnesium-46%
Zinc-37
Vitamin C-41%

Note: the reason for the high nutrient content is the use of instant breakfast, which is fortified. If you have more than one fortified food in a day, such as instant breakfast and a fortified cereal PLUS a prenatal vitamin, you can have too much of some vitamins and minerals.

Variations:

1. Omit peanut butter and add 1/2 teaspoon peppermint flavoring. 2. Add 1/2 frozen banana.

2. Use vanilla instant breakfast and add frozen unsweetened berries, frozen pineapple and banana or peaches.

Diabetic Variation:

Use sugar-free Instant Breakfast.

Diabetic Exchanges:

2 Skim Milk

Pina Colada Frappe'

2 Servings

1/2 cup frozen pineapple

1/2 frozen banana

1 cup plain non-fat yogurt

1/2 teaspoon coconut flavor

2 teaspoons of sugar or 1 packet
of Equal, optional

1. Blend all and serve.

Nutrient Analysis per Serving:

127 calories

7 g protein

25 g carbohydrate

0 g fat

1 g fiber

Key Nutrients:

Potassium-23%

Calcium-20%

Vitamin C-14%

Vitamin B6-12%

Magnesium-12%

Diabetic Exchanges:

1 Fruit, 3/4 Skim Milk

Raspberry Surprise Shake

2 Servings

1 cup plain non-fat yogurt or 1 cup skim milk

2 fresh peaches or nectarines, peeled, sliced, and frozen

1/2 of 1-10 ounce package frozen sweetened raspberries (or strawberries)

1. Blend all and serve.

Nutrient Analysis per Serving:
- 174 calories
- 8 g protein
- 36 g carbohydrate
- 0 g fat
- 3 g fiber

Key Nutrients:
- Vitamin B12-31%
- Potassium-27%
- Vitamin C-26%
- Magnesium-11%

Diabetic Variation:

Use unsweetened fruit and add Equal to taste.

Nutrient Analysis:
- 135 calories
- 8 g protein
- 26 g carbohydrate
- 0 g fat
- 3 g fiber

Diabetic exchanges:
- 1 Fruit, 1/2 Milk

Very Berry Shake

2 Servings

1 cup frozen unsweetened berries, any combination

1 cup plain non-fat yogurt or skim milk

3 tablespoons all-fruit strawberry spread (or 1 tablespoon sugar)

1 teaspoon vanilla

1. Blend all and serve.

Nutrient analysis per serving:

125 calories

7 g protein

25 g carbohydrate

2 grams fiber

0 g fat

Key Nutrients:

Vitamin C-45%

Vitamin B12-31%

Potassium-20%

Calcium-19%

Diabetic Exchanges:

1 Fruit, 1/2 Milk

Strawberry Bread

My friend Peggy gave me this recipe, which she made for my baby shower. Serve with fat-free cream cheese whipped with strawberry fruit spread.

1-15 Slice Loaf

1 cup flour, sifted

1/2 cup oats

1/4 cup sugar

1/4 cup vegetable oil

1-10 ounce package of frozen strawberries, thawed and drained

1 egg

1 teaspoon baking soda

1 1/2 teaspoon cinnamon

1/2 cup chopped pecans, optional

1. Preheat oven to 350° F.

2. Combine first 3 ingredients; set aside. Combine oil, sugar, and egg. Mix well. Stir in dry ingredients, Mix until just moistened.

3. Puree strawberries and add to batter. Add nuts if desired.

4. Pour into lightly oiled 9 x 5 pan and bake for 50-60 minutes.

Nutrient Analysis per Serving:

117 calories

4 g fat

19 g carbohydrate

Key Nutrients:

This bread has a small amount of most nutrients.

Diabetic Exchanges:

1 Starch, 1 Fat

"Thrive on Five" Bread

I started out with a basic zucchini bread recipe and came up with a bread that contains 5 different fruits and vegetables!

1-15 Slice Loaf

1 cup each grated carrot and zucchini

1/2 cup each whole wheat flour, white flour and wheat germ

1 egg

1/4 cup vegetable oil

1/2 cup crushed pineapple in juice, drained well

1/2 cup applesauce

1/4 cup brown sugar

2 teaspoons baking soda

1 teaspoon baking powder

1/2 cup raisins

1/3 cup molasses

1/2 teaspoon cinnamon

1/4 teaspoon cloves

1/4 teaspoon ginger

1. Preheat oven to 350° F.

2. Mix together all dry ingredients and set aside. Mix together oil, eggs, and molasses. Add vegetables.

3. Gradually add dry ingredients into egg mixture. Mix until just moistened.

4. Pour into 9 x 5 inch loaf pan that is lightly oiled or sprayed with non-stick spray.

Nutrient Analysis per Serving:
- 136 calories
- 3 g protein
- 23 g carbohydrate
- 5 g fat
- 2 g fiber

Key Nutrients:
- Manganese-24%
- Vitamin A-17%
- Iron-7%

Diabetic Exchanges:
- 1 Starch, 1 Fat (Plus a tiny portion of Fruit and Vegetable)

Tropical Pudding

Women who don't tolerate milk will enjoy this dessert.

4 Servings

1 package vanilla instant pudding

1/2 cup orange juice

1 cup plain non-fat yogurt

1/2 cup crushed pineapple, well drained

1/2 teaspoon coconut flavor

1. Mix juice into pudding mix with wire whisk. Stir in yogurt and coconut extract. Follow package directions for mixing time.

2. Stir in pineapple. Chill at least 30 minutes.

Garnish with pineapple ring or fresh pineapple cube.

Nutrient Analysis per Serving

   157 calories

   4 g protein

   36 g carbohydrate

   0 g fat

Key Nutrients for Both Variations:

   Vitamin B12-35%

   Vitamin C-22%

   Calcium-10%

Diabetic Variation:

   Substitute sugar-free instant pudding for regular pudding.

Nutrient Analysis:

   86 calories

   3.5 protein

   18 g carbohydrate

   0 g fat

Diabetic exchanges:

   1/3 Starch, 1/2 Fruit, 1/3 Skim Milk

Yogurt Fruit Parfait

4 Servings

4 cups plain non-fat or low-fat
yogurt

2 cups strawberries or any fruit

3-4 tablespoons all fruit spread,
or 1 1/2 tablespoon sugar

1. Mix yogurt with fruit spread.

2. Spoon 1/4 cup yogurt in parfait dish. Spoon over 1/2 cup yogurt and top with remaining fruit.

Nutrient Analysis per Serving:

167 calories

13 g protein

27 g carbohydrate

<1 g fat

2 g fiber

Key Nutrients

Vitamin C-63%

Calcium-38%

Folate-10%

Diabetic Exchanges:

1 Skim Milk, 1 Fruit

Menus and Recipes for the Second Trimester

Menus You Will Find In This Chapter:

♦ A Month of Breakfast Ideas
♦ Menus for a Hungry Appetite
♦ I Could Cook All Day Menus
♦ Company's Coming! Menus
♦ Recipes for the Second Trimester

A Month of Breakfast Ideas

♦ Peanut butter on toast with banana
♦ Frozen Nutri-Grain waffles topped with blueberries
♦ Vanilla yogurt with Health Valley Granola, Bran muffin
♦ Oat bran cereal with strawberries
♦ Eggs frittata, milk
♦ Apple Date Bran Muffins (page 242), mixed fresh fruit salad, milk
♦ Orange slices, wheat berry english muffin with Farmer's cheese
♦ Leftover pizza, apple slices, milk

♦ French French Toast (page 276), broiled grapefruit, milk
♦ Microwaved scrambled eggs with lowfat cheese, mushrooms and tomato slices, toast, milk
♦ Krusteaz Oat Bran Belgium Waffles with peaches
♦ Cantaloupe and Cottage cheese, Blueberry bagel
♦ Bran cereal with mixed dried fruit, milk
♦ Oatmeal with raisins, peanut butter on graham crackers, milk
♦ Poached egg and ham on english muffin, tangerine, milk
♦ Mango, Quick and Healthier Pancakes (page 283), yogurt
♦ Bran muffin, honeydew, milk
♦ Spiced peaches, Vegetarian Breakfast Tacos (page 336), milk
♦ "Thrive on Five Bread" (page 260) with fat-free cream cheese, hot cocoa
♦ Breakfast Pancakes with Raspberry Sauce (page 269), milk
♦ Hot wheat cereal with chopped dried figs, milk

- Yogurt Fruit Parfait (page 262), cinnamon toast triangles, milk

- Melted Swiss cheese on rye bread, apple pieces, milk

- Canteloupe, wheat toast with peanut butter, milk

- Vegetable juice, boiled eggs, wheat bagel, milk

- Cheerios, banana, milk

- Ham and cheese melted on corn muffin, fresh pear, milk

- Peanut butter and honey on whole wheat bread, kiwi and peaches, milk

- Banana Ginger Shake (page 254), oat bran toast

- Raspberry Surprise Shake (page 257), poppy seed muffin

- Very Berry Shake (page 258), Strawberry Bread (page 259)

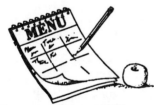

Menus for a Hungry Appetite

Mixed green salad
Stuffed Eggplant Creole (page 287)
Wheat bagette
Frozen yogurt with berries

Vegetable juice
French French Toast (page 276)
Mixed fruit salad

Leek and Potato Soup (page 278)
Savory Oven Fried Chicken
(page 285)
Carrots Antibes (page 245)
Wheat rolls
Updated Fruit Betty (page 292)

Salad with grated carrot, red cabbage, garbanzo beans and corn
Pasta with Quick Alfredo Sauce
(page 248)
Garlic bread
Tropical Pudding (page 261)

Raw veggies with Ranch yogurt dip
Tortellini with Pesto Sauce
Wheat rolls
Chocolate Mocha Cake
(page 271) with strawberries

Caesar salad
Spinach Stuffed Shells (page 331)
Green beans
Hard rolls
Frozen melon balls

Coleslaw with pineapple
Vegetarian Chili (page 336)
Home baked tortilla chips (page 243)
Sugar Cookies and frozen yogurt

Chicken and Shrimp with Fruit Salsa
(page 310)
Broccoli and carrot stir fry
Roasted New Potatoes (page 329)
Strawberry Bread (page 259)

Pina Colada Frappe (page 256)
Breakfast Pancakes (page 269)
with Raspberry Sauce
Turkey sausage slices

Black Bean Dip with Homemade Tortilla Chips (page 306)
Jicama and orange salad
Bean and Cornbread Bake
(page 305)
Yogurt Fruit Parfait (page 262) with Pound cake

Creamy Broccoli Soup (page 246)
Greek Island Pita Pockets (page 277)
Banana pudding

Three bean salad
Linguine with Cheese Basil Sauce
(page 270)
Herbed dinner rolls
Sunshine Sorbet (page x)

Homemade Cream of Tomato Soup
Hoppin' John (page 317)
Cheese cornbread rolls
Strawberry ice-milk with blueberries

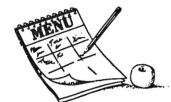

Company's Coming! Menus

Company Fondue (page 272)

Spinach Stuffed Shells (page 331)
Garlic bread sticks
Tossed salad
Frozen blueberry yogurt with raspberries

Chicken with Dijon Sauce
(page 313)
Brown rice with steamed vegetables
Wheat rolls
Updated Fruit Betty (page 292)

Apricot Glazed Chicken (page 303)
Steamed asparagus with lemon
Rice-wheat berry pilaf or quinoa
Mixed fruit salad
Apple Date Bran Muffin (page 242)

Mixed green salad
Spanish Steak Roll with
Sauteed Vegetables (page 286)
Potatoes Marie Louise (page 281)
Fruit Sorbet

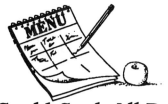

I Could Cook All Day Menus

Sesame Beef (page 330)
Oriental Noodles
Stir fried vegetables
Tangy Salad (page 288)

Cream of Chicken-Wild Rice Soup
(page 273)
Turkey Pot Pie (page 290)
Pumpkin Roll (page 282)

Grilled pork loin chops
Ratatouille (page 327) over
rice or bulgur
Apple Date Bran Muffins (page 242)
Frozen yogurt fruited sundae

Orange glazed Cornish hens
Thanksgiving Sweet Potatoes
(page 289)
Green beans almondine
Pumpkin Parfait (page 250)

Salmon en Papillote with julienne
vegetables (page 284)
Spaghetti Squash with warm
tarragon vinaigrette
Country sourdough bread
Peaches with Caramel Creme Sauce
(page 308)

Coleslaw
Quick Grilled Fish (page 326)
Carrots Antibes (page 245)
Wild rice pilaf
Chocolate Mocha Cake (page 271)
with Raspberries and Cream

Crepes: (page 274)
Ham and Cheese Crepes
Spinach and Cheese crepes
Fruit crepes with yogurt

Minute Minestrone (page 280)
Fettucini with Quick Alfredo Sauce
(page 248)
Sorbet

Veal Piccata with Roasted Red Pep-
per and Cream Sauce (page 335)
Spinach Pasta with vegetables
Apple tart

Leg of Lamb (page 279)
Green beans and lima beans
Roasted New Potatoes (page 329)
Fresh melon

Rocky Mountain Quesadillas
(page 251)
Ole' Kale and Pork Soup (page 323)
Lowfat cheesecake with raspberries

Second Trimester Recipes

These recipes were developed for the
eating moods of the second trimester. Most women feel their best during these months, so the recipes are
hearty and require a bit more time in
the kitchen that recipes for the other
trimesters.

Basic Bean Cooking

Soaking

Quick Soak:

Add 6-8 cups hot water to 1 pound
of beans. Heat, boil for 2 minutes; set
aside and cover; let soak 1 hour.

Overnight Soak:

Add 6 cups cold water to 1 pound
dry beans. Let soak overnight or at
least 6 hours in a cool place, not
refrigerated.

After soaking, drain the soak water
and rinse the beans before adding
more water for cooking.

Cooking Methods

Standard Way:

Place beans in large pot with 6 cups
hot water. Boil gently with lid tilted
until desired tenderness is reached.

Savory Way:

Place beans in large pot. Add 3 cups
hot water, 2 teaspoons onion salt, 1/
4 teaspoon garlic salt, 1/4 teaspoon
white pepper and 1 tablespoon
chicken stock base or 3 consomme'
cubes. Boil gently with lid tilted until
desired tenderness is reached. Add
water as needed to keep beans covered.

General Tips for Cooking Beans:

♦ Simmer beans slowly; cooking too fast and stirring frequently breaks skins.

♦ Add a tablespoon or two of oil to prevent foaming.

♦ Acid slows down cooking. Add tomatoes, vinegar, etc., last.

♦ At high altitudes, beans take longer to cook.

♦ When cooking in hard water, add 1/8 teaspoon to 1/4 teaspoon baking soda (no more) per pound of beans to shorten cooking time.

♦ When cooking large limas for casseroles and stews which require longer cooking, avoid overcooking. To puree or mash, cook until soft.

♦ Some old time recipes call for cooking unsoaked limas with meats, vegetables etc. This is acceptable. However soaking and discarding soak water improves flavor and digestibility and shortens cooking time. Nutrient loss is minimal.

♦ Long, slow cooking in water is essential for rehydration and digestibility of dry beans.

♦ Microwave ovens can be used for reheating cooked or canned beans.

Source: *Favorite Recipes of Four Generations featuring California's Large Lima Beans,* by the Large Lima Council of the California Dry Bean Advisory Board

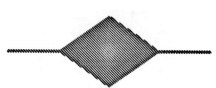

Dry Bean Arthrimetic

1 lb package
= 2 cups beans
= 5 cups soaked beans
1-15 1/2 oz. can
= 1 2/3 cups beans

Basic Black Beans

Black beans often fill my craving for something creamy and rich that sticks to my ribs. It can easily be turned into soup or a dip. I often eat it with cheese melted on top with fresh tomatoes for lunch. Or make a soft taco or tostado out of it. If you don't have time to make beans from scratch, keep a stock of canned beans on hand.

10 Servings

4 cloves garlic

3 medium shallots or 1 onion, chopped

1 teaspoon each cumin and chili powder

1/2 teaspoon pepper

2-3 pieces turkey bacon or ham (optional)

1. Soak beans overnight or use quick soak method. Discard soak water.

2. Combine all ingredients in large pot. Cover with water.

3. Cook 4-6 hours, or until beans are tender.

Nutrient Analysis per 2/3 cup Serving:
  201 calories
  14 g protein
  34 g carbohydrate
  1 g fat
  6 g fiber
Key Nutrients:
  Folate-64%
  Magnesium-37%
  Zinc & Iron-12%

Diabetic Exchanges:
  2 1/2 Starch, 1 Lean Meat

Variations:

1. "Refried" Black Beans

To 2 cups cooked beans, add 1-2 cloves garlic, cumin and salt to taste. Mash by hand or in food processor or blender.

2. To make soup, while blending, add chicken broth until desired consistency is reached.

Breakfast Pancakes with Raspberry Sauce

Margo Marrow won first place in the bread category with this dish in the Delicious and Nutritious Recipe Contest.   She has a special interest in nutrition since she works for the WIC program, a nutrition program for pregnant women and children. Her recipe shows her love of good food and nutrition. The variety of grains boosts the nutrient and fiber content and the raspberry sauce is high in vitamin C.

3 Servings

Pancakes

3/4 cups soy-wheat pancake flour (or use 1/4 cup soy flour and 1/2 cup wheat flour)

1/4 cup each corn meal, oatmeal and white flour

3 egg whites

3/4 cup skim evaporated milk or skim milk

1/2 cup orange juice

Margarine or canola oil to grease griddle

Raspberry Sauce

1-10 ounce package frozen raspberries (unsweetened) or 1 1/4 cup fresh berries

3 tablespoons sugar

1 tablespoon cornstarch

1 teaspoon vanilla

1/3 cup any juice (orange, apple or cranberry)

Pancakes:

1. Lightly beat egg whites. Add milk, flours and orange juice. Using paper towel, lightly grease pan with oil or spray with non-stick spray.

2. Pour 3-inch pancakes using about 1 full tablespoon for each.

3. Serve on plates kept hot in the oven.

Raspberry sauce

1. Strain thawed berries, reserving juice. Heat berries in saucepan to simmering.

2. Dissolve cornstarch in cold juice. Add with sugar to simmering Raspberry juice. Stir occasionally to prevent sticking.

3. Cook until slightly thick and clear. Add vanilla and berries.

4. Serve warm over pancakes.

Nutrient Analysis per Serving:

298 calories
12 g protein
58 g carbohydrate
2 g fat
5 g fiber

Key Nutrients:

Vitamin C-32%
Magnesium-20%
Calcium-13%

Diabetic Variation:

Omit sugar and use 1/3 cup diluted frozen juice concentrate instead of regular juice in sauce.

Nutrient Analysis:

292 calories
13 g protein
55 g carbohydrate
2 g fat
5 g fiber

Key Nutrients:

Vitamin C-90%
Potassium-31%
Folate-20%

Diabetic Exchanges:

2 Starch, 1 Fruit, 1/2 Skim Milk

Cheese Basil Sauce

4 Servings

1 cup lowfat cottage cheese

1/4 cup parmesan cheese (preferably freshly grated)

1 cup plain nonfat yogurt

1/4 cup prepared pesto sauce
(can usually be purchased in
produce department)

2 teaspoons tarragon vinegar

freshly ground pepper

salt

1. Combine all ingredients in
food processor or blender.

2. Blend until smooth, adding
more or less yogurt according to
desired thickness.

3. Pour into microwave safe
bowl and heat 2 minutes on
medium high. Or cook slowly over
stove until hot.

Nutrient Analysis per Serving:
179 calories
15 g protein
8 g carbohydrate
9 g fat

Key Nutrients:
Vitamin B12-36%
Calcium-20%
Potassium-14%

Diabetic Exchanges:
1/2 Skim Milk, 1 1/2 Lean
Meat, 1 Fat

Chocolate Mocha Cake

Just because you're pregnant doesn't mean you want to give up your chocolate! Just make it a little healthier! This cake is so moist, it reminds me of chocolate cheesecake, and just a small piece is enough.

15 Servings

1 3/4 cups flour

1/2 cup brown sugar, packed

1/4 cup canola oil

3/4 cup evaporated skim milk

1/4 cup cocoa powder

1/2 cup applesauce

1 cup strong decaffeinated coffee

1 teaspoon baking powder

1 teaspoon baking soda

1 teaspoon vanilla

1. Preheat oven to 375° F.

2. Mix all ingredients until well blended, about 1-2 minutes with electric mixer.

3. Pour into an 8 x 8 inch or 9 inch round cake pan that has been lightly greased and floured.

4. Bake 35-40 minutes.

Serve sprinkled with powdered sugar or with lowfat frozen yogurt and strawberries for a special treat!

Nutrient Analysis per Serving:
  155 calories
  3 g protein
  26 g carbohydrate
  4 g fat
Key Nutrients:
  Potassium-11%
  Thiamin-10%
  Calcium-6%

Diabetic Exchanges:
  2 Starches

Company Fondue

The first time I had this was at a gathering of co-workers. It was great fun because everyone brought a small portion of the meal, but there was really no work involved; just a lot of good food! For a last minute company meal, I can't think of a faster meal to put together.

8 Servings

6 cups chicken or beef broth

2 ounces each of beef tenderloin, chicken and scallops per person, or any combination of meats

1 pound of spinach, washed and trimmed

2 lb fresh mushrooms, washed and trimmed

1. Cut beef and chicken into 1 inch pieces. Heat broth. Pour into fondue pot or crock pot.

2. Arrange beef and vegetables on separate platters.

3. Guests cook meat and vegetables to desired doneness and dip in sauces.

4. When everyone is finished eating, pour a dash of sherry or sherry vinegar into the broth and divide it among the guests.

Serve with noodles or brown rice and tossed green salad.

Dipping Sauces

1. Teryiaki Sauce

2. Dijon Cream Sauce

Mix 1/2 cup plain nonfat yogurt with 1/2 cup lowfat sour cream and 1-2 tablespoons dijon mustard.

3. Heat 1/2 cup fruit spread (apricot or plum) with 1 tablespoon soy sauce and 1-2 teaspoons vinegar.

4. Horseradish mayonnaise.

Mix 1 tablespoon white horseradish with 1/2 cup lowfat mayonnaise.

5. Honey mustard sauce

6. Steak sauce/barbecue sauce

Nutrient Analysis per Serving:

(not including broth or sauces)

259 calories

41 g protein

3 g carbohydrate

9 g fat

Key Nutrients:

Zinc-20%
Vitamin B6-20%
Folate-17%
Iron-17%

Diabetic Exchanges:

5 1/2 Lean Meat, 1/2 Vegetable

Cream of Chicken-Wild Rice Soup

Stella Riley Bender, winner of local and national cooking contests, allowed me to use this recipe.

6 Servings

1 cup chopped fresh mushrooms plus 12 mushroom slices

2 chicken breast halves, skinned

1 teaspoon fines herbes (or assortment of mixed herbs)

6 whole peppercorns

1/4 cup uncooked wild rice

1 celery stalk, finely chopped

1 small onion, chopped

1 carrot, finely chopped

1/4 cup cornstarch or 1/2 cup flour

1-12 oz. can evaporated milk

Salt and pepper to taste

1. Simmer chicken in 3 cups of water with herbs and peppercorns. Cook until tender, about 45 minutes.

2. Cool. Pull chicken off bones; set aside. Strain broth and reserve.

3. Cook wild rice in 1 1/2 cups water until tender. Do not drain; let set, covered until needed.

4. In large saucepan, combine celery, carrots, onion, and mushrooms, reserving slices of mushroom for garnish. Add 1/3 cup water and cook over low heat until vegetables are tender-crisp, about 5 minutes.

5. Stir in cornstarch or flour and salt, add 1 cup of reserved chicken broth, continuing to stir until thick.

6. Add rest of broth, chicken and cooked rice in it's liquid. (If you like a thicker soup, don't use all the water from the rice.) Simmer 15 minutes to blend flavors.

7. Add evaporated milk, salt and pepper; heat and serve. Garnish with fresh mushroom slices.

Note: Pheasant can be substituted for chicken.

Nutrient analysis per serving:
206 calories
14 g protein
22 g carbohydrate
7 g fat
2 g fiber

Key Nutrients:
Vitamin A-33%
Niacin-21%
Calcium-15%

Diabetic Exchanges:
1 Starch, 1 Lean Meat, 1/2 Vegetable, 1/2 Whole Milk, 1/2 Fat

Crepe Dinner

I had to include one of our family favorites. Crepes are versatile; you can have them for breakfast, an elegant lunch, dinner or desert. Have the left-overs as a snack. Or host a "Make Your Own Crepe Party!"

10-12 Servings

Batter:

2 cups flour

2 cups skim or evaporated skim milk

3 eggs (or substitute 2 egg whites for each or all eggs to increase protein content)

2 teaspoons canola oil

1/8 teaspoon salt

1/2 teaspoon dry active yeast, optional (my husband says this is how they make them in France, though most recipes here don't call for any leavening.)

Optional: 1 teaspoon vanilla and 2 tablespoons sugar

1. Beat eggs and oil. Add flour and milk alternately. Beat until smooth. Let stand several minutes.

2. Using ladle, pour 2-3 tablespoons of batter into heated 10-inch non-stick skillet that has been sprayed with cooking spray. It is essential to have a pan that is in good shape without nicks or scratches. After pouring, quickly rotate the pan so that the batter covers the pan.

3. Cook over medium to medium-high heat until one side starts browning. Turn over and cook briefly on other side.

4. Fill immediately, or place between pieces of waxed paper

or foil to use later or freeze.

5. Unused batter may be kept several days. Let the batter sit at room temperature a few minutes and beat well before using.

Crepe Dinner (continued)

Fillings:

Breakfast:

- ◆ Peanut Butter and banana
- ◆ Berries and strawberry fruit spread
- ◆ Ham and cheese
- ◆ Margarine and sugar or honey
- ◆ Applesauce and cinnamon

Lunch or Dinner:

- ◆ Spinach filling from "Spinach Stuffed Shells" (page 331)
- ◆ Ham and Swiss Cheese, topped with "Dijon Sauce" (page 313)
- ◆ Chicken and mushrooms topped with thick cream of mushroom soup.

- ◆ Ratatouille (page 327) and Mozzarella cheese
- ◆ Salmon Pate (page 252) with cucumbers
- ◆ Sauteed or steamed shrimp and scallops with white sauce

Dessert:

- ◆ Peaches with Caramel Creme Sauce (page 308)
- ◆ Fresh fruit with vanilla yogurt
- ◆ Frozen nonfat chocolate yogurt topped with raspberries
- ◆ Margarine and sugar or honey
- ◆ Vanilla frozen yogurt and blueberries with heated strawberry all-fruit spread

Nutrient Analysis per Serving:

(2 crepes-unfilled)

119 calories

4.5 g protein

2 g fat

Key Nutrients:

Contains small amounts of all nutrients

Diabetic Exchanges:

1 1/2 Starch, 1/2 Fat

French French Toast

When you're married to someone from another country, you find out which ethnic foods are "real." Though our "french" toast doesn't exist in France, my husband's mother does remember eating this dish as a child. It's great for those with a hearty appetite or for those who need to gain more weight.

2 Servings

6 slices of stale French bread

(or 3-4 slices regular bread)

2 large eggs or 4 egg whites

3 tablespoons milk

2 ounces ham

2 ounces Swiss cheese

Salt and Pepper to taste

1. Mix eggs, milk, salt and pepper. Soak bread pieces in egg mixture. Spray pan with non-stick spray.

2. Place bread in pan and cook over medium-heat for several minutes. Turn over and add ham and cheese to each piece. Cook several more minutes, and remove when cheese is melted.

Nutrient Analysis per Serving:
    380 calories
    27 g protein
    16 g fat
    1 g fiber
Key Nutrients:
    Vitamin B12-55%
    Vitamin A-22%
    Zinc-18%
Diabetic Exchanges:
    2 Starch, 3 Medium-fat Meat, 1 Fat

Greek Island Pita Pockets

This mimics the flavor of a gyro sandwich, with less fat.

4 Servings

1 lb boneless pork loin or loin chops

4 pieces of whole wheat pita bread

1 clove garlic, minced

1/2 cup lemon juice

1 teaspoon dry oregano

1 tablespoon dijon mustard

1 tomato, chopped

Leaf lettuce, shredded

1. Cut pork into 1/2 slices.

2. Mix together remaining ingredients and place in ziploc bag or glass container. Add pork and marinate at least 1 hour.

3. Stir fry 3-5 minutes until pork is no longer pink and is thoroughly cooked. Stuff meat, lettuce and tomato inside pita bread. Top with Cucumber Yogurt Sauce.

Cucumber Yogurt Sauce

1/2 cup plain lowfat yogurt

1/2 small clove garlic (or less if you can't tolerate garlic well. You may just want to put a few dashes of garlic powder)

1/4 teaspoon oregano

1 teaspoon lemon juice

1/2 cucumber peeled and chopped

1/8 teaspoon salt

1. Place ingredients in food processor or blender and process until cucumbers are finely chopped but not pureed. Or, chop cucumber more finely by hand and mix all other ingredients in.

Nutrient Analysis per Serving:
417 calories
38 g protein
26 g carbohydrate
15 g fat
2 g fiber

Key Nutrients:
Thiamin-82%
Niacin-46%
Vitamin B6-24%
Zinc-19%

Diabetic Exchanges:
2 Starch, 4 Medium-fat Meat

Leek and Potato Soup

When you taste this, you may swear it has ham in it–it doesn't!
This soup is great on a fall or winter day with cheese toast and fresh fruit.

16 Servings

2 pounds of leeks

4 medium carrots

8 potatoes

2 cups evaporated skim milk

Salt and pepper to taste

1. Peel potatoes and carrots. Cut leeks down the center and rinse thoroughly. Cut all vegetables into 1-2" pieces.

2. Place all vegetables into large pot of hot water. Bring to a boil and simmer, covered for 45 minutes, or until potatoes and carrots are tender. (since carrots take longer to cook, you may want to give them a head start in the pot)

3. Drain 90% of the water off. Puree in batches in blender with small amount of milk in each batch.

4. Place all pureed soup in large bowl. Stir well, adding additional milk if needed.

Nutrient Analysis per Serving:

141 calories

6 g protein

30 g carbohydrate

0 g fat

3 g fiber

Key Nutrients:

Vitamin A-74%

Vitamin B6-24%

Folate and Vitamin C-17%

Diabetic Exchanges:

1 Starch, 1 1/2 Vegetable, 1/2 Skim Milk

Leg of Lamb

If not for my husband, I may never have had the joy of discovering leg of lamb. The French usually eat it with flagolet, (a legume,) green beans, and some type of potato. The leftovers are good cold with Dijon mustard or as a sandwich on an onion roll. Bon Appetit!

---

1 Leg of lamb, with or without bone

4-6 garlic cloves, peeled and sliced into 2-3 pieces

1 1/2 teaspoons each: Rosemary, Oregano, Thyme, Marjoram

or 3-4 teaspoon Herbs de Province (found in gourmet shop)

1. Preheat oven to 450° F.

2. Cut small slits in leg. Insert garlic clove pieces as deep as possible into the slits.

3. Sprinkle outside of leg with spices.

4. Turn oven down to 325° F.

5. Bake 30 minutes per pound. If you prefer pink or rare meat, reduce cooking time to 15 or 20 minutes per pound. Internal temperature should be 175-180 for well done and 160-165 for medium rare.

Serve with pan juices or mint jelly. We eat ours plain.

Nutrient Analysis per 4 oz. Serving:

217 calories

32 g protein

0 g carbohydrate

9 g fat

Key Nutrients:

Zinc-46%

Iron-16%

Folate-14%

Diabetic Exchanges:

4 Lean Meat

Minute Minestrone

4 Servings

5 ounces frozen spinach, thawed, or cooked and minimal amount of water, not drained

1-8 ounce can tomato sauce

1-14 1/2 ounce can diced tomatoes

1 cup green beans

1 cup garbanzo or kidney beans

3/4 to 1 cup cooked pasta

1 cup water

1/2 teaspoon onion powder

1/2 teaspoon garlic powder

1 teaspoon Italian spices

1/2 teaspoon dried basil

1 teaspoon dried or 2 teaspoons fresh parsley

1. Combine all ingredients in a 1 1/2 quart saucepan.

2. Simmer 10-15 minutes, until heated. Add more water for a thinner soup.

Variation:

Omit green beans and spinach and add 1-10 ounce package frozen mixed vegetables package to soup. Cook until vegetables are done.

Nutrient Analysis per Serving
   182 calories
   9 g protein
   36 g carbohydrate
   2 g fat
Key Nutrients:
   Vitamin A-51%
   Vitamin C-46%
   Potassium-41%

   Iron-15%
Diabetic Exchanges:
   1 1/2 Starch, 3 Vegetables, 1/2 Fat

Potatoes Marie Louise

This is another favorite at our house; it's a great way to include more vegetables in your diet!

18 Servings

10 medium potatoes (about 7 ounces each), peeled and cubed

5 medium carrots, peeled and sliced

1 to 1/2 cups skim evaporated milk

2 tablespoons soft margarine

Salt and pepper to taste

1. Place carrots and potatoes in large pot; cover with water. Cook 45 minutes to 1 hour, or until both are tender.

2. Drain, place vegetables in large bowl. Whip with electric beater; add milk, margarine, and seasoning. Add more milk until desired consistency is reached.

Nutrient Analysis per Serving:
   127 calories
   3 g protein
   26 g carbohydrate
   4 g fat
   2 g fiber

Key Nutrients:
   Vitamin A-70%
   Potassium-23%
   Vitamin C-12%

Pumpkin Roll

Mary H. Dudley, M.D. a practicing physician, developed this recipe. It won second place for desserts in a local recipe contest.

12 Servings

2 eggs plus 2 egg whites
1/2 cup honey
1/3 cup pumpkin
1 teaspoon lemon juice
3/4 cup whole wheat flour
1 teaspoon baking powder
2 teaspoons cinnamon
1/2 teaspoon nutmeg
1/2 teaspoon salt
1 cup chopped walnuts

Filling:

8 oz. yogurt cheese (or fat-free cream cheese)
1/2 cup honey
1 tablespoon vanilla
Garnish: powdered sugar

1. Beat eggs for 5 minutes; beat in honey, pumpkin and lemon juice. Combine dry ingredients and add to pumpkin mixture.

2. Spread on well greased 15 x 10 x 1 inch pan. Top with 1 cup finely chopped walnuts.

3. Bake at 375 for 15-20 minutes. Cool 5 minutes; only then turn onto dish towel sprinkled with powdered sugar.

4. Roll into jelly roll shape. Cool. Unroll.

5. Combine filling ingredients. Spread over cake. Roll up and keep chilled (Also freezes well.)

Yogurt Cheese:

This is an excellent nonfat replacement for high fat items like cream cheese, mayonnaise and sour cream. You can make it into a sweet cream or a spicy dip!

Makes 8 ounces

♦ Place 16 ounces of plain nonfat yogurt (without added gelatin) in a colander lined with coffee filters. Place over a bowl and cover top.
♦ Refrigerate for 18-24 hours (The longer it drains, the thicker it gets.) Discard liquid and store Yogurt Cheese in a covered container until ready to use.

Nutrient Analysis per Serving:

214 calories
8 g protein
33 g carbohydrate
7 g fat
2 g fiber

Key Nutrients:

Vitamin A-21%
Selenium-15%
Vitamin B12-14%
Magnesium-13%

Diabetic Variation

In cake, reduce honey to 1/4 cup. Omit honey from filling and substitute 1/3 cup orange juice concentrate and Equal to taste.

Nutrient Analysis:

160 calories
8 g protein
19 g carbohydrate
7 g fat
2 g fiber

Diabetic Exchanges:

1 Starch, 1 1/2 Fat

Quick and Healthier Pancakes

I developed this recipe for those who aren't quite ready for 100% whole grain pancakes, but yet are beyond "all white" pancakes.

4 Servings

1 cup biscuit mix

1/2 cup oatmeal

1/2 cup wheat germ

4 Tablespoons molasses

1/2 cup 1% milk (or lowfat yogurt)

1 tsp cinnamon

1 egg or 2 egg whites

1. Mix all ingredients together just until well blended.

2. Spray pan with non-stick spray or use small amount of margarine. Pour about 1/3 cup of batter for each pancake.

3. Cook over medium heat until bubbles form on top and batter looks "set."

4. Turn and cook briefly until to desired browness.

Fruity Variation: After pouring batter, add raisins and/or thinly sliced bananas on top of batter. Gently push into batter. Cook as usual. This makes the pancake sweet so you can cut down or omit the syrup. The leftovers make a good snack, too!

Nutrient Analysis per serving:
  289 calories
  10 g protein
  8 g fat
  3 g fiber
Key Nutrients:
  Magnesium-20%
  Zinc-19%
  Iron 17%
  Riboflavin-17%
  Calcium-16%

Diabetic Exchanges:
  3 Starch, 1 1/2 Fat

Salmon en Papillote

The beauty of fish is that it cooks so quickly. This is "a dash of this and a dash of that" recipe–use your imagination! This dish is traditionally cooked in parchment paper; I use aluminum foil. Some people like to add a few teaspoons of dry white wine or tarragon vinegar for more flavor. Salmon is a good source of omega-3 fatty acid, which is important for the development of your baby's nervous system and brain.

4 Servings

1- (2) pound whole salmon

Lemon slices

Lemon pepper

Dill, preferably fresh

Garlic powder

Aluminum foil or parchment paper

Julienne zucchini and carrots (optional)

1. Preheat oven to 400° F. Cut off head and remove skin from salmon. Place in a piece of foil or paper that is large enough to "wrap" the fish in.

2. Sprinkle the inside and outside of fish with spices. Add or delete any spices according to your mood. Top with several very thin lemon slices.

3. Bring the ends of the paper together above the fish and roll over. Crimp the sides and ends so that fish is enclosed in an almost air-tight package.

4. Place on cookie sheet and bake for 15 minutes per inch of thickness of fish.

5. Serve the fish still in it's baking paper, so your guests can open their package and enjoy the aroma.

Nutrient analysis per serving:

331 calories

46 g protein

0 g carbohydrate

14 g fat

Key Nutrients:
Selenium-80%
Niacin-84%
Magnesium-19%

Diabetic Exchanges:
6 1/2 Lean Meat

Savory Oven Fried Chicken

4 Servings

4 chicken breasts, boned and skinned or 1-2 pound broiling chicken, quartered with skin and fat removed.

1/3 cup fat-free Italian dressing

1/2 cup crushed bran flakes or crushed oat cereal

2 tablespoons parmesan cheese

1/2 teaspoon each garlic powder, basil, oregano, onion powder, and rosemary

1. Preheat oven to 375° F.

2. Marinate chicken in Italian dressing for at least 10 minutes, but preferably longer.

3. Mix crumbs with spices. Dip each piece of chicken into crumb mixture or shake in a bag.

4. Arrange chicken on a rack over cookie sheet.

5. Bake for 50-60 minutes.

Serve with bulgar wheat pilaf or brown rice.

Nutrient analysis per serving:
   231 calories
   37 g protein
   7 g carbohydrate
   5 g fat
   1 g fiber

Key Nutrients:
   Vitamin B6-38%
   Potassium-17%
   Zinc-10%

Diabetic exchanges:
   1/2 Starch, 5 Lean Meat

Spanish Steak Roll with Sauteed Vegetables

Sandy Collins won first place with this recipe in the 1991 National Beef Cookoff®. I'm sure you'll agree that it's delicious! You may want to omit the chilies if you can't tolerate spicy foods.

6 Servings

1 1/2 pound boneless beef top sirloin steak, cut 1 inch thick
1 teaspoon garlic powder, divided
1/4 teaspoon freshly ground black pepper
2 teaspoons vegetable oil, divided
1 teaspoon butter
3/4 teaspoon salt, divided
1 each red and green bell pepper, cut lengthwise into strips
1 small white onion, thinly sliced
1 cup sliced fresh mushrooms
1 tablespoon sour cream or low-fat yogurt
1/3 cup chopped walnuts
1/4 teaspoon chili powder
1-4 ounce can chopped green chilies
Lemon slices
Cilantro Sprigs

1. Pound boneless beef top sirloin steak to about 1/4 inch thickness. Sprinkle with 1/2 teaspoon garlic powder and pepper. Heat 1 teaspoon oil and butter in 12-inch heavy frying pan over medium-high heat until hot.

2. Panfry steak 5-7 minutes for medium-rare doneness, turning once. Remove steak to heated platter; sprinkle with 1/2 teaspoon salt. Keep warm.

3. Add remaining 1 teaspoon oil to frying pan. Add red and green peppers, opinion, mushrooms and walnuts. Cook 2 minutes, stirring frequently. Add remaining 1/2 teaspoon garlic powder, 1/4 teaspoon salt and chili powder; continue cooking 2 minutes, stirring frequently.

4. Spread steak with sour cream; top with chilies. Starting at long side, roll up steak jelly-roll fashion; secure with 6 wooden picks. Spoon vegetables around steak roll; garnish with lemon slices and cilantro springs. To serve, carve steak roll between wooden picks; remove and discard wooden picks.

Nutrient analysis per serving:

320 calories
37 g protein
7 g carbohydrate
16 g fat
2 g fiber

Key Nutrients

Vitamin C-58%
Zinc-52%
Magnesium-18%
Iron-15%

Diabetic Exchanges:

5 Lean Meat, 1 Vegetable

Reprinted with permission, 1991 National Beef Cookoff®

Stuffed Eggplant Creole

When my husband made this while I was pregnant, I could hardly eat it due to the cayenne pepper. This recipe is toned down so most should tolerate it!

4 Servings

2 small eggplants (1 lb each)

1 tablespoon vegetable oil

1 pound shrimp, crawfish, ground beef, or tofu (or a combination)

1 clove garlic, crushed

1/4 cup each: finely chopped onion, green pepper and celery

1-14 1/2 ounce can tomatoes, undrained

1/4 teaspoon dried thyme

1 cup dried bread crumbs

1/2 cup lowfat sour cream or plain nonfat yogurt

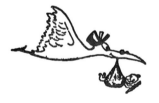

1. Preheat oven to 375° F. Wash eggplant; cut in half lengthwise. Place in large pan. Cover with water. Bring to a boil and cover. Simmer 15 minutes. Drain and cool.

2. Scoop out pulp from eggplant taking care to leave 1/4 inch of the shell intact.

3. In skillet, heat vegetable oil. Saute garlic with either beef, seafood or tofu. Add vegetables and cook 5 minutes over low, stirring occasionally.

4. Stir in tomatoes, salt, thyme, and tabasco if desired. Add 1/2 of bread crumbs. Add eggplant pulp and sour cream. Stir.

5. Stuff mixture back into 4 eggplant shells. Top with remaining bread crumbs.

6. Place in baking dish and bake 30 minutes.

Nutrient Analysis per Serving:

347 calories

29 g protein

37 g carbohydrate

9 g fat

6 g fiber

Key Nutrients:
Vitamin C-35%
Magnesium-25%
Iron-19%
Zinc-15%

Diabetic Exchanges:
1 1/2 Starch, 3 Lean Meat, 3 Vegetable, 1 Fat

Tangy Salad

My neighbor Gwen Shaw often serves this to her family. Even picky children should enjoy this. It's like a waldorf salad, but tastier.

4 Servings

1 green apple, peeled and chopped

1 large carrot, peeled and thinly sliced

1 celery stalk, chopped

1 medium orange, peeled, seeded and sectioned (or use 1-11 ounce can mandarin oranges, drained)

4 tablespoons raisins

2 tablespoons chopped walnuts

4 pieces of leaf lettuce

Dressing

3/4 cup plain nonfat or lowfat yogurt

1 1/2 tablespoons honey

1 tablespoon lemon juice

1/4 teaspoon each of cinnamon and nutmeg

Fresh mint or orange twists for garnish

1. Combine dressing ingredients in small bowl. Set aside.

2. Wash and drain lettuce. Peel 4 whole leaves off and line each plate.

3. Combine fruits and vegetables. Toss with dressing. Divide between plates. Garnish with orange slice and/or mint sprig.

Nutrient Analysis per Serving:

170 calories

5 g protein

30 g carbohydrate

3 g fat

3 g fiber

Key Nutrients:

Vitamin A-67%

Vitamin C-37%

Potassium-19%

Diabetic Variation:

Substitute 2 packets of Equal for honey.

Nutrient Analysis:

145 calories

5 g protein

23 g carbohydrate

3 g fat

3 g fiber

Diabetic Exchanges:

1 Fruit, 1 Vegetable, 1/2 Fat

Thanksgiving Sweet Potatoes

Have thanksgiving anytime with this variation of a classic french dish!

6 Servings

3 medium sweet potatoes, thinly sliced

2 tablespoons margarine, melted

2 tablespoons brown sugar

1 teaspoon minced ginger root or prepared ginger root in a jar

1. Pre-heat oven to 400° F.

2. Spray a 9-inch glass pie plate with cooking spray.

3. Toss potatoes with 1 tablespoon margarine, sugar and ginger.

4. Place potatoes in an overlapping circle around the bottom of the pie plate, adding a layer around the edge of the plate. Brush the remaining margarine on top.

5. Cover with aluminum foil and place a heavy weight such as an iron skillet or cake pan. Bake on the bottom rack for 30 minutes. Remove foil and bake another 30 minutes, or until potatoes are brown and carmelized.

Nutrient Analysis per Serving:
  126 calories
  1 g protein
  18 g carbohydrate
  2 g fiber

Key Nutrients:
  Vitamin A-158%
  Vitamin C-20%
Diabetic Exchanges:
  1 Starch, 1 Fat

Turkey Pot Pie

A great way to use those holiday leftovers. Divide into individual micro-wave/freezer containers for your own "pot pies to go."

4 Servings

4 medium carrots, peeled and
   sliced

1 tablespoon oil

2 green onions, thinly sliced

1 clove garlic, minced

3 tablespoons flour

1 cup hot chicken broth

2 cups diced turkey meat, skin
   removed

1/2 cup frozen peas, thawed

1/2 cup evaporated skim milk

2 tablespoons chopped parsley

1/4 teaspoon each: thyme, salt
   and pepper

4 Whole Grain Biscuits (1/2 can)

1. Preheat oven to 375° F. Place carrots in microwave dish with 1/4 cup hot water and cover. Cook 5-7 minutes on High. Drain and set aside.

2. Heat oil in non-stick pan. Saute green onion and garlic; cook until soft.

3. Whisk in flour and cook 1 minute. Stir in chicken broth gradually and cook stirring constantly until thickened, about 5 minutes.

4. Stir in remaining ingredients. Pour into pie pan or baking dish.

5. Arrange 4 pieces of biscuit dough over "pie." (You can bake remaining biscuits in the oven on a cookie sheet.) Bake 15-20 minutes or until biscuits are browned.

Nutrient Analysis per Serving:
   346 calories
   29 g protein
   31 g carbohydrate
   12 g fat
   5 g fiber

Key Nutrients:
   Vitamin A-247%
   Potassium-30%
   Vitamin B6-25%
   Zinc-19%

Diabetic Exchanges:
   1 Starch, 3 Lean Meat, 2 Vegetable, 1/2 Fat

Turkey with Hoisin Sauce

I've found turkey breast even more versatile than chicken breast. It's larger, so you have the option of making a roast, slicing it into "filets" or "scallopini" (as in veal) or slicing it thin for stir-fry. Another benefit–it is often less expensive than boneless chicken breast!

4 Servings

1 pound turkey cutlets, or turkey tenderloin, sliced in 1/2" slices

2 teaspoons canola oil

1 clove garlic, minced

2 green onions, chopped

2 tablespoons soy sauce

2 tablespoons frozen orange juice concentrate, thawed

1 tablespoon hoisin sauce (found in the oriental section of your grocery)

1 teaspoon cornstarch

1. Heat oil in non-stick pan over medium-high heat.

2. Add garlic. Saute for 1-2 minutes.

3. Add turkey and saute for 2-3 minutes per side. Remove and keep warm.

4. Add green onion to pan and saute briefly. In a small bowl, mix cornstarch with 1/2 cup water. Add this mixture to pan along with orange juice, soy sauce and hoisin sauce. Bring to a boil and cook until slightly thickened.

5. Pour sauce over turkey and serve.

Serve with brown rice and stir-fried vegetables.

Nutrient Analysis per Serving:

197 calories

34 g protein

3 g carbohydrate

4 g fat

Key Nutrients:

Niacin-50%

Vitamin B6-29%

Vitamin B12-20%

Diabetic Exchanges:

5 Lean Meat

Updated Fruit Betty

This is another of Stella Bender's recipes. What I love about it is that it cooks so quickly in the microwave! This dish is great by itself or as a topping on frozen yogurt. This was originally an apple crisp, but when I didn't have apples once, I added pears and peaches. Many people preferred the mixed fruit version to the apple crisp.

12 Servings

4 heaping cups of sliced, cored apples and or pears
(about 3-4 medium)

1-16 ounce can peaches canned in juice, drained (or you can use 5 cups apples and omit all other fruits)

3 1/2 tablespoons flour

1 1/2 teaspoons cinnamon

3/4 cup apple juice concentrate, thawed, (pick one with vitamin C)

3/4 cup water

3 tablespoons honey

1 cup old fashioned oats

1/4 cup whole wheat flour

3 tablespoons brown sugar

2 tablespoons margarine, cut in tiny pieces (easier to do when partly frozen or very cold)

2 tablespoons sesame seeds, optional

1. Mix 3 1/2 tablespoons flour with cinnamon. Toss with all fruit. Pour fruit into 1 1/2 quart microwave safe dish.

2. Combine water, juice concentrate and honey. You may have to heat mixture briefly (1 minute) in microwave so honey will mix completely.) Pour over fruit and toss gently.

3. Mix flour, oats, brown sugar, and sesame seeds, if desired. Sprinkle over fruit. Place margarine pieces evenly over top. Cook in microwave on High for 8 minutes. Turn 1/2 turn and continue cooking 6-8 minutes.

4. Let set 30-45 minutes to allow all of the liquid to be absorbed.

Nutrient Analysis per Serving:
140 calories
25 g carbohydrate
3 g protein
4 g fat
4 g fiber

Key Nutrients:
Vitamin C-43%
Magnesium-11%
Thiamin-9%
Diabetic Exchanges:
1 Starch, 1 Fruit, 1 Fat

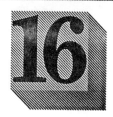

Menus and Recipes for The Third Trimester

Menus You Will Find In This Chapter:

♦ Menus from the Grocery Deli
♦ Using Leftovers with Flair
♦ Meals in Minutes
♦ Feel Full Menus
♦ Vegetarian Budget Menus
♦ Third Trimester Recipes

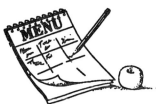

Menus from the Grocery Deli

Most foods in these menus are from the deli; some are from other parts of the grocery store. Some menus don't include a fruit; add your favorite.

Note:

Because there have been a small number of cases of Listeriosis, a type of food poisoning, associated with delicatessen foods, the Food and Drug Administration has advised that "pregnant women may choose to avoid these foods or to thoroughly reheat cold cuts before eating." See page 197 for more information.

Cool Supper for a Hot Summer Night

———
Pasta salad with ham
Greek salad
Fresh fruit

Ole!

———
Bean burrito
Guacamole
Fiesta cole slaw

———
Roasted chicken
Mashed potatoes/potato salad
Carrot raisin salad

———
Stir fry vegetables
Chicken skewers
Chinese slaw
Frozen yogurt

Ready to make pizza
Marinated vegetables
Fruit salad

Celery, broccoli and carrots with dip
Spaghetti and meatballs
Fruit sorbet

Tropical seafood pasta salad
Melba toast
Waldorf salad

Meatless Meals

Baked beans
Pea salad with cheese
Ambrosia salad

Cheese manicotti
Ratatouille
Jello with fruit
Garlic bread

Spinach quiche
Tossed salad
Fresh fruit

Carrot raisin salad
Ham and Swiss cheese on rye
Vanilla pudding with banana

Coleslaw
BBQ chicken
Potato salad

Cucumber and tomato salad
Meatloaf
Twice baked potato
Blueberries

Shrimp fried rice
Green pepper steak
Chinese coleslaw

Boiled shrimp
Pasta with pesto sauce
Fresh fruit salad

At Your Own Risk Due To Spiciness!

Cajun chicken breast
Red cabbage
Rice pudding

Sloppy Joe's
California slaw
Ambrosia salad

Beef tamales
Chile rellenos
Spanish rice

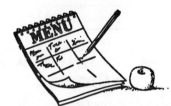

Using Leftovers with Flair

Day 1

Tossed salad
Grilled chicken
Rotini pasta
Steamed zucchini and yellow squash

Day 2

Colorado Stuffed Bell Peppers
(page 311)
(cook black beans in crock
pot during day)
Cornbread
Fresh fruit salad over
vanilla frozen yogurt

Day 3

Lunch
Grilled chicken (from day 1)
in Pita Pocket with
vinaigrette or Spinach salad
with grilled chicken

Day 4

Bridget's Garden Salad (page 244)
(using rotini pasta from day 1 and
leftover veggies)

Day 5

Black bean soup with cheese
Cornbread
Tomato/Avocado slices,
fat-free Italian dressing

Day 6

Beef fajitas
Guacamole Dip (using leftover
tomato and avocado from day 5)
Lettuce, tomato, reduced fat cheese

Day 7

Salmon en Papillote (page 284)
Steamed vegetables
Easy Microwave Potatoes (page 314)
Sorbet

Day 8

Lunch
Tossed salad with leftover fajita
strips, canned kidney beans, and
cheese, Homemade Tortilla Chips
(page 243)

Day 9

Linguine with salmon and parmesan
cheese (using fish from day 7)
Crusty wheat bread
Coleslaw
Fruit salad

Day 10

Baked Chicken
(from grocery deli if in a hurry)
Mom's Mashed Potatoes (page 323)
(use potatoes from day 7)
or Potatoes Marie Louise (page 281)
Green beans
Tangerine

Day 11

Curried chicken salad over spinach
leaves (from day 10) in pita pocket
Fresh melon or kiwi

Day 12

Grilled fish
Grilled bananas
Grilled corn and zucchini

Day 13

Fish on a Kaiser roll (from day 12)
Tossed salad with vinaigrette
Bell pepper and corn salad (leftover
from day 12)

Day 14

Company's Coming

Shrimp cocktail
Company Fondue (page 272)
Spinach and mushrooms

Day 15

Ratatouille (page 327) over
Brown Rice with poached egg
Kiwi and peaches over
angel food cake

Day 16

Chicken with Dijon Sauce
(page 313)
Pasta with steamed vegetables
Updated Fruit Betty (page 292)

Day 17

Ratatouille and cheese on Boboli
Bread (from day 15)
Tossed salad
Frozen melon balls

Day 18

Lunch
Pasta or Romaine lettuce Salad with
Dijon Chicken (from day 16)
Frozen vanilla yogurt with Fruit
Betty as topping

Day 19

Vegetarian Chili (page 337)
Coleslaw
Sunshine Sorbet (page 333)

Day 20

Vegetarian Tacos or Taco Salad (use
chili from day 18)
Tossed salad
Peaches with Caramel Creme Sauce
(page 333)

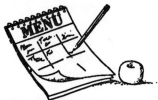

Meals in Minutes

Wonton Cup of Soup
Turkey with Hoisin Sauce (page 291)
Instant brown rice with snow peas
Frozen banana

Canned split pea soup
Microwave grilled cheese sandwich
Tomato slices
Fresh fruit

Bean tostadas with lettuce and
tomato
Frozen yogurt with strawberries

Scallop and shrimp stir-fry
Microwave baked potato
Carrot sticks
Fresh peach

Salad with smoked turkey, cherry
tomatoes, romaine lettuce
Breadsticks
Fresh orange

Three bean salad (canned) with
cheese
Leftover Cream of Chicken-Wild Rice
Soup (page 273)
Strawberries and banana slices

Minute steak on wheat bun
Spinach salad
Banana pudding

Minute Minestrone (page 280)
Turkey and cheese sandwich on
wheat roll
Apple

Turkey with Hoison Sauce
(page 291)
Kid's Carrots (page 318)
Spinach pasta twists

Raw vegetables with fat-free cream
cheese
Hoppin' John (page 317)
Very Berry Shake (page 258)

Apricot Glazed Chicken (page 303)
Easy Microwave Potatoes with
Italian seasoning (page 314)
Delightful Spinach (page 247)

Creamy Asparagus Soup (page 246)
Quick Grilled Fish (page 326)
Pasta
Tropical Pudding (page 261)

Crustless Quiche (page 312)
French Bread
Frozen grapes
Sugar cookies

Honeydew Soup (page 316)
Salad with leftover grilled chicken
Tabouli salad (made with bulgur)
Strawberry ice milk

Pea Salad (page 249)
Tomato soup
Wheat toast

Pita Pizza (page 324)
Tossed salad
Yogurt with berries

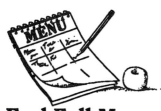

Feel Full Menus

These menus give you the very most nutrition per bite when you can't eat much!

Spanish Steak Roll (page 286)
Delightful Spinach (page 247)
Bulgur pilaf

Leg of Lamb (page 279)
Green Beans
Potatoes Marie Louise (page 281)
Raspberries

Sesame Beef (page 330)
Stir fried bell peppers and tomatoes
Mom's Mashed Potatoes (page 321)
Pumpkin Parfait (page 250)

Black Bean and Corn Salad
(page 243)
Homemade Tortilla Chips
Fresh orange

Stuffed Eggplant Creole (page 287)
Brown rice or quinoa
Sunshine Sorbet (page 333)

Creamy Broccoli Soup (page 246)
Spinach Stuffed Shells (page 331)
Bread sticks
Mango slices

Chicken and Shrimp with Fruit Salsa
(page 310)
Carrots Antibes (page 245)
Barley pilaf

Veal Piccata with Roasted Red Pepper and Cream Sauce (page 335)
Whole wheat pasta
Frozen melon balls and banana slices

Crustless Quiche (page 312)
Wheat bagette
Updated Fruit Betty (page 292)

Spanish Steak Roll with Vegetables
(page 286)
Roasted New Potatoes (page 329)
Canteloupe

Apricot Glazed Chicken (page 303)
Romaine lettuce salad
Pina Colada Frappe' (page 256)

Creamy Asparagus Soup (page 246)
Lentil Tomato Loaf (page 319)
Tangy Salad (page 288)

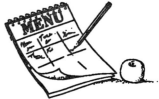

Best Bite Snacks:

These snacks have the most nutrients per calorie.

Rocky Mountain Quesadillas
(page 251)

Favorite Snack Cake (page 315)

Black Bean Dip with homemade tortilla chips (page 306)

Very Berry Shake (page 258)

Raspberry Surprise Shake (page 257)

Stuffed Figs(page 52)

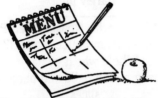

Vegetarian Budget Menus

The following two weeks of sample menus and recipes come from an article by Ruth Ransom, R.D. in Vegetarian Journal Reports.   I modified them slightly to adapt to the special nutrient needs of pregnancy. The first week uses foods that require ingredients found in your pantry and that require little preparation. The second week introduces meals using some common recipes.

Another recommended vegetarian cookbook for busy people is: Meatless Meals for Working People-- Quick and Easy Vegetarian Recipes, available from the Vegetarian Resource Group, P.O. Box 1463, Baltimore MD 21203.

These menus use 2% lowfat milk, and added fats that you might add but aren't written in, such as margarine or oil. The menus average 2200 calories, and assume serving sizes such as 1 1/2 cups of cereal or soup, 1/2 to one cup fruit, 1/2 cup to 1 cup of vegetables, 2 Tb peanut but-

ter, 1 cup milk, etc. Unlike other menus, the beverages are included because they have been included in calculating calories and nutrients.

Week 1

Monday

Breakfast

Quick and Healthier Pancakes
(page 283)
Fruit salad
Milk

Lunch

Tomato soup
Grilled cheese on whole wheat bread
Apple

Dinner

Vegetable stew or Vegetarian Chili
(page 337)
Cornbread muffins
Coleslaw
Watermelon
Milk

Snacks

Crackers with peanut butter
Milk

Tortilla chips with bean dip
Tomato juice

Tuesday

Breakfast

Total Raisin Bran
Banana
Milk

Lunch:

Peanut butter and apples slices on
whole wheat bread
Carrot and raisin salad
Milk

Dinner

Cheese omelette with vegetables (a
good way to use leftovers)
Wheat toast
Broiled tomato halves
Roasted New Potatoes or Home
Fries (page 329)

Snacks

Ginger snaps
Milk

Canned pear with Cottage cheese
Fruit juice

Wednesday

Breakfast

Oatmeal with dry fruit and molasses
Biscuit
Milk

Lunch

Black Bean and Corn Salad
(page 243)
Ice milk with Updated Fruit Betty
(page 292)

Dinner

Hoppin' John (page 317)
Cornbread
Collard greens or spinach
Tomato and cucumber salad
Plums

Snacks

Popcorn
Milk

Pina Colada Frappe' (page 256)
Graham crackers

Thursday

Breakfast

Hard boiled eggs
Wheat toast
Grapefruit
Milk

Lunch

Pita Pizza (page 324)
Tossed salad
Pineapple chunks

Dinner

Creamy Broccoli Soup (page 246)
Colorado Stuffed Bells (page 311)
Fresh pear
Milk

Snacks

Cheese and crackers

Apple bran muffin, milk

Friday

Breakfast

Hot wheat cereal
Peanut butter & banana on toast
Milk

Lunch

Mock Egg Foo Young (page 320)
Brown rice or bulgur
Stir-fried spinach
Frozen fruit

Dinner

Lentil Tomato Loaf (page 319)
Wheat bread or rolls
Tossed salad
Peach halves

Snacks

Oatmeal cookies
Milk

Brown rice pudding with raisins

Saturday

Breakfast

Cheese toast
Cinnamon applesauce
Milk

Lunch

Peanut butter and fruit spread on
whole wheat bread
Celery/carrot sticks
Apple
Milk

Dinner

Spaghetti with mushrooms, zucchini
and Parmesan cheese
Kid's Carrots (page 318)
Garlic bread
Fruit salad
Milk

Snacks

Hot cocoa
Fig bars

Very Berry Shake (page 258)
Favorite Snack Cake (page 315)

Sunday

Breakfast

Vegetarian Breakfast Tacos
(page 336)
Mango slices
Milk

Lunch

Macaroni and cheese
Sliced tomatoes
Rye toast
Banana
Milk

Dinner

Lentil Soup
Cabbage Salad
Strawberry Bread with
light cream cheese (page 259)
Fresh orange

Snacks

Frozen yogurt sundae

Granola bar
Milk

Week 2

Monday

Breakfast

French toast with strawberries
Milk

Lunch

Leek and Potato Soup (page 278)
Wheat biscuits or wheat English
muffins
Celery with lowfat cream cheese
Frozen grapes
Milk

Dinner

Ratatouille (page 327)
Macaroni, black beans and corn
Kiwi slices

Snacks

Graham crackers with peanut butter
Milk

Cheese toast

Tuesday

Breakfast

Eggs on English muffin
Fresh orange
Milk

Lunch

Grilled Swiss cheese and sauerkraut
on rye bread
Potato salad
Fresh apple

Dinner

Oat Nut Burgers (page 322)
or Carrot Cutlets (page 309)
Mixed vegetables
Wheat rolls
Fruit cocktail
Milk

Snacks

Bran muffin
Milk

Fat-free Cream Cheese Dip
Cauliflower and carrot sticks
Wheat crackers

Wednesday

Breakfast

Cheese grits
Canteloupe
Wheat toast

Lunch

Tofu Spread (page 334) on wheat
roll with lettuce, tomato and sprouts
Carrot and pineapple salad

Dinner

Rigatoni Combination (page 328)
Steamed green beans
Wheat garlic toast
Fresh fruit salad
Milk

Snacks

Tangerine
String cheese

Leftover veggies and beans in wheat
tortilla with cheese
Milk

Thursday

Breakfast

Whole grain cereal
Sliced peaches
Milk

Lunch

Sliced avocado, cheese, tomato and
lettuce on wheat bread
Salad
Plums
Milk

Dinner

Bean and Cornbread Bake
(page 305)
Coleslaw
Strawberries over angel food cake
Milk

Snacks

Yogurt with fruit

Refried vegetarian beans
Homemade tortilla chips or toasted
pita bread triangles

Friday

Breakfast

Poached eggs
Cinnamon Raisin Bagels
Apple juice
Milk

Lunch

Minute Minestrone (page 280)
Cottage cheese with raw vegetables
Cornbread
Grapes

Dinner

Broccoli and Tofu Stir Fry
(page 307)
Chinese noodles or brown rice
Pineapple Slices

Snacks

Crackers & peanut butter
Milk

Granola bar
Milk

Saturday
Breakfast

Oatmeal
Raisins/prunes
Toast
Milk

Lunch

Grilled cheese sandwich
Potato salad
Tomato slices
Watermelon
Milk

Dinner

Pasta with frozen vegetables and
Quick Alfredo Sauce (page 248)
Spinach salad
Garlic bread
Milk

Snacks

Yogurt Fruit Parfait (page 262)

Vegetarian nachos made with Guiltless Gourmet Chips
Vegetable juice

Sunday
Breakfast

Frozen waffles
Frozen strawberries
Milk

Lunch

Navy bean soup
Crackers
Carrot/celery sticks
Chocolate Mocha Cake (page 271)
Milk

Dinner

Stuffed Cabbage (page 332)
Three bean salad with
cherry tomatoes
Melon

Snacks

Popcorn
Juice

Banana
Peanut butter
Milk

THIRD TRIMESTER RECIPES

Apricot Glazed Chicken

You can make this chicken in a flash and serve it to family or friends.

4 Servings

4 chicken breast halves, skinned and boned

2 teaspoons margarine

1/3 cup apricot or peach all fruit spread

2 teaspoons fresh grated ginger (I buy ginger already grated in a jar)

1 1/2 tablespoons tarragon wine vinegar or other flavored vinegar

1/4 cup chopped cashews

1. Rinse chicken and pat dry. Melt margarine in non-stick pan.

2. Saute chicken over medium heat for 8-10 minutes. Remove chicken and keep warm. Sprinkle with salt and pepper. Reserve juices in pan.

3. Stir preserves, vinegar, and ginger into pan juices. Cook over medium heat hot.

4. Spoon glaze over chicken breasts. Sprinkle with cashews.

Nutrient Analysis per Serving:

240 calories

28 g protein

11 g carbohydrates

9 g fat

Key Nutrients:
Niacin-70%
Vitamin B6-24%
Magnesium-14%
Diabetic Exchanges:
4 lean meat, 1 fruit

Commit to the Bean Routine!

Dry beans are a nutritional gold-mine for today's mom-to-be! They are high in protein, complex carbohydrate and fiber, low in fat, and full of important nutrients. They make a great main dish when you can't tolerate meat. To top it all off, beans will save you money on your food budget; you can save time by using canned beans.

One cup of cooked dried beans provides 27% of a pregnant woman's need for protein, 25% of the requirement for manganese, 18% of the requirement for iron, and 31% of the requirement for folacin. Plus, they provide about 9 grams of fiber (20-35 grams per day is recommended.)

Beating Bean Bloat

One common concern about beans is that they can cause gas. A University of California, Berkeley study reported greater intestinal tolerance after three weeks of eating beans regularly. Here are some tips for getting your body adjusted to the bean routine!

1.   Build up your body's tolerance. Eat small servings at first, and then increase your intake slowly.

2.   Soaking and cooking your beans properly can break down starches, making them more digestible.

3.   Chewing well and slowly assists digestion and can minimize the problem.

4.   Drinking enough fluids helps your digestive system handle the increased dietary fiber.

From "Good Health is Habit Forming...- Commit to the Bean Routine", American Dry Bean Board

Bean and Cornbread Bake

This one dish meal is easy and high in fiber too. Serve with a spinach salad and fresh fruit.

6 Servings

1-16 ounce can pinto beans, drained

1-16 ounce can kidney, black beans or blackeyed peas, drained

(any combination will work!)

1/4 cup each: chopped green pepper, onion, and celery

2 tablespoons ketchup

1-8 ounce can tomato sauce

1 teaspoon dry mustard

1 small package (7 to 8 1/2 ounces) cornbread mix

1/4 cup grated cheddar cheese

(1/4 cup green chiles-optional)

1. Preheat oven to 375° F. Mix together all but last three ingredients. Pour into baking dish that has been lightly oiled or sprayed with non-stick spray.

2. Prepare cornbread according to package directions, adding cheese and chiles if desired. Pour over beans.

3. Bake for 30-35 minutes or until cornbread is golden brown.

Nutrient Analysis per Serving:
   338 calories
   18 g protein
   53 g carbohydrate
   7 g fat
   3 g fiber

Key Nutrients:
   Folate-37%
   Potassium-29%
   Magnesium-22%
   Iron-11%
Diabetic Exchanges:
   3 1/2 Starch, 1 High-fat Meat

Black Bean Dip

When you taste this, you won't believe it's so easy. You can whip it up for your next drop-in guests in about 5 minutes.

16 servings

1-16 ounce can black beans, drained (reserve liquid as needed)

1 tablespoon vinegar (may want to experiment with different flavors)

2 cloves garlic, minced or mashed

1/2 teaspoon salt

1. Blend ingredients in blender. Serve either warm or at room temperature with toasted pita bread pieces, wheat crackers or home baked tortilla chips.

Nutrient analysis per 2 tablespoon Serving:
- 33 calories
- 2 g protein
- 0 fat
- 1 g fiber

Key Nutrients:
- Folate-9%
- Magnesium-5%
- Potassium-4%

Diabetic Exchanges:
- 1/2 Starch

Broccoli and Tofu Stir Fry

4 Servings

2 teaspoons peanut or canola oil

1-2 teaspoons grated fresh ginger
   (or press through garlic press)

2 cloves garlic, minced

3 green onions, chopped

1 bunch broccoli, coarsely
   chopped

1 tablespoon vinegar

1/4 teaspoon sesame oil

1 tablespoon hoisin sauce

3 tablespoons soy sauce

1/4 cup water

1 pound firm tofu, cubed

1. Heat peanut oil in non-stick pan. Add ginger, garlic and green onions and saute 2 minutes. Add broccoli and stir-fry until broccoli is tender-crisp.

2. Mix together vinegar, sesame oil, hoisin sauce, soy sauce and water; set aside. Add tofu to broccoli and stir fry two more minutes. Add sauce mixture and continue cooking until warmed through.

Nutrient Analysis per Serving:

   222 calories

   22 g protein

   12 g carbohydrate

   12 g fat

   2 g fiber

Key Nutrients:
   Vitamin C-60%
   Iron-41%
   Calcium-21%
   Zinc-13%

Diabetic Exchanges:
   3 Lean Meat, 2 Vegetable, 1/2 Fat

Caramel Creme Sauce

The original of this recipe (which I had at a French restaurant) was "sinfully" sweet and buttery. This version is just as good, but a little healthier for you. Serve it over fresh peaches, over frozen yogurt or crepes.

8 Servings

1/3 cup plus 2 tablespoons plain nonfat yogurt

1/3 cup packed brown sugar

1 tablespoon margarine

1 tablespoon water

1. Melt margarine. Add sugar and let bubble for 1 minute. Add water and yogurt and cook just until heated.

Nutrient Analysis per Serving:

54 calories

1 g protein

1 g fat

Key Nutrients:

Contains small amounts of all nutrients.

Diabetic Variation:

Substitute 4 packets of Equal for brown sugar and add 1 teaspoon caramel flavor (available from Watkins.)

Nutrient Analysis:

22 calories

2 g carbohydrate

1 g protein

1 g fat

Diabetic Exchanges:

1 Free Food

Carrot Cutlets

This recipe is modified from a recipe in *Meatless Meals for Working People*, by Debra Wasserman and Charles Stahler, *Vegetarian Resource Group*

4 Servings

2 cups cooked brown rice or millet

1 small onion, chopped

1 tablespoon oil (if you fry)

1 tablespoon. chopped fresh parsley

1 cup carrots, cooked and mashed

1 tablespoon water or soy milk

2 tablespoon corn starch

3/4 cup wheat germ

1 tablespoon canola oil

1. Mix all ingredients except oil.

2. Form small patties and fry in oil or in non-stick pan over medium heat until brown on both sides.

Serve plain or with sauteed onions and mushrooms.

Nutrient Analysis per Serving:

302 calories

10 g protein

10 g fat

7 g fiber

Key Nutrients:

Vitamin A-181%
Zinc-29%
Vitamin B6-24%
Folate-23%

Diabetic Exchanges:

3 Starch, 1 Vegetable, 2 Fat

Chicken and Shrimp with Fruit Salsa

My friend Debbie Russell is a wizard in the kitchen. She has won regional and national cooking contests. This is one of her winners.

6 Servings

Marinade

1/4 cup mild picante sauce
1 tablespoon lime or lemon juice
1 tablespoon soy sauce
1/2 teaspoon ground coriander
1/2 teaspoon grated fresh ginger root
1 clove garlic, crushed
1 pound large shrimp, shelled and deveined
1 pound boneless, skinless chicken breasts, cut into pieces

Fruit Salsa:

1/2 cup diced peaches
1/2 cup diced pineapple
1/2 cup diced green apple
1/2 cup diced red bell pepper
2 tablespoon chopped green onion
1 teaspoon lime or lemon juice
1 teaspoon sugar
Garnish: 12 thin slices pineapple or peaches; cilantro or parsley sprigs

1. In dish or plastic bag, combine picante sauce, lime juice, soy sauce, coriander, ginger and garlic. Add shrimp and chicken, turning to coat well. Cover dish or close bag and marinate at least 30 minutes in refrigerator.

2. In small bowl, combine salsa ingredients except for garnish. Cover and set aside.

3. Drain shrimp and chicken. Thread shrimp and chicken alternately on skewers. Broil chicken and shrimp over medium-hot coals or broil at 400 until shrimp turns pink and chicken is cooked–7-10 minutes, basting often with marinade. Or stir-fry.

4. Serve with fruit salsa on the side of dish. Garnish with pineapple or peach slices and cilantro or parsley.

Variation:

Serve with Peanut Butter Sauce instead of Fruit Salsa

1/2 cup plain nonfat yogurt
2 teaspoons peanut butter
1/2 teaspoon dijon mustard
1/8 teaspoon Worcestershire sauce

Combine yogurt, peanut butter, dijon mustard, and Worcestershire sauce; mix well.

Nutrient Analysis per Serving:

With Fruit Salsa
279 calories
36 g protein
18 g carbohydrate
7 g fat
1 g fiber

Key Nutrients:

Selenium-90%
Niacin-68%
Vitamin C-30%
Vitamin B6-26%

Diabetic Exchanges:

5 Lean Meat, 1 Fruit, 1/2 Vegetable

Nutrient Analysis per Serving:

with Peanut Butter Sauce
247 calories
37 g protein
4 g carbohydrate
8 g fat

Key nutrients

Selenium-92%
Niacin-68%
Vitamin B6-24%
Magnesium-16%

Diabetic Exchanges:

5 Lean Meat

Colorado Stuffed Peppers

4 Servings

1 cup cooked brown rice

3 Roma tomatoes or 2 medium tomatoes, chopped coarsely

1 clove garlic, minced

2 green onions, chopped

1/4 medium red onion, finely chopped

1/2 sweet red pepper, chopped

1 1/2 cups cooked black beans

1/4 cup plus 2 teaspoons reduced-fat cheddar cheese, grated

2 teaspoons olive or canola oil

4 bell peppers, cored and seeded.

1. Saute onions, garlic and red pepper in oil until cooked to desired tenderness. (The less the tomato and pepper are cooked the more vitamin C they retain)

2. Add brown rice, black beans, and 1/4 cup cheese to pan and gently stir until warm and cheese is melted. Meanwhile, steam whole peppers in microwave. Fill with bean mixture. Top with 1 1/2 teaspoon of cheese.

To increase protein content, add some lean meat, chicken, tofu or more cheese.

Nutrient Analysis per Serving:
237 calories
12 g protein
37 g carbohydrate
7 g fat
5 g fiber

Key Nutrients:
Vitamin C-106%
Selenium-32%
Folate-30%
Magnesium-27%
Diabetic Exchanges:
2 Starch, 1/2 Medium-fat Meat, 1 1/2 Vegetable, 1 Fat

Crustless Quiche

I love quiche, but hate making the crust, so I whipped this up one night for a quick and satisfying dinner. Serve with a generous salad, crusty wheat rolls and fruit sorbet.

4 Servings

5 large eggs

1 cup evaporated skim milk

1-10 ounce package of spinach, thawed or cooked and drained

4 ounces part-skim mozzarella or reduced-fat cheddar cheese (or use a mixture)

1 teaspoon Italian seasoning

1/3 teaspoon salt

1/4 teaspoon garlic powder

1. Preheat oven to 350° F.

2. Beat eggs, milk, and spices together until frothy. Add spinach and cheese and mix well.

3. Pour into 10 inch pie plate that has been sprayed with cooking spray. Bake for 45-50 minutes.

Variation: Use 1 cup of any leftover vegetables. Or saute grated carrots and zucchini briefly before using. Add soy sauce instead of salt and add water chestnuts to give it an oriental flavor.

Nutrient Analysis per Serving:

225 calories

21 g protein

10 g carbohydrate

11 g fat

Key Nutrients:

Vitamin A-76%

Calcium-38%

Folate-25%

Zinc-15%

Diabetic Exchanges:

2 Medium Fat Meat, 1/2 Skim Milk, 1 Vegetable

Dijon Sauce

4 Servings

1/2 cup lowfat sour cream

1/2 cup plain nonfat yogurt

1-2 tablespoons Dijon mustard

salt, pepper and garlic powder to taste

1. Mix all together. Heat over low heat until very warm. If serving with cooked meat, heat with pan juices.

Variation:

Omit sour cream and use all nonfat or lowfat yogurt.

Nutrient Analysis per Serving:
48 calories
2 g protein
3 g fat

Key Nutrients:
Contains a small amount of all nutrients

Diabetic Exchanges:
1/4 skim milk, 1/2 fat

Easy Microwave Potatoes

With the help of a microwave, the potato can be a very quick and nutritious side dish!

Potatoes, any amount cut into 1
   inch pieces
2 tablespoons water
Salt and pepper to taste

1. Cook potatoes on high for 5 minutes. Rotate dish. Cook 5 more minutes on high. Continue cooking until fork can easily pierce through potato.

Variations:

1. Italian: Add Italian spices before cooking and parmesan cheese and the last few minutes of cooking.

2. German: Add sauteed onions, bacon bits the last few minutes of cooking. Sprinkle with vinegar and toss.

Nutrient Analysis per Serving: (1
medium potato)
   178 calories
   4 g protein
   41 carbohydrate
   0 g fat
   2 g fiber

Key Nutrients:
   Potassium - 38%
   Vitamin C - 36%
   Vitamin B6 - 26%

Favorite Snack Cake

This is one of my son's favorite snack cakes. Unfortunately, it's also our dog's favorite–the first time I made it he found the cake on the counter and finished it off!

12 Servings

1 1/4 cups whole wheat flour

1/2 cup oatmeal

1/4 cup cornstarch

1 3/4 cups applesauce (use the type fortified with vitamin C)

1/2 cup blackstrap molasses

2 tablespoons canola oil

1 large egg

1 teaspoon baking soda

1 teaspoon each ground ginger and cinnamon

1/2 teaspoon ground cloves

1/2 teaspoon salt

1. Preheat oven to 325° F. Mix together all dry ingredients and spices.

2. In a separate bowl combine eggs, oil, molasses and applesauce.

3. Gradually add egg mixture to dry ingredients.

4. Pour batter into a greased and floured 9 x 9 pan (in a pinch you can also use a 9" pie plate.)

5. Bake 45 minutes, or until knife inserted in middle comes out clean. Let cool on wire rack.

Nutrient Analysis per Serving:
129 calories
2 g protein
25 g carbohydrate
3 g fat
2 g fiber

Key Nutrients:
Potassium-23%
Iron-9%
Calcium-8%

Diabetic Exchanges:
1 1/2 Starch, 1/2 Fat

Honeydew Soup

Eat this as a snack or an appetizer on a warm summer evening.

2 Servings

1/2 medium honeydew melon,
   pureed (about 1 1/4 cup)

1/2 cup plain nonfat yogurt

1 tablespoon sugar

1/2 teaspoon vanilla

1. Blend together melon, yogurt and sugar in blender until smooth. Garnish with sliced strawberries and mint.

Nutrient Analysis per Serving:
   114 calories
   4 g protein
   26 g carbohydrate
   0 g fat
Key Nutrients:
   Vitamin C-61%
   Potassium-30%
   Vitamin B12-15%

Diabetic Variation:
   Omit sugar and substitute 1 1/2 packets of Equal, if desired.
Nutrient Analysis:
   91 calories
   4 g protein
   21 g carbohydrate
   0 g fat
Diabetic Exchanges:
   1 Fruit, 1/2 Skim Milk

Hoppin' John

This southern classic can be made in a flash with canned beans and quick cooking brown rice or bulgur.

4 Servings

2-16 ounce cans red kidney beans or blackeyed peas

2 cups cooked brown rice or bulgur

6 ounces lean ham, chopped

1/4 teaspoon onion powder

pepper and salt to taste

1 tablespoon fresh parsley, chopped

Red onion, optional

1. Combine beans with liquid, rice, ham and spices. Cook over medium heat, stirring frequently.

2. Serve topped with parsley and chopped onion if desired. If you can't tolerate raw onion, cook it with the beans.

Nutrient Analysis per Serving:

262 calories

17 g protein

39 g carbohydrate

4 g fat

2 g fiber

Key Nutrients:

Selenium-89%

Zinc-17%

Vitamin B6-16%

Diabetic Exchanges:

2 1/2 Starch, 1 1/2 Lean Meat

Kid's Carrots

You're never too young to get in the kitchen! That philosophy paid off for 12 year old Andy Hawk, who placed 3rd in the vegetable category of the Delicious and Nutritious Recipe Contest. His recipe won't keep you in the kitchen long, though!

5 Servings

1-1 pound package of frozen baby
   carrots

2 tablespoons honey

1 tablespoon minced fresh or 1
   1/2 teaspoons dried mint

1. Cook carrots according to package directions. Drain.

2. Stir in honey to coat carrots. Stir in mint. Serve.

Nutrient Analysis per Serving:
   48 calories
   1 g protein
   19 g carbohydrate
   0 g fat
   3 g fiber
Key Nutrients:
   Vitamin A-167%
Diabetic Exchanges:
   1/4 Starch, 1 Vegetable

Lentil Tomato Loaf

This recipe is from *Meatless Meals for Working People.*

6 Servings

2 cups cooked lentils

2 cups tomato sauce

1/2 cup onions, chopped

1/2 cup celery, chopped

3/4 cup rolled oats

1/2 teaspoon garlic powder

1/4 teaspoon Italian seasoning

1/4 teaspoon celery seed

Salt and pepper to taste

1/2 cup chopped nuts, optional

1. Pre-heat oven to 350° F.

2. Mix ingredients and place in loaf pan which is lightly oiled or sprayed with non-stick spray.

3. Bake 45 minutes.

Nutrient Analysis per Serving:
    146 calories
    9 g protein
    27 g carbohydrate
    1 g fat
    5 g fiber
Key Nutrients:
    Folate-33%
    Vitamin C-18%
    Vitamin B6-12%
    Zinc-9%
Diabetic Exchanges:
    1 1/2 Starch, 1/2 Lean Meat, 1
    Vegetable

Mock Egg Foo Young

This recipe is modified from a recipe in *Meatless Meals for Working People*

3 Servings

10 ounces tofu, crumbled

2 finely chopped green onions

1/2 garlic clove, minced or garlic powder to taste

1 1/2 teaspoons soy sauce

4 tablespoons corn meal

1 carrot, finely grated

1 tablespoon sesame seeds

1/4 teaspoon oregano

1 teaspoon canola oil

Salt and pepper to taste

1. Stir all ingredients together until well blended.

2. Form patties and cook in small amount of oil until lightly browned.

Nutrient Analysis per Serving:

216 calories

17 g protein

12 g fat

4 g fiber

Key Nutrients:

Vitamin A-89%

Iron-35%

Magnesium-36%

Calcium-17%

Diabetic Exchanges:

1 Starch, 2 Lean Meat, 1/2 Vegetable

Mom's Mashed Potatoes

8 Servings

2 pounds cooked new potatoes with skin (see Easy Microwave Potatoes page 314)

1 cup or more evaporated skim milk

1 teaspoon Molly McButter Sour Cream and Chive Flavor

Salt and pepper to taste

1. Place potatoes in blender with milk and Molly McButter, salt and pepper. Puree until creamy, adding more milk if necessary.

Nutrient Analysis per Serving:
143 calories
5 g protein
31 g carbohydrate
<1 g fat
3 g fiber

Key Nutrients:
Potassium-30%
Vitamin C-25%
Vitamin B6-18%

Diabetic Exchanges:
2 Starch

Oat Nut Burgers

This recipe is modified from a recipe in *Meatless Meals for Working People*. When I had my "picky eater" friends try this, they wanted seconds!

3-4 Servings

2/3 cups rolled oats

2/3 cups chopped cashews (or other nuts)

1 onion chopped

3 stalks celery, chopped

2 carrots, grated (or use 1 carrot and 1/2 small zucchini, grated)

1/4 cup each whole wheat flour and water.

1 teaspoon soy sauce (optional) and salt and pepper to taste

1. Mix all ingredients. Season to taste with salt, pepper or soy sauce.

2. Shape into 6 burgers.

3. Cook in lightly oiled pan (or pan sprayed with non-stick spray) until brown on both sides. Or broil in oven.

Nutrient Analysis per Serving:
189 calories
7 g protein
25 g carbohydrate
8 g fat
4 g fiber

Key Nutrients:
Vitamin A-49%
Magnesium-25%
Zinc-11%

Diabetic Exchanges:
1 1/2 Starch, 1 Vegetable, 1 1/2 Fat

Ole' Kale and Pork Soup

8 Servings

1 teaspoon canola oil

1 medium onion, chopped

1 clove garlic, minced

16 ounces pork loin or loin
    chops, trimmed of all fat and
    cut into 1 inch cubes

5 cups water

1 bunch fresh kale, trimmed and
    cut into 1 inch pieces

1-16 ounce can whole peeled
    tomatoes

5 roma tomatoes, halved and
    sliced,
    or 3 medium tomatoes,
    chopped

1 1/2 teaspoons ground cumin

3/4 teaspoon chili powder

1-15 ounce can hominy

1/2 can tomato paste

Salt, pepper, and hot pepper
    sauce, to taste

1. In saucepan, heat oil over medium heat. Add onion, garlic and pork. Cook about 10 minutes, stirring occasionally.

2. Place pork in large microwave safe dish. Add water. Cook 5 minutes on High. Add kale. Cook 5 minutes on High.

3. Add tomatoes, spices, hominy and tomato paste; cook 15 minutes on High, or until kale is to desired tenderness. Add more tomato paste for thicker soup.

Serve with homemade corn chips and guacamole.

Vegetarian Variation:

Substitute tofu or pinto beans for the pork.

Nutrient Analysis per Serving:
   229 calories
   19 g protein
   19 g carbohydrate
   9 g fat
   4 g fiber

Key Nutrients:
   Vitamin C-49%
   Thiamin-40%
   Vitamin A-40%
   Vitamin B6-18%

Diabetic Exchanges:
   1/2 Starch, 2 Medium-fat Meat,
   2 Vegetables

Pita Pizzas – Italiano

The beauty of these quick pizzas is that they can be made with almost any bread: english muffins, tortillas, Boboli bread or even French bread!

4 Servings

1 cup lowfat cottage cheese

1 tablespoon Italian seasoning

2 ounces part-skim mozzarella cheese

4 whole wheat pita bread

(or 4 whole grain english muffins,

 cut in half)

1/2-3/4 cup prepared spaghetti sauce

6 artichoke hearts or 1/2 cup sliced steamed red and yellow bell peppers

1/3 cup canned or steamed fresh mushrooms

1. Puree cottage cheese and seasoning in blender or food processor.

Spread 2-3 tablespoons sauce on each pita or on 2 english muffin halves.

2. Top with 1/4 cup of cottage cheese and 1/2 oz. of mozzarella. Add 3 artichoke halves, or several pepper strips and mushrooms. Broil until cheese is bubbling.

Nutrient Analysis per Serving:
   243 calories
   18 g protein
   29 g carbohydrate
   6 g fat
   3 g fiber

Key Nutrients:
   Calcium-19%
   Thiamin-15%
   Vitamin C-10%
Diabetic Exchanges:
   1 1/2 Starch, 1 1/2 Medium-fat Meat, 1 Vegetable

Pita Pizzas – Ole!

My interviews with pregnant women showed that although many have trouble with heartburn, they still crave and eat mexican foods. Here is a mexican version of pita pizza.

1 cup lowfat cottage cheese

1 tablespoon taco seasoning mix

2 ounces reduced-fat cheddar cheese

1/2 cup salsa, chopped tomatoes or pico de gallo (a mix of tomatoes, onion, lemon juice and cilantro)

1/2 avocado for garnish

1. Follow directions for Pita Pizza Italiano, substituting ingredients to the left. Garnish with 2 thin avocado slices.

Variation: Quick Calzone

1. Substitute 8 whole grain canned biscuits for pita bread.

2. Combine two pieces of biscuit dough. Roll or pat out into a circle, as thin as possible. Add filling and sauce. Fold over and seal edges.

3. Broil until cheese bubbles. Serve with additional sauce.

Nutrient Analysis per Serving:
226 calories
15 g protein
25 g carbohydrate
7 g fat
3 g fiber
Key Nutrients:
Potassium-15%
Calcium-13%
Vitamin C-10%
Diabetic Exchanges:
1 1/2 Starch, 1 1/2 Lean Meat,
1 Vegetable, 1/2 Fat

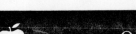
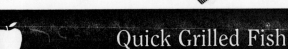

Quick Grilled Fish

I never enjoyed thick pieces of fish until I started marinating them. Marinating adds flavor and keeps it moist. Now we have fish cooked this way at least twice a month!

1 pound halibut or other "steak' cut fish

1/2 cup vinaigrette or fat-free Italian dressing (experiment with different flavored dressings)

1. Pour fish and dressing into ziploc bag. Marinate at least 1 hour; the longer the better.

2. Grill approximately 10 minutes per inch of thickness at thickest part. Or broil at 450° F for same amount of time. Fish is cooked when opaque and flakes easily with fork.

Nutrient Analysis per Serving:
  158 calories
  23 g protein
  <1 g carbohydrate
  6 g fat
Key Nutrients
  Selenium-81%
  Vitamin B12-55%
  Magnesium-29%
Diabetic Exchanges:
  3 Lean Meat

Ratatouille

My husband introduced me to this wonderful dish. It is very versatile. You can serve it over rice with cheese as a main dish, as a side dish, or as a topping on your pizza or potato. In Europe it is often served with a fried egg on top!

8 Servings

4 garlic cloves, crushed

8 tomatoes, cut into quarters

3 zucchini, sliced

1 eggplant, peeled and cut into 1 inch cubes

1 cup sliced mushrooms

1 teaspoon oregano

1 teaspoon basil

1 teaspoon salt

1/4 teaspoon pepper

1 tsp olive oil

1. Brown eggplant in oil in non-stick pan. When tender, add garlic and cook until tender.

2. Add remaining ingredients. Cook over medium heat until vegetables are tender, stirring frequently.

3. Reduce heat, cover and simmer 10-15 minutes.

4. Remove cover and continue cooking until most of the liquid has evaporated.

Variations:

Add chopped red and bell peppers, and sliced black olives.

Quick Method: Use 16 oz. can of tomatoes and 1/4 cup tomato paste instead of fresh tomatoes.

Nutrient analysis per serving:

58 calories

2 g protein

12 g carbohydrate

1 g fat

4 g fiber

Key nutrients:

Vitamin C-40%

Potassium-29%

Folate-9%

Diabetic exchanges:

2 Vegetables

Rigatoni Combination

This recipe is from *Meatless Meals for Working People.*

4 Servings

4 cups cooked rigatoni shells, macaroni or other pasta

1 onion, chopped

1 clove garlic, minced

1/2 green pepper, chopped

olive or vegetable oil

1 small can tomato sauce

1-1 lb can kidney beans, drained

1/4 teaspoon salt

1/2 teaspoon chili powder (or to taste)

pepper to taste

2 cups lowfat cottage cheese (optional)

1. Saute onions, garlic and green pepper 4-5 minutes or until soft.

2. Stir in tomato sauce, kidney beans, soy sauce, salt, chili powder and a pinch of black pepper.

3. Simmer several minutes to heat through. Stir in pasta.

4. Serve as is or add 1/2 cup cottage cheese to each serving to make a lasagna like dish.

Nutrient Analysis per Serving:
287 calories
12 g protein
1 g fat
7 g fiber
Key Nutrients:
Thiamin-25%
Vitamin C-25%
Iron-12%
Diabetic Exchanges:
3 1/2 Starch, 1 Vegetable

Roasted New Potatoes

Like fried foods, but not the fat that comes with it? Try these crispy roasted potatoes. The secret is the high oven temperature.

4 Servings

1 pound new potatoes or baking potatoes, well scrubbed

1-2 cloves garlic, crushed

1 tablespoon olive oil

1/2 teaspoon salt

1 teaspoon dried rosemary or 2 teaspoons fresh rosemary, chopped

1. Preheat oven to 450° F.

2. Cut potatoes into 1 inch pieces. Toss in a bowl with oil, rosemary and garlic.

3. Spread out on a cookie sheet. Roast about 30 minutes until potatoes are tender and brown, turning once halfway through cooking.

Variations:

1. Slice potatoes into 1/4 inch slices to make home fries, or even thinner for homemade potato chips.

2. Use thinly sliced sweet potatoes dusted with cinnamon for a sweet snack chip.

3. Cut into thin, long strips for french fries.

Nutrient Analysis per Serving:
144 calories
26 g carbohydrate
2 g protein
4 g fat
3 g fiber

Key Nutrients:
Vitamin C-24%
Vitamin B6-16%
Riboflavin-10%

Diabetic Exchanges:
2 Starch, 1 Fat

Sesame Beef

This recipe was modified from a recipe in the 1991 National Beef Cookoff®.

6 Servings

2 pounds boneless top sirloin

Marinade:

1/4 cup each rice wine or white vinegar and soy sauce

2 tablespoons dark sesame oil

1 tablespoon granulated sugar

1 teaspoon each: fresh minced ginger and baking soda

2 teaspoons cornstarch

Sauce:

8 oz. beef broth

2 tablespoons cornstarch

1/2 cup packed light brown sugar

1/4 cup hoisin sauce

1 1/2 tablespoons sesame seeds

1 tablespoon teriyaki baste and glaze

1/2 tablespoon molasses

1 clove garlic, minced

1 tablespoon dark sesame oil

1 large head Romaine lettuce, shredded

Sesame seeds

Crushed red pepper pods or hot chili paste, optional

1. Slice beef into 1 inch strips, removing all fat.

2. Mix together marinade ingredients. Toss with beef and store in plastic bag, turning occasionally. Marinate at least 30 minutes, but preferably overnight.

3. Drain marinade. Cook beef quickly in non-stick pan, adding small amount of oil if needed. Keep warm.

4. Reserve 2 tablespoons broth; mix with cornstarch and set aside. Mix remaining broth with other sauce ingredients.

5. In same pan that beef was cooked in, add garlic and 1/2 teaspoon oil. Saute 1 minute. Add sauce mixture; bring to a boil. Add broth-cornstarch mixture. Cook over medium heat until thickened, stirring occasionally.

6. Arrange lettuce on platter. Top with meat and drizzle with sauce or serve sauce on the side.

Nutrient Analysis per Serving:

503 calories
46 g protein
30 g carbohydrate
21 g fat

Key Nutrients:

Zinc-65%
Vitamin B6-31%
Iron-22%
Folate-16%

Diabetic Variation:

Because of high sugar content, limit sauce to 1 1/2 teaspoons and count as "free."

Nutrient Analysis

for meat and lettuce only
386 calories
46 g protein
21 g fat
2 g carbohydrate

Diabetic Exchanges

6 1/2 Lean Meat, 1 Vegetable

Spinach Stuffed Shells

I recently discovered large pasta shells. I used to stuff manicotti shells, but got discouraged when the shells often ripped as I was stuffing them.

Shells can be the busy woman's elegant meal!

4 Servings

1/2 pound large pasta shells, cooked until still slightly firm or al dente', and drained

1-10 ounce package frozen spinach, cooked or thawed and well drained

1 cup cottage cheese

1/3 cup parmesan cheese, preferably freshly grated

1/2 cup grated mozzarella cheese

1/4 teaspoon garlic powder, or to taste

Grated mozzarella and parmesan cheese for garnish

Pink Sauce

1/2 cup lowfat cottage cheese

5 whole canned tomatoes, drained

2 teaspoons Italian seasoning

1/4 teaspoon each salt and pepper, or to taste

Shells

1. Mix all ingredients except shells until well blended.

2. Stuff each shell with some of spinach mixture.

Sauce

1. Mix sauce ingredients in food processor or blender. Spoon small amount over shells and heat in oven or microwave until warm. Garnish with extra cheese.

2. If you choose to refrigerate or freeze until ready to use, store sauce and shells in separate containers.

Nutrient Analysis per Serving:

247 calories

23 g protein

23 g carbohydrate

7 g fat

Key Nutrients:
Vitamin A-57%
Vitamin B12-41%
Calcium-28%
Folate-21%

Diabetic Exchanges
1 Starch, 2 Lean Meat, 1 1/2 Vegetable

Stuffed Cabbage

This recipe is modified from a recipe in *Meatless Meals for Working People*.

6-8 Servings

1 head cabbage, steamed

2 cups apple juice

1 1/2 pounds tofu, crumbled

2 tablespoons oil

1 cup raisins

1-6 ounce can tomato paste

1 teaspoon cinnamon

1/2 teaspoon salt

1/2 teaspoon allspice

1. Preheat oven to 375° F. After cabbage has cooled, separate leaves. Mix together the other ingredients, stuff the leaves and roll up.

2. Place in baking pan with apple juice. Bake for 30 minutes

Nutrient Analysis per Serving:
    307 calories
    20 g protein
    40 g carbohydrate
    13 g fat
    5 g fiber
Key Nutrients:
    Iron-45%
    Magnesium-43%
    Vitamin C-32%
    Folate-12%
Diabetic Exchanges
    1/2 Starch, 2 Lean Meat, 1 Vegetable, 1 1/2 Fruit, 1 Fat

Sunshine Sorbet

The beauty of this dessert is that is made entirely of fruit with no added sugar or thickener!

5 Servings

1-20 ounce can crushed pineapple, in it's own juice

1 ripe banana, sliced

3 nectarines, peeled and sliced or

1 cup canned peaches in it's own juice

1 cup strawberries, fresh or frozen unsweetened

2 teaspoons freshly grated orange or lemon rind

Fresh mint

1. Freeze fruit before preparing. Thaw pineapple enough to slice into chunks.

2. Place all fruit in food processor, and process until smooth. Scrape down sides occasionally.

3. Serve immediately garnished with mint sprigs or place in 8 x 8 pan and freeze. Thaw enough to break into chunks. Process again in food processor and store in airtight freezer container.

Nutrient Analysis per Serving:

112 calories

1.2 g protein

<1 g fat

2 g fiber

Key Nutrients:

Vitamin C-36%

Pottassium-19%

Vitamin B6-10%

Diabetic exchanges:

2 Fruit

Tofu Spread

This recipe is from *Meatless Meals for Working People.*

6 Servings

16 ounce tofu

1 stalk celery

1 dill pickle, chopped or 1/4 cup
   dill or sweet relish

1 tablespoon mustard

1/2 cup lowfat mayonnaise

1/4 teaspoon garlic powder

10 small stuffed olives

1. Slice celery into eight strips lengthwise and then thinly slice crosswise. Mince dill pickle and slice olives as thinly as possible.

2. Crumble tofu with your fingers and add remaining ingredients. Mash and mix or blend.

Nutrient Analysis per Serving:
182 calories
12 g protein
7 g carbohydrate
13 g fat
1 g fiber

Key Nutrients:
Iron-27%
Magnesium-22%
Calcium-13%

Diabetic Exchanges:
1/2 Starch, 1 Lean Meat, 2 Fat

Veal Piccata with Roasted Red Pepper Sauce

4 Servings

16 ounces veal loin

3 tablespoons lemon juice

1/2-1 clove garlic, crushed

1. Marinate veal in lemon juice and garlic for at least 1 hour.

2. Cook over medium-high heat or grill to desired doneness.

3. Serve with Roasted Red Pepper and Cream sauce, which can be made ahead and refrigerated.

Variation:

Turkey tenderloin or chicken breast can also be used.

Roasted Red Pepper and Cream Sauce

1/2 green onion, chopped (if you can't tolerate onions, just use the top.

1 heaping cup roasted red bell peppers (can be bought in a jar)

2 tablespoons white wine vinegar (can be flavored)

1/3 cup parsley (or use 2 fresh spinach or lettuce leaves)

1/3 cup nonfat yogurt or reduced fat sour cream.

Dash cayenne pepper (optional)

1. Puree in food processor or blender. Place in microwave safe dish and heat on Medium-High 2 minutes.

2. Fold in yogurt or sour cream. Return to microwave for 30 seconds on high. Stir and serve over meat.

Nutrient Analysis per Serving:
301 calories
39 g protein
5 g carbohydrate
12 g fat

Key Nutrients:
Vitamin C-44%
Zinc-32%
Vitamin B-6-19%

Diabetic Exchanges:
5 1/2 Lean Meat, 1 Vegetable

Vegetarian Breakfast Tacos

Linda Hood developed this recipe, which won first place for entrees in a local recipe contest. Although "mexican food" often brings to mind high fat, this recipe is lower in fat, but full of flavor. This is not a real spicy recipe, however you may make it very mild by reducing garlic and onion, using mild salsa (or simply chopped tomatoes with lemon juice and onion powder). You can also use parsley instead of cilantro.

4 Servings

- 2 teaspoons olive or canola oil
- 1 small clove garlic
- 1/2 cup each chopped onion and green pepper
- 1 medium potato, chopped
- 1 small zucchini, chopped
- 1 medium tomato, chopped
- 1 egg plus 2 egg whites (or 3 whole eggs)
- 1 cup mexican salsa
- 4 Whole wheat flour or corn tortillas
- 4 ounces shredded part-skim mozzarella cheese
- 1 tablespoon chopped cilantro or parsley
- Salt and pepper to taste

1. In oil, saute garlic, onion and green pepper. Add potato and zucchini. Stir until tender. Push veggies aside and scramble eggs in the middle of skillet, gradually stir in vegetables.

2. Add tomato and heat thoroughly. Season with cilantro, salt and pepper.

3. Steam tortillas on top of mixture in covered skillet. Fill tortillas with vegetable-egg mixture. Fold over. Spoon salsa over and sprinkle cheese on top.

Nutrient Analysis per Serving:
- 255 calories
- 16 g protein
- 27 g carbohydrate
- 10 g fat
- 3 g fiber

Key Nutrients:
- Vitamin C-51%
- Calcium-20%
- Vitamin B12-17%

Diabetic Exchanges:
- 1 1/2 Starch, 1 1/2 Lean Meat, 1 Vegetable, 1 Fat

Vegetarian Chili

Dr. R.L. Ohlsen Jr. developed this recipe. He began making meatless chili to help lower his cholesterol. If you're craving something south of the border, but don't want meat, this recipe's for you. (The beans add protein.)

6 Servings

2 tablespoons canola oil

1 medium onion diced

1 bell pepper, diced

1 cup fresh mushrooms, sliced

2 cups tomatoes, fresh cut into wedges, or canned, drained

2 stalks celery (about 1/2 cup chopped)

2 cups cooked wheat bulgur

2 cups cooked red or pinto beans

2-3 tablespoons chili powder (or to taste)

Garlic powder to taste

Salt and pepper to taste

1. In heavy skillet or sauce pan, saute onion, pepper, mushrooms tomatoes and celery in a little oil until tender.

2. Add bulgar, beans, chili powder and garlic powder. Bring to a boil for 5 minutes, then reduce to simmering for 45 minutes to 1 hour. Extra water may be needed depending on how much juice is made by the vegetables. Additional tomatoes can be added.

3. The amount of salt needed will depend on if you used canned or fresh tomatoes.

4. Add jalapeno pepper if desired.

5. For maximum flavor, refrigerate a day before serving to let flavors blend.

Nutrient Analysis per Serving:
    191 calories
    9 g protein
    35 g carbohydrate
    3 g fat
    9 g fiber

Key Nutrients:
    Vitamin C-48%
    Vitamin B6-27%
    Iron-10%
Diabetic Exchanges:
    2 Starch, 1 Vegetable, 1/2 Fat

References

Chapter 2: Contemplating Pregnancy

1. MRC Vitamin Study Research Group. *Lancet.* July 1991;338:131.
2. Willett WC. *American Journal of Public Health* . May 1992;82,(5):666.
3. McMannus-Kuller J. *Journal of Perinatal and Neonatal Nursing* .1990;3(4):73.
4. Pennington J, Young BE. *Journal of the American Dietetic Association* .1991;2:179.
5. International Food Information Council. *Food Insight;Current Topics in Food Safety and Nutrition.* March/April 1992:1.
6. Lambert-Lagace' L. *The Nutrition Challenge for Women.* City:Bull Publishing;1990:9.
7. Naeye R. *American Journal of Clinical Nutrition* .1990;52:273.
8. "Our Environment", *Better Homes and Gardens Magazine.* May 1992:128.
9. Shortbridge L. *Journal of Perinatal and Neonatal Nursing.* 1990;3(4):1.
10. Proceedings of the National Academy of Sciences. December 1991;88:11003.
11. International Food Information Council, *Food Insight;Current Topics in Food Safety and Nutrition.* May/June 1992:6.
12. Wilson J. *The Pre-Pregnancy Planner.* Garden City, N.Y:Doubleday & Co. Inc;1986:70.
13. Lindbohm ML, et al. *American Journal of Public Health* .1991;81:1029.
14. Shortbridge L. *Journal of Perinatal and Neonatal Nursing* . 1990;3(4):1.
15. Cochrane C. *The Practitioner* . March 1992;236:300.
16. Ries CP, et al. *Journal of the American Dietetic Association* . 1987;87:463.
17. American College of Obstetricians and Gynecologists, *Planning for Pregnancy, Birth and Beyond.* Washington, D.C.:ACOG;1990:10.

Chapter 3: The Knowledgeable Pregnancy–What Every Woman Needs to Know

1. International Food Information Council and the American Dietetic Association *How Are Kids Making Food Choices?* July 1991.
2. Committee on Diet and Health, National Research Council. *Diet and Health:Implications for Reducing Chronic Disease Risk.* Washington DC:National Academy Press;1989:514-515.
3. Ibid:514.
4. Ibid:678.
5. Abrams B, et al. *Obstetrics & Gynecology.* 1989;74 (4):577.
6. News Release. Office of Public Information, University of California, Berkeley. May 1992.
7.*Diet and Health*:205-206.
8. Committee to Study the Prevention of Low Birthweight, Division of Disease Prevention and Health Promotion, Institute of Medicine. *Preventing Low Birthweight.* Washington DC:National Academy Press;1985:1.
9. Williams M, et al. *American Journal of Obstetrics and Gynecology.* July 28 1991;165(1):28.
10. American Heart Association. *The American Heart Association Diet–An Eating Plan for Healthy Americans.* 1991.
11. *Diet and Health*:515.
12. Whitney E , Sizer F. *Nutrition;Concepts and Controversies.* St. Paul, MN:West Publishing Company;1988:188.
13. Subcommittee on Nutritional Status and Weight Gain During Pregnancy. *Nutrition During Pregnancy* . Washington DC:National Academy Press;1990:324.
14. Bailey L. *Nutrition Today.* September/October 1990:12.
15. The Centers for Disease Control. *Journal of the American Medical Association.* September 4, 1991;266(9):1190.
16. *Diet and Health*:71
17. Sandstead H., *Food and Nutrition News.* January/February 1992:1.
18. *Diet and Health*:422.
19. Ibid:73.
20. *Nutrition During Pregnancy*:15.

21. Ibid:254, 16.
22. *Nutrition During Pregnancy*:17.
23. MRC Vitamin Study Research Group. *Lancet* July 1991;338:131.
24. Profet M. Personal communication. Division of Biochemistry and Molecular Biology, Barker Hall, University of California, Berkeley, CA 94720. June, 1992.
25. Belizan J, et al. *New England Journal of Medicine*. November 14, 1991;325:1399.
26. Villar J, Repke J. *American Journal of Obstetrics and Gynecology*. 1990;103:1124 .
27. Marcoux S, et al. *American Journal of Epidemiology*. June 15, 1991;133(12):1266.
28. Greeley A. *FDA Consumer*. July/August 1991:27-28.
29. *Nutrition During Pregnancy*:322.
30. Hallberg L, et al. *American Journal of Clinical Nutrition*. 1991;53:112.
31. Federick J, Anderson ABM. *British Journal of Obstetrics and Gynaecology*. 1976;83:342.
32. Department of Health, Education and Welfare. *Smoking and health;report of the surgeon general*. 1979. Washington DC:U.S. Department of Health and Welfare;DHHS (PHS) DHEW publication 79-50066.
33. Meyer MB, Tonascia JA. *American Journal of Obstetrics and Gynecology* . 1977;128:494.
34. *Nutrition During Pregnancy*:394.
35. Greeley A. 28.
36. Franklin D. *Hippocrates*. September 1991:33.
37. Heins H. *American Baby*. May 1992:16.
38. Eliason M, and Williams J, *Journal of Perinatal and Neonatal Nursing* . 1990;3(4):65.
39. *Diet and Health*:450.
40. Rosenthal R. *The New York Times Magazine*. February 4, 1990:30.
41. Ibid.
42. Rosenberg L, et al. *Journal of the American Medical Association*. 1982;247:1429.
43. International Food Information Council. *Food Insight;Current Topics in Food Safety and Nutrition*. May/June 1992:6.
46. Jacobson M, et al. *Safe Food;Eating Wisely in a Risky World*. Los Angeles:Living Planet Press;1991:45.
47. *The Boston Globe*. December 13, 1989:1.
48. Sullivan K. The *Journal of Perinatal and Neonatal Nursing* . 1990;3(4):12 .
49. Ibid.
50. Haines P, et al. *Journal of the American Dietetic Association* . June 1992;92:698.

Chapter 4: The First Trimester

1. Subcommittee on Nutritional Status and Weight Gain During Pregnancy. *Nutrition During Pregnancy* . Washington DC:National Academy Press;1990:430.
2. Food and Nutrition Board *Recommended Dietary Allowances*. 10th ed. Washington DC:National Academy Press;1989.
3. *Nutrition During Pregnancy*:386.
4. Rose D, et al. *American Journal of Clinical Nutrition*. September 1991(54):520 .
5. Position Statement of the American Diabetes Association. *Diabetes Care*. April 1992;(15)Suppl 2:23.
6. Committee on Diet and Health, National Research Council. *Diet and Health:Implications for Reducing Chronic Disease Risk*. Washington DC:National Academy Press;1989:678.
7. Profet M. Personal communication, June 1992.

Chapter 5: The Second Trimester

1. Subcommittee on Nutritional Status and Weight Gain During Pregnancy. *Nutrition During Pregnancy* . Washington DC:National Academy Press;1990:12.
2. Position of the American Dietetic Association:Vegetarian Diets-Technical Support Paper. *Journal of the American Dietetic Association*. 1988;88(3):352.
3. Food and Nutrition Board *Recommended Dietary Allowances*. 10th ed. Washington DC:National Academy Press;1989.
4. Ibid.

5. Deehr M. *American Journal of Clinical Nutrition.* January 1990;51(1):95.
6. VillarJ, et al. *Obstetrics and Gynecology.* 1988;71(5):697.
7. Solomons NW, et al. *American Journal of Clinical Nutrition.* 1985;41:199.
8. Lee CM, Hardy C. *American Journal of Clinical Nutrition* . 1989;49:840.
9. Recker R, et al. *American Journal of Clinical Nutrition.* 1988;47:93.
10. Whitney E , Sizer F. *Nutrition;Concepts and Controversies.* St. Paul, MN:West Publishing Company;1988:248.
11. CSPI Staff. *Nutrition Action Healthletter.* May 1992:11.

Chapter 6: The Third Trimester

1. Food and Nutrition Board *Recommended Dietary Allowances.* 10th ed. Washington DC:National Academy Press;1989:163.
2. Subcommittee on Nutritional Status and Weight Gain During Pregnancy. *Nutrition During Pregnancy* . Washington DC:National Academy Press;1990:265.
3. Roshon MS, Hagen RL. *Journal of Abnormal Child Psychology.* 1989;17:349.
4. Behar D, et al. *Nutrition and Behavior.* 1984;74:876 .
5. Position of the American Dietetic Association:Appropriate Use of Nutritive and Non-Nutritive Sweeteners, *Journal of the American Dietetic Association* . 1987;87:1869.

Chapter 7: Vegetarian Eating

1. Burr ML, et al. *American Journal of Clinical Nutrition.* 1982;36:873.
2. Phillips RL, et al. *American Journal of Epidemiology.* 1980;112:296.
3. Sacks F, et al. *Journal of the American Medical Association.* 1985;254:1337.
4. Cooper RS, et al. *Atherosclerosis.* 1982;43:71.
5. Reisin E, et al. *New England Journal of Medicine.* 1978;298:1.
6.West KM, Kalbfleisch JM. *Diabetes.* 1971;20:99.
7. Marsh AG, et al. *Journal of the American Dietetic Association.* 1980;76:148.
8. Pixley F, et al. *British Medical Journal.* 1985;l 291:11.
9. Gear JS, et al. *The Lancet.* 1979;1:511.
10. Committee on Diet and Health, National Research Council. *Diet and Health:Implications for Reducing Chronic Disease Risk.* Washington D.C:National Academy Press;1989:78-9.
11. Pike R, Brown M. *Nutrition, An Integrated Approach.* New York:John Wiley and Sons;1975:792.
12. Food and Nutrition Board *Recommended Dietary Allowances.* 10th ed. Washington DC:National Academy Press;1989:176.
13. Haddad J. *New England Journal of Medicine.* April 30, 1992; 326(18):1213. Letter.
14. Freeland-Graves J, et al. *Journal of The American Dietetic Association.* December 1980;77:655.
16. Position of the American Dietetic Association:Vegetarian Diets. *Journal of the American Dietetic Association.* 1988;88(3):351.

Chapter 8: Special Care for High Risk Pregnancies

1. American Diabetes Association, *Diabetes and Pregnancy:What to Expect.* Alexandria VA:American Diabetes Association;1989:15.
2. Kitzmiller J. *Journal of the American Medical Association.* 1991;265:731.
3. *Diabetes and Pregnancy:What to Expect.* 39.
4. American College of Obstetricians and Gynecologists, *Planning for Pregnancy*, Birth and Beyond. Washington, D.C.:ACOG;1990:133.
5. Ibid.
6. Krall L, Beaser RS. *Joslin Diabetes Manual.* 12th ed. Philadelphia:Lea and Febiger;1989:236.
7. Ruggiero L, et al. *Diabetes Care.* 1990;13:441.
8. *Diabetes and Pregnancy:What to Expect.* 42.
9. DiGiacomo JE, Hay Jr WW. Metabolism. February 1990;39 (2):193.
10. American Diabetes Association, *Gestational Diabetes and Pregnancy:What to Expect.* Alexandria VA:American Diabetes Association Inc;1989:12.

11. Ibid:16.

12. Ibid:14-15.

13. Ibid:14.

14. Ibid:13

15. Spears B. Telephone interview. April 1992.

16. Jovanovic-Peterson L, Peterson C. *Diabetes* . December 1991;40, Suppl 2:179.

17. Spears B. Telephone interview. April 1992.

18. Committee on Diet and Health, National Research Council. *Diet and Health:Implications for Reducing Chronic Disease Risk.* Washington D.C:National Academy Press;1989:473.

19. Position Statement of the American Diabetes Association;Use of Noncaloric Sweeteners. *Diabetes Care* . March 1991;14, Suppl 2:28.

20. London R. *The Journal of Reproductive Medicine.* 1988;33(1):17.

21. American Academy of Pediatrics, Committee on Nutrition, *Final Report, Task Force on the Dietary Management of Metabolic Disorders.* December 1985:35-38.

22. Jacobson M, et al. *Safe Food;Eating Wisely in a Risky World.* Los Angeles:Living Planet Press;1991151-165.

23. Black R. Personal communication. March 1992.

24. *Gestational Diabetes:What to Expect.* 12.

25. *Working Group Report on High Blood Pressure in Pregnancy,* High Blood Pressure Education Program. Washington DC: US Department of Health and Human Services;1991. NIH Publication 91-3029.

26. Ibid:6

27. Eskenazl B, et al. *Journal of the American Medical Association.* July 10 1991;266(2):237.

28. Villar J, Repke, J. *American Journal of Obstetrics and Gynecology* . 1990;103:1124.

29. Belizan J. *New England Journal of Medicine* . November 14 1991;325:1390.

30. Working Group Report on High Blood Pressure in Pregnancy. 14.

31. Ibid:2-3.

32. Ibid:29.

33. Ibid:6.

34. Subcommittee on Nutritional Status and Weight Gain During Pregnancy. *Nutrition During Pregnancy* . Washington DC:National Academy Press;1990:12.

35. Pederson AL. *Journal of the American Dietetic Association.* 1989;5:642.

36. *Nutrition During Pregnancy.* 212.

37. Olds S, et al. *Maternal Newborn Nursing;A Family Centered Approach.* 2nd ed. Menlo Park, CA:Addison-Wesley Publishing;1984:182.

38. Dubois S, et al. *American Journal of Clinical Nutrition.* 1991;53:1397.

39. Cambell D, et al. *Acta Genetica Gemellologica.* 1982;32:221.

40. Sassoon D, et al. *Obstetrics & Gynecology.* May 1990;75(5):817.

41. Collins MS, Bleyl JA. *American Journal of Obstetrics and Gynecology.* June 1990;162(6):1384.

42. Ales KL, et al. *Surgery, Gynecology and Obstetrics.* September 1990;17(3):209.

43. Berkowitz G. *New England Journal of Medicine* . March 8, 1990;322(10):659.

44. Ales KL, et al. op. cit.

45. Berkowtiz G. op. cit.

46. Hales D, Johnston T. *Intensive Caring* . New York:Crown;1990:36.

47. The Rand Youth Poll, *The Marketing Charecteristics of American Teenagers,* New York, NY, 1990.

48. National Adolescent Student Health Survey, *A Report on the Health of America's Youth.* 1989;US Department of Health and Human Services, Public Health Service.

49. Schneck M, et al. *Journal of the American Dietetic Association* . 1990;4:555.

50. *Nutrition During Pregnancy* :10.

51. Hediger M, et al. *Obstetrics and Gynecology* . July 1989;74 (1):6.

Chapter 9: Considering Breastfeeding

1. Subcommittee on Nutritional Status during Lactation et al. *Nutrition during Lactation*. Washington DC:National Academy Press;1990:169.
2. La Leche League International Staff, *The Womanly Art of Breastfeeding*. 4th rev ed. Franklin Park, IL:La Leche League International;1987:8.
3. *Healthy People 2000*. Washington DC:US Department of Health and Human Services;1991. DHHS (PHS) publication 91-50212:379.
4. Crase B. Personal communication. May 1992.
5. Nafziger, S. Reprinted with permission of author, from Community Network Newsletter. First quarter 1992;Pueblo, Colorado.
6. Crase B. Personal communication. May 1992.
7. Ibid:
8. Krebs N. Presentation; Colorado Dietetic Association Annual Meeting. May 14, 1992.
9. Krebs N. Personal communication. June 1992.
10. *Nutrition During Lactation* :74.
11. Strode MA. *Acta Paediatrica Scandinavica* . 1986;75:222.
12. Butte N et al. *American Journal of Clinical Nutrition*. February 1984;39:296.
13. *Recommended Dietary Allowances*. 10th ed.
14. *Nutrition During Lactation*. 219.
15. *Recommended Dietary Allowances*. 10th ed.
16. Chandr RK, Hamed A. *Annals of Allergy* . 1991;67:129.
17. *Nutrition During Lactation*:168.
18. *Nutrition During Lactation*:14.
19. Mathur NB. *Acta Paediatrica Scandinavica* . 1990;79:1039.
20. Lucas A, et al. *Lancet*. 1992;339:261.
21. Little RE, et al. *New England Journal of Medicine*. 1989;321:425.
22. Mennella J. *New England Journal of Medicine*. 1991;325:981.
23. *Nutrition During Lactation*:177.
24 Ibid:171.
25. *Environmental Nutrition*. June 1992;15(6):1.
26. *Nutrition during Lactation*:171.
27. *Nutrition and the MD* . March 1992;18(3):3.
28. Ibid.
29. Merchant K et al. *American Journal of Clinical Nutrition* . 1990;52:280.
30. Nommsen L, et al. *American Journal of Clinical Nutrition*. 1990;53:457.
31 .Hayslip C, et al. *Obstetrics and Gynecology* . April 1989;73(4):588.
32. Koetting C, Wardlaw G. *American Journal of Clinical Nutrition*. 1988;48:1479.
33. Hreshchyshyn M, et al. *American Journal of Obstetrics and Gynecology*. 1988;159:318.
34. Chan G, et al. *American Journal of Clinical Nutrition*. 1987;46:319.
35. Rogan WJ, et al. *American Journal of Public Health*. 1986;76(2):172.
36. Crase B. Personal communication. May 1992.
37. *The Womanly Art of Breastfeeding*:348.
38. Ibid:233.
39. Nafziger S. Personal communication June1992.
40. *Recommended Dietary Allowances*. 10th ed.:163.
41. Lovelady C, et al. *American Journal of Clinical Nutrition*. 1990;52:103.
42. Siskind V, et al. *American Journal of Epidemiology*. August 1989;130(2):229.

Chapter 10: Now That You Can See Your Feet Again... Or The First Weeks With Baby

1. *Pediatrics*. December 1989;84(6):114.
2. Policy statement; The use of whole cow's milk in infancy. *American Academy of Pediatrics News*. May 1992:18.
3. Shannon M, Graef J. *New England Journal of Medicine* . January 9, 1992;326(2)137. letter.

4. Dishman RK, ed. *Exercise Adherence.* Champaign, IL:Human Kinetics;1988.

5. Fischman-Havstad L, Marston AR. *British Journal of Clinical Psychology.* 1984;23:265.

6. Edell BH, et al. *Addictive Behavior.* 1987;12:63.

7. Sternberg B, Relapse in weight control: definitions, processes, and prevention strategies. In: Marlatt GA, Gordon JR, eds. *Relapse Prevention.* New York:Guilford Press;1985:52.

8. International Food and Information Council, *Food Insight;Current Topics in Food Safety and Nutrition.* March/April 1992.

9. Greene G, et al. *Obstetrics and Gynecology* . May 1988;71(5):701.

Chapter 11: Fitting Fitness In

1. American College of Obstetricians and Gynecologists, *Planning for Pregnancy, Birth and Beyond.* Washington, D.C.:ACOG;1990:77, 82.

2. Jovanovic-Peterson L, Peterson C. *Diabetes.* December 1991;40, Suppl 2:179.

3. *Nutrition and the MD* . April 1992;18(4):7.

Chapter 12: Stocking the Pregnant Kitchen

1. The Food and Drug Administration, FDA Backgrounder;*Food labeling reform:a progress report.* November 1991.

2. Committee on Diet and Health, National Research Council. *Diet and Health:Implications for Reducing Chronic Disease Risk.* Washington D.C:National Academy Press;1989:676.

3. American Heart Association, *The AHA Diet-An Eating Plan for Healthy Americans.* 1991.

4. *Diet and Health:*676.

5. *Consumer Reports On Health.* March 1992:18.

6. *Nutrition Action Healthletter.* January/February 1992:11.

7. Whitmire D. Telephone interview. June 1992.

8. Stone M. Presentation;Colorado Dietetic Association Annual Meeting. May 17, 1992.

9. *National Council Against Health Fraud Newsletter.* January/February 1990:5.

11. Smith G. *The Safety of Beef.* Presentation at the National Beef Cook Off, Colorado Springs, CO. September 23, 1991.

12. Dairy Industry Coalition. *Facts About BST and Milk Safety.*

13. Daughaday WH, Barbano DM. *Journal of The American Medical Association.* 1990;264:1003.

16. Wilson LW. *Producing Leaner Beef More Efficiently* . Presentation at Pennsylvania State University. 1989.

14. Kendall P. Telephone interview. June 1992.

15. National Pork Producers Council. *Today's Pork in Foodservice.* 1988:6.

17. Texas A & M University. *Growth Promoting Hormones, A Scientific Review,* January 1989.

18. Baker K. Personal communication, June 1992.

19. *Consumer Reports Magazine.* February 1992. 57(2):106.

20. Bolger M. Telephone interview. May 1992.

21. The Food and Drug Administration, *FDA Consumer.* April 1992:5.

22. Harsila J. Telephone interview. May 1992.

23. Nettleton J. *Eat Fish and Seafood Twice Twice a Week:It can Make a Difference.* National Fisheries Institute, Arlington VA.

24. Jacobson M, et al. *Safe Food;Eating Wisely in a Risky World.* Los Angeles:Living Planet Press;1991:13.

25. Ruddon K. Telephone interview. American College of Obstetricians and Gynecologists Information Office. May 1992.

26. Wilson M. Personal communication. May 1992.

27. Messenger T. Telephone interview. April 1992.

RECOMMENDED READING

As you may know there are many, many good books about health and nutrition. It was difficult to pick out just a few:

Pregnancy

Pre-Conceptions; What You Can Do Before Pregnancy to Help You Have a Healthy Baby, Nora Tannenhaus, Contemporary Books
Your Pregnancy Month by Month, Glade B. Curtis M.D., Fischer Books
Drugs, Vitamins, Minerals in Pregnancy, Ann Karen Henry, Pharm D, Jill Feldhausen M.S., R.D., Fisher Books
Essential Exercises for the Childbearing Year, Elizabeth Noble, Houghton Mifflin Company
Pregnancy & Childbirth, The Complete Guide for a New Life, Tracy Hotchner, Avon Books.
What to Expect When You're Expecting, Arlene Eisenberg et al., Workman Publishing
The Complete Mothercare Manual; An Illustrated Guide to Pregnancy Birth and Childcare Through Age Five, Rosalind Ting M.D., Herbert Brant MD, and Kennth Holt MD, Consultants, Prentice Hall Press
To order a large variety of birth and parenting books by mail:
Birth and LIfe Bookstore, P.O. Box 70625, Seattle WA, 98107, 206-789-4444

High Risk Pregnancy

Getting Pregnant and Staying Pregnant, Overcoming Infertility and Managing your High Risk Pregnancy, Diana Raab B.S., R.N., Hunter House
When Pregnancy isn't Perfect, Laurie Rich, Penguin Books
Intensive Caring, Diane Hales and Timothy Johnson MD, Crown
Having Twins; A Parent's Guide to Pregnancy, Birth and Early Childhood, Elizabeth Noble, Houghton Mifflin Co.
Pregnancy Bedrest, Susan Johnston MSW and Deborah Kraut MILR, Henry Holt and Co.

Teen Pregnancy and Parenthood

Teens Parenting Series: *Your Pregnancy and Newborn Journey*, Jeanne Warren Lindsay and Jean Brunelli, PHN; and *Your Baby's First Year*, Jeanne Warren Lindsay Morning Glory Press
Surviving Teen Pregnancy: Your Choices Dreams and Decisions, Shirley Arthur, Morning Glory Press,
The Challenge of Three-Generation Living, Jeanne Warren Lindsay, Morning Glory Press, 714-828-1998

Parenthood

Dr. Mom's Parenting Guide: Commonsense Guidance for the Life of Your Child, Marrianne Neifert MD, Dutton and *Dr Mom; A Guide to Baby and Child Care*, Marianne Neifert MD et al. Signet
Parenting with Love and Logic, Foster W. Cline and Jim Fay, Navpress, A Ministry of The Navigators
Baby Product Basics, The Busy Person's Guide to Baby Products on a Budget, R. Rolle-Whatley, Sandcastle Publishing, (213)-255-3616
Black Fatherhood: The Guide to Male Parenting, Impact! Publications, (310)-677-6311
Meditations for New Mothers, Beth Wilson Saavedra, Workman Publishing
Without Spanking or Spoiling: A Practical Approach to Toddler and Preschool Guidance, Elizabeth Crary, Parenting Press, 1-800-992-6657
The Sleep Book for Tired Parents, Becky Huntley, Parenting Press, 1-800-992-6657
Getting Your Child to Sleep...and Back to Sleep, Tips for Parents of Infants, Toddlers and Preschoolers, and many other books by Vicki Lansky, 1-800-255-3379
Any books by parenting experts Penelope Leach, T. Berry Brazelton or William Sears
What to Expect the First Year, Arlene Eisenberg et al., Workman Publishing

Good Morning Merry Sunshine; A Father's Journal of His Child's First Year, Bob Green, Penguin Books

Pregnancy and Parenting Books with a touch of humor
From Here to Maternity, Carol Weston, Little
The Pregnant Husband's Handbook, Jeff Justice, Strawberry Patch, 1-800-875-7242
*You Know You're A New Parent When..*Jeff Justice and Diane Pfeifer, Strawberry Patch, 1-875-7242
The Thirteen Months of Pregnancy; A Guide for the Pregnant Father, Bill Atalla, Oddly Enough, (707)-833-1222

Feeding your Infant and Child
The Womanly Art of Breastfeeding, La Leche League International, 1-800-La Leche
The Nursing Mother's Companion, Kathleen Huggins, Harvard Common Press
Child of Mine; Feeding with Love and Good Sense, by Ellyn Satter R.D., MSW, Bull Publishing
How to Feed Your Kid-But Not Too Much, Ellyn Satter RD, MSW, Bull Publishing
Feeding Your Baby From Conception to Age Two by Louise Lambert-Lagace', Surrey Books

General Nutrition
Opening The Door to Good Nutrition, Marion Franz MS, RD Betsy Kerr Hedding RD, MPH and Gayle Leitch BS, DCI Publishing
The Nutrition Challenge for Women, Louise Lambert Lagace', Surrey Books
The Restaurant Companion, Hope Warshaw MS, RD, Surrey Books
Every Woman's Guide to Nutrition, Judith Brown, University of Minnesota Press
Eating on the Run, by Evelyn Tribole M.S., R.D., Human Kinetics Publishers
The Real Life Nutrition Book; Making the Right Choices Without Changing Your Life-Style, Susan Finn PhD, RD, and Linda Stern Kass, Penguin Books
The Fast Food Diet: Quick and Healthy Eating on the Run, Mary Donkersloot R.D., Simon & Schuster
The Food Pharmacy, Jean Carper, Bantam Books

Cookbooks

General-Healthy
Quick & Healthy; Recipes and Ideas by Brenda Ponichtera R.D., ScaleDown, (503)-386-7272
Mexican Light Cooking, Kathi Long, Putnam Publishing Group
The Guiltess Gourmet Goes Ethnic, Judy Gilliard and Joy Kirkpatric RD, DCI Publishing
The American Heart Association Low Fat-Low Cholesterol Cookbook, Scott Grundy MD, editor, Times Books
For Goodness' Sake, An Eating Well Guide to Lowfat Cooking, Terry Joyce Blonder, Camden House
The Best of Sunset-Light and Healthy Cookbook, Sunset Publishing Co.
Cooking Light Cookbook Series, Oxmoor House
The American Diabetic Association and the American Dietetic Association Family Cookbook (4 volumes)
Seafood
Seafood, A Collection of Heart Healthy Recipes and *Light Hearted Seafood* and *Seafood A to Z* both by Janis Harsila and Evie Hansen, National Seafood Educators, P.O. Box 60006, Richmond Beach, WA 98160, (206)-546-6410.

Vegetarian
The Vegetarian Mother and Baby Book, Rose Elliott, Pantheon
Life's Simple Pleasures; Fine Vegetarian Cooking for Sharing and Celebration, by Karen Mangum, Pacific Press Publishing Association

Indian Recipes for a Healthy Heart From the Kitchen of Mrs. Lakbani, Fahil Publishing Co., (310)-541-8099
Laurel's Kitchen, Laurel Robertson, Carol Flinders and Brian Ruppenthal, Ten Speed Press
Moosewood Cookbook, The Enchanted Broccoli Forest and *Still Life with Menu Cookbook,* all by Molly Katzen, Ten Speed Press
Simply Vegan by Debra Wasserman and Reed Mangels, PhD, Vegetarian Resource Group
Meatless Meals for Working People, Debra Wasserman and Charles Stahler, Vegetarian Resource Group

Diabetic Cookbooks
The All New Cookbook for Diabetics and Their Familes, Oxmoor House
Better Homes and Gardens Diabetic Cookbook, Better Homes and Gardens Books
The Microwave Diabetes Cookbook, Betty Marks, Surrey Books
The Art of Cooking for the Diabetic, Mary Abbott Hess R.D., M.S., and Katherine Middleton, Signet Books
The Guiltless Gourmet Goes Ethnic; Italian, French, Spanish and Cajun Cuisine for the Health Conscious Cook, Judy Gilliard and Joy Kirkpatrick R.D.

Diabetes
Gestational Diabetes: Guidelines for a Safe Pregnancy and Healthy Baby, Marion Franz MS, RD, Nancy Cooper and Lucy Mullen, DCI Publishing
Diabetes: What to Expect and *Gestational Diabetes: What to Expect,* The American Diabetes Association, 1-800-ADA-DISC
Exchanges for All Occasions-Meeting the Challenge of Diabetes, by Marion Franz, DCI Publishing

Weight Control
Living Lean by Choosing More, The Eight Week Weight Loss Program that Can Change Your Life, Cheryl-Jennings-Sauer, Taylor Publishing Co.
The New American Diet, Sonja Connor MS, RD and William Connor MD, Simon & Schuster
The Choose to Lose Diet; A Food Lovers Guide to Permanent Weight Loss, Dr. Ron and Nancy Goor and Katherine Boyd RD
Diets That Work For Weight Loss and Medical Needs, Deralee Scanlon RD with Larry Straus, Lowell House

OTHER RESOURCES
Phone numbers:
National Organization of Mothers of Twins Clubs-505-275-0955
Triplet Connection-209-474-3073/0885
Twin Services (counseling and referrals) 510-524-0863
Sidelines 714-497-2265 (support for those experiencing a high risk pregnancy) The Confinement Line 703-941-7183 (offers a support network for women on bed rest)
Consumer Product Safety Commission-800-638-2772
Vegetarian Resource Group-410-VEGE

Newsletters and Magazines
Tufts University Diet and Nutrition Letter
Environmental Nutrition, The Professional Newsletter of Diet, Nutrition and Health
University of California, Berkeley Wellness Letter
Nutrition Action Health Letter, Center for Science in the Public Interest, Washington DC
Vegetarian Journal, Vegetarian Resource Group
Eating Well Magazine
Cooking Light Magazine
American Health Magazine
Hippocrates Magazine

Index

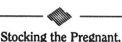

Recipe Index

Computerized Nutrition Analysis Form

Fill out this form to receive a computer analysis of your diet compared to the Recommended Dietary Allowances for pregnancy. Your printout will include analysis of your diet for over 30 nutrients including calories, protein, fat, carbohydrate, cholesterol and fiber. If you are doing a 1 day analysis, write down what you eat in a "typical" day. If you are doing a 3 day analysis, which gives you a better picture of your average eating habits, write down 1 weekend day and 2 week-days of food eaten. (See order form on next page.)

Directions for filling out form:

Write down everything you eat and drink (except water) in a 24 hour period. Please be as specific as possible in listing foods including serving size and how the food was prepared (fried, baked, etc.) Also don't forget to include extras such as margarine, oil and salad dressings. Please include descriptions such as 2% (for milk) low- fat, fat-free, etc.

Please reproduce this form for each day or more as needed. Send with order form on the next page.

Food	Amount	How Prepared

The Eating Expectantly Order Form

Order additional copies of Eating Expectantly or computerized nutrition analysis of your diet by mail, phone or fax!

Please send me: Total

_____ copies of Eating Expectantly @ $13.95 $_____

_____ I want to share the gift of good nutrition with
friends! Send 3 copies @ 11.95 each   **$ 35.85**

_____ days of computerized nutrition analysis
@ $5.00 per day (see form on previous page) $_____

Shipping and Handling:

$2.50 per book; $1.00 for each additional book. $_____

Colorado residents add sales tax–4.00% $_____

Colorado Springs residents add sales tax–6.5% $_____

TOTAL ENCLOSED $_____

Please enclose a check, money order or charge to your credit card:

Visa # _____ Expiration date_____

Master Card# _____ Expiration date_____

Name as it appears on on Card _____

Signature _____

Ship to:

Name: _____

Address: _____

Mail to:

Fall River Press
PO Box 62578 · Colorado Springs, CO 80962-2578

OR

Phone your order to *1-800-284-MOMS* , OR
FAX your order using this form to *1-719-594-6124*

The Eating Expectantly Order Form

Order additional copies of Eating Expectantly or computerized nutrition analysis of your diet by mail, phone or fax!

Please send me: Total

_____ copies of Eating Expectantly @ $13.95 $_____

_____ I want to share the gift of good nutrition with
             friends! Send 3 copies @ 11.95 each   **$ 35.85**

_____ days of computerized nutrition analysis
             @ $5.00 per day (see form on previous page) $_____

Shipping and Handling:

$2.50 per book; $1.00 for each additional book. $_____

Colorado residents add sales tax–4.00% $_____

Colorado Springs residents add sales tax–6.5% $_____

TOTAL ENCLOSED $_____

Please enclose a check, money order or charge to your credit card:

Visa # _____ Expiration date_____

Master Card# _____ Expiration date_____

Name as it appears on on Card _____

Signature _____

Ship to:

Name: _____

Address: _____

Mail to:

Fall River Press
PO Box 62578 · Colorado Springs, CO 80962-2578

OR

Phone your order to *1-800-284-MOMS* , OR
FAX your order using this form to *1-719-594-6124*